AGROBIODIVERSITY, SCHOOL GARDENS AND HEALTHY DIETS

This book critically assesses the role of agrobiodiversity in school gardens and its contribution to diversifying diets, promoting healthy eating habits and improving nutrition among schoolchildren as well as other benefits relating to climate change adaptation, ecoliteracy and greening school spaces.

Many schoolchildren suffer from various forms of malnutrition and it is important to address their nutritional status given the effects it has on their health, cognition, and subsequently their educational achievement. Schools are recognized as excellent platforms for promoting lifelong healthy eating and improving long-term, sustainable nutrition security required for optimum educational outcomes. This book reveals the multiple benefits of school gardens for improving nutrition and education for children and their families. It examines issues such as school feeding, community food production, school gardening, nutritional education and the promotion of agrobiodiversity, and draws on international case studies, from both developed and developing nations, to provide a comprehensive global assessment.

This book will be essential reading for those interested in promoting agrobiodiversity, sustainable nutrition and healthy eating habits in schools and public institutions more generally. It identifies recurring and emerging issues, establishes best practices, identifies key criteria for success and advises on strategies for scaling up and scaling out elements to improve the uptake of school gardens.

Danny Hunter is a senior scientist at Bioversity International.

Emilita Monville-Oro is Country Director for the Philippines at the International Institute of Rural Reconstruction (IIRR).

Bessie Burgos is the former Programme Head of research and development at the Southeast Asian Regional Center for Graduate Study and Research in Agriculture (SEARCA).

Carmen Nyhria Rogel is a program specialist in research and development at SEARCA.

Blesilda Calub is a university researcher at the University of the Philippines Los Baños.

Julian Gonsalves is a senior program advisor at the International Institute of Rural Reconstruction (IIRR).

Nina Lauridsen is a research fellow at Bioversity International.

Issues in Agricultural Biodiversity
Series editors: Michael Halewood and Danny Hunter

This series of books is published by Earthscan in association with Bioversity International. The aim of the series is to review the current state of knowledge in topical issues associated with agricultural biodiversity, to identify gaps in our knowledge base, to synthesize lessons learned and to propose future research and development actions. The overall objective is to increase the sustainable use of biodiversity in improving people's well-being and food and nutrition security. The series' scope is all aspects of agricultural biodiversity, ranging from conservation biology of genetic resources through social sciences to policy and legal aspects. It also covers the fields of research, education, communication and coordination, information management and knowledge sharing.

Published titles:

Farmers' Crop Varieties and Farmers' Rights
Challenges in Taxonomy and Law
Michael Halewood

Tropical Fruit Tree Diversity
Good practices for *in situ* and on-farm conservation
Edited by Bhuwon Sthapit, Hugo A.H. Lamers, V. Ramanatha Rao, and Arwen Bailey

Farmers and Plant Breeding
Current Approaches and Perspectives
Edited by Ola T. Westengen and Tone Winge

Agrobiodiversity, School Gardens and Healthy Diets
Promoting Biodiversity, Food and Sustainable Nutrition
Edited by Danny Hunter, Emilita Monville-Oro, Bessie Burgos, Carmen Nyhria Rogel, Blesilda Calub, Julian Gonsalves, and Nina Lauridsen

For more information about this series, please visit: https://www.routledge.com/Issues-in-Agricultural-Biodiversity/book-series/ECIAB

AGROBIODIVERSITY, SCHOOL GARDENS AND HEALTHY DIETS

Promoting Biodiversity, Food and Sustainable Nutrition

Edited by Danny Hunter, Emilita Monville-Oro, Bessie Burgos, Carmen Nyhria Rogel, Blesilda Calub, Julian Gonsalves, and Nina Lauridsen

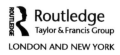
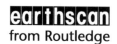

First published 2020
by Routledge
2 Park Square, Milton Park, Abingdon, Oxon OX14 4RN

and by Routledge
52 Vanderbilt Avenue, New York, NY 10017

Routledge is an imprint of the Taylor & Francis Group, an informa business

© 2020 Bioversity International

All rights reserved. No part of this book may be reprinted or reproduced or utilised in any form or by any electronic, mechanical, or other means, now known or hereafter invented, including photocopying and recording, or in any information storage or retrieval system, without permission in writing from the publishers.

Trademark notice: Product or corporate names may be trademarks or registered trademarks, and are used only for identification and explanation without intent to infringe.

British Library Cataloguing-in-Publication Data
A catalogue record for this book is available from the British Library

Library of Congress Cataloging-in-Publication Data
Names: Hunter, Danny, editor. | Monville-Ora, Emilita, editor. | Burgos, Bessie, editor. | Rogel, Carmen Nyhria, editor. | Calub, Blesilda, editor. | Gonsalves, Julian F., 1949– editor. | Lauridsen, Nina, editor.
Title: Agrobiodiversity, school gardens and healthy diets: promoting biodiversity, food and sustainable nutrition / edited by Danny Hunter, Emilita Monville-Ora, Bessie Burgos, Carmen Nyhria Rogel, Blesilda Calub, Julian Gonsalves, and Nina Lauridsen.
Description: Abingdon, Oxon; New York, NY: Routledge, 2020. | Includes bibliographical references and index.
Identifiers: LCCN 2019046968 (print) | LCCN 2019046969 (ebook) | ISBN 9780367148850 (hardback) | ISBN 9780367148867 (paperback) | ISBN 9780429053788 (ebook)
Subjects: LCSH: School gardens—Case studies. | Agrobiodiversity. | School children—Food. | Children—Nutrition. | Sustainable agriculture.
Classification: LCC SB55 .A47 2020 (print) | LCC SB55 (ebook) | DDC 631.5/8—dc23
LC record available at https://lccn.loc.gov/2019046968
LC ebook record available at https://lccn.loc.gov/2019046969

ISBN: 978-0-367-14885-0 (hbk)
ISBN: 978-0-367-14886-7 (pbk)
ISBN: 978-0-429-05378-8 (ebk)

Typeset in Bembo
by codeMantra

CONTENTS

List of figures   *xi*
List of tables   *xv*
List of boxes   *xvi*
Acknowledgements   *xviii*
List of contributors   *xx*
List of abbreviations   *xxxviii*

1 School gardens: multiple functions and multiple outcomes   1
   Julian Gonsalves, Danny Hunter, and Nina Lauridsen

2 Schools as a system to improve nutrition   33
   Stineke Oenema, Lesley Drake, Kaia Engesveen, Andrea Polo Galante, Danny Hunter, David Ryckembusch, Luana Swensson, and Florence Tartanac

3 Strategies for integrating food and nutrition in the primary school curriculum   48
   Maria Theresa M. Talavera and Aileen R. de Juras

4 Linking school gardens, school feeding, and nutrition education in the Philippines   62
   Emilita Monville-Oro, Imelda Angeles-Agdeppa, Irish P. Baguilat, Julian Gonsalves, and Mario V. Capanzana

5 School gardens in Nepal: design, piloting, and scaling   77
   Dhruba Raj Bhattarai and Pepijn Schreinemachers

6 Trees nurture nutrition: an insight on how to
   integrate locally available food tree and
   crop species in school gardens   86
   Stepha McMullin, Barbara Stadlmayr, Erick Ngethe,
   Brendah Wekesa, Ken Njogu, Agnes Gachuiri, Ben Mbaya,
   Agnes Katiwa, and Ramni Jamnadass

7 The role of school gardens as conservation networks for
   tree genetic resources   105
   Francesca Grazioli, Muhabbat Turdieva, and Chris J. Kettle

8 The impact of school gardens on nutrition outcomes in
   low-income countries   115
   Pepijn Schreinemachers, Ray-yu Yang, Dhruba Raj Bhattarai,
   Bal Bdr Rai, and Mamounata Sandaogo Ouedraogo

9 Parent engagement in sustaining the nutritional gains
   from School-Plus-Home Gardens Project and school-
   based feeding programmes in the Philippines: the case
   of the Province of Laguna   126
   Blesilda Calub, Leila S. Africa, and Bessie Burgos

10 Scaling up the integrated school nutrition model in the
   Philippines: experiences and lessons learned   142
   Emilita Monville-Oro, Imelda Angeles-Agdeppa,
   Irish P. Baguilat, Julian Gonsalves, and Mario V. Capanzana

Case study

C1 The Stephanie Alexander Kitchen Garden Foundation Program   159
   Stephanie Alexander Kitchen Garden Foundation

C2 Reviving local food systems in Hawai'i   171
   Nancy Redfeather and Elizabeth Cole

C3 Food Plant Solutions: School gardens in Vietnam   178
   Karalyn Hingston and Natalie Ching

C4 Preserving local cultural heritage through capacity
   building for girls in the Moroccan High Atlas   185
   Pommelien Da Silva Cosme

C5	Learning gardens cultivating health and well-being – stories from Australia *Peter Dawe, Anthea Fawcett, and Torres Webb*	193
C6	African leafy vegetables go back to school: farm to school networks embrace biodiversity for food and nutrition in Kenya *Aurillia Manjella, Alessandra Grasso, and Victor Wasike*	208
C7	Grow to learn – learning gardens for Syrian children and youth in Lebanon *Nina Lauridsen*	215
C8	School gardens (*māra*): today's learning spaces for Māori *Nick Roskruge*	222
C9	Intergenerational transfer of knowledge and mindset change through school gardens among indigenous children in Meghalaya, North East India *Melari Shisha Nongrum*	231
C10	*Laboratorios para la Vida*: action research for agroecological scaling through food- and garden-based education *Bruce G. Ferguson and Helda Morales*	238
C11	Agrobiodiversity education: the inclusion of agrobiodiversity in primary school curricula in Xiengkhouang Province, the Lao People's Democratic Republic *Chinda Milayvong, Kevin Kamp, and Manivanh Aliyavong*	246
C12	*Katakin kōṃṃan jikin kallib ilo jikuul* – Republic of the Marshall Islands School Learning Garden Program *Koh Ming Wei and Samuel Bikajle*	257
C13	Where the wild things are *Ayfer Tan, Neşe Adanacioğlu, Saadet Tuğrul Ay, Malek Batal, Hala Ghattas, and Salma Talhouk*	267
C14	Slow Food 10,000 gardens – cultivating the future of Africa *Reguli Damas Marandu, John Kariuki Mwangi, Samson Kiiru Ngugi, and Edward Mukiibi*	276

C15 The integration of food biodiversity in school curricula
through school gardens and gastronomy in Brazil 283
*Ana Rosa Domingues dos Santos, Nádia Lúcia Almeida
Nunes, Alessandra Santos dos Santos, Camila Neves Soares
Oliveira, Lidio Coradin, Daniela Moura de Oliveira Beltrame,
and Neio Lúcio de Oliveira Campos*

Index *293*

FIGURES

1.1	The multiple benefits of school gardens	2
1.2	Sustainability is enhanced with seed saving practices, which are now a special feature of the Philippine government's school garden programme	5
1.3	School gardens across the Philippines now feature crop museums where local agrobiodiversity is demonstrated. School gardens serve as a platform for self-learning for parents, students, and the local community	12
1.4	Green leaf manure (with *Gliricidia*) helps to feed soil microbial life, to regenerate soils, to store moisture, and to store carbon in the soils in school gardens	16
1.5	School garden activity with children from the Khasi community in Mulieh, Jaintia Hills, Meghalaya	18
1.6	*Dar Taliba* students in the garden on their way to plant vegetable seedlings which they cultivate	20
4.1	An example of a lighthouse school	65
4.2	Integrated school nutrition model	66
4.3	An example of a bio-intensive garden	67
4.4	Photo of recipes with indigenous vegetables	68
4.5	Photo of a nutrition education activity in a school	69
5.1	Example of the standard garden design with crop calendar	79
5.2	School gardening activities in Ramechhap district of Nepal	82
5.3	School gardening activities in Ramechhap district of Nepal	82
6.1	Based on the original methodology developed by World Agroforestry, a Fruit Tree Portfolio – providing for year-round harvest of at least one fruit rich in vitamins A or C, illustrated by a calendar wheel	91

xii Figures

6.2 An example of a Food Tree and Crop Portfolio for Ngobit, Laikipia County, Kenya. This portfolio provides a recommendation for a diversity of socio-ecological suitable indigenous/underutilized and exotic food trees and crops (vegetables, pulses, and staples) that can be cultivated for addressing year-round food harvest and providing key micronutrients (iron, folate, vitamins A and C) in local diets 93
6.3 Project sites and counties where food tree and crop portfolios have been developed, and school garden locations used as demonstration sites in Kenya (Shalom Primary School, Ngobit, Laikipia County; Yikiatine Primary School and Makutano DEB Primary School, Machakos County. World Agroforestry/Food Trees Project.) 94
6.4 4K Club pupils standing in front of their 'Talking Wall' at school painted with the diversity of healthy foods they have sown in their communal garden 97
6.5 School children participating in a training module on tree planting and management 97
6.6 Customized food and nutrition education training tools developed by programme partners for use in schools and with communities 99
7.1 Dr Dorohova is explaining to schoolchildren technology of artificial cross-breeding of fruit trees used to create a new plant in a school orchard 112
9.1 Operational model of the School-Plus-Home Gardens Project (S+HGP) 128
9.2 Trends in the percentage of SBFP repeaters among partner schools from school years 2016–2019 136
10.1 IIRR's scaling up framework 144
10.2 Research conceptual and theoretical framework 146
10.3 Multi-scalar scaling up strategy 147
10.4 Distribution of LSs in Region IV-A 149
10.5 Crop museum 149
10.6 School visits/exchanges 151
10.7 Package of information, education, and communication materials 153
10.8 Adoption at national scale through DepEd National 155
C1.1 Students and raised beds in Sunshine North Primary School's kitchen garden 161
C1.2 Students from Deans Marsh Primary School are sharing a meal with pasta and vegetables from the garden 163
C1.3 Primary students from Wyndham are learning about cutting vegetables and discovering that it is better to have good sharp knives 164
C2.1 Students at the Māla'ai Culinary Garden cutting morning snack (right) and girls studying a taro leaf (Kalo i ke Kumu) 172
C2.2 Some of the youngest participants in the lo'i (taro patch) 173

C2.3	Students at Ke Kula 'o 'Ehunuikaimalino Public Charter School ku'i the kalo into poi.	174
C2.4	Students at Hōnaunau Elementary School Garden appreciating their morning snack of fruit and cassava, and each other!	177
C3.1	Exploring the picture guide during a training session for teachers	180
C3.2	An example of one of the school gardens	181
C3.3	Students examining the soil	182
C4.1	The Dar Taliba ethnobotanical school garden design from above	187
C4.2	Dar Taliba students planting seedlings in the greenhouse	188
C4.3	Students during a plant and vegetable distribution	190
C5.1	Potential benefits of gardens	194
C5.2	Torres (right) with students from Tagai State College School Community in the Torres Strait	199
C5.3	The Aboriginal learning space and garden. Illustration: Luciano Valeo	201
C5.4	Cultural learning, gardening and leadership in action at Wiridjiribin Nura	202
C5.5	Diverse tropical planting garden (left) and Shepherdson College's Award winning 'Water-wise' food garden and play area (right). Both from Nov 2014	205
C6.1	A selection of ALVs in Kenya. From the left corner: cowpea leaves (*Vigna unguiculata*), African nightshade (*Solanum nigrum*), Ethiopian kale (*Brassica carinata*), spider plant (*Cleome gynandra*), jute mallow (*Corchorus olitorius*), amaranth (*Amaranthus*), slender leaf (*Crotalaria brevidens*), and moringa (*Moringa oleifera*)	209
C6.2	Aurillia with Nakayo and classmates at Mundika Special School	211
C6.3	Students in Busia proudly showing their mandala garden	212
C7.1	The theoretical part of the workshop in Sa'adnayel takes place in the outdoor classroom under a tent canvas where the participants and the trainer can seek cover from the sun while exchanging knowledge (2018)	217
C7.2	Learning garden pre-workshop for children and youth from the local community in Bar Elias, Beqaa Valley. Placed in groups around tables with pens and papers, the attendees had to draw their hopes and dreams for the upcoming garden, which later came to frame the design for this garden (2016)	217
C7.3	The participants and local trainer, Walid, wrapping up a day of hard work in Sa'adnayel after nursing and cultivating their blooming garden (2018)	220
C8.1	Waihi (later Motunui) School (*Rohe o Ngāti Rahiri*) Taranaki. 1915	223
C8.2	*Kura Kaupapa* children assisting with planting native plants around a māra near Whanganui (Putiki). An example of biodiversity in the garden	225
C8.3	Māori Pre-School known as *Kohanga Reo* (language nest) establishing their version of a container garden	226

C8.4	Māra kai produce (and Sarah Puha), Hauiti marae hui, Uawa/Tolaga Bay, East Coast, North Island, New Zealand	229
C9.1	School Garden activity at Nongnah, South West Khasi Hills	234
C9.2	Agrobiodiversity walk at Nongtraw, East Khasi Hills, with the children (left) and Ibanjalis Rani explains about the wild edibles she has collected during the Agrobiodiversity walk at Nongtraw, East Khasi Hills (right)	235
C9.3	Children showcase wild edibles gathered during the agrobiodiversity walk at Nongtraw, East Khasi Hills	236
C10.1	Good food plate created by Lupita Rivera Alcázar, a student in Juan Marcos Mendoza's science class at a preparatory school near the border of Chiapas and Tabasco	240
C10.2	Educators in LabVida training learn to harvest (Figure C10.2a), plant, and cook with (Figure C10.2b) amaranth seed. Amaranth is a nutrient-dense pseudo-grain and vegetable historically grown in much of Mexico. The Spanish suppressed its use in the colonial era because of the religious significance of amaranth-seed figurines for the Aztecs	241
C11.1	Xiengkhouang Province in Laos	247
C11.2	Schematic of the ABD curriculum development process and approval	250
C11.3	Ms Bouaphan is teaching on importance of ABD	250
C11.4	Students learning to make Lao sweet 'Khao Tom'	251
C11.5	Traditional medicinal plants collected from school garden	252
C12.1	Aerial view of the reef and Islets	257
C12.2	Atoll agroforest	260
C12.3	Compost pile with layer of copra cake	262
C12.4	Teachers engaged in cooking	263
C13.1	Student chefs cooking with wild edible plants	270
C13.2	Student presenting a poster about wild edible plants at the Foça Science Education Festival	270
C13.3	Children enjoying hummus sandwiches and fresh carrots prepared by community women	273
C14.1	Molo Street Children Community Garden in Nakuru county, Kenya. Credit: Slow Food International Archive	277
C14.2	Planting seedlings in the Kibubuti Primary School Garden in Kiambu county, Kenya. Credit: Slow Food International Archive	279
C14.3	Schoolchildren with yams in the Nkosi Memorial School Garden in Mukono district, Uganda. Credit: Aimie Eliots	280
C15.1	Students working at the vegetable garden	286
C15.2	Example of a tiny space consortium vegetable production	287
C15.3	Food presentation activity	288
C15.4	Traditional recipes cooking workshop	289
C15.5	Toddlers learning about the benefits of fruits	289

TABLES

3.1	Most common SHCN problems by country	50
4.1	Savings on expenses in a 120-day feeding cycle in sentinel schools	70
4.2	Savings on expenses in a 200-day feeding cycle in sentinel schools	70
4.3	Total number of children that can benefit from the garden produce shared to SBFP in the three sentinel schools	71
4.4	Results of soil analysis in the three sentinel schools	73
4.5	Garden use as platform for learning and sharing nutrition and environment information in 58 lighthouse schools	74
4.6	Integration of garden visitation in different learning areas of 36 lighthouse schools for SY 2016–2017	75
4.7	Use of gardens as learning venues in different learning areas of the sentinel schools for school year 2016–2017 and 2017–2018	75
5.1	Standard cropping calendar used for the Nepal school gardens	80
6.1	Nutrient composition of selected tree and shrub foods (expressed per 100 g edible portion (EP) of fresh weight)	89
8.1	Data collected for the study	118
8.2	Impact of the school garden intervention on nutrition outcomes in Bhutan, Nepal, and Burkina Faso, average treatment effects showing marginal effects at means	120
9.1	Home gardening experience of the respondent households	130
9.2	Changes in vegetable consumption among households of undernourished students from the start to the end of the project	137
9.3	Feedback from parents about benefits derived from and challenges faced in participating in school gardens and having their own home gardens	137
C10.1	Examples of agrobiodiversity-related content in each of LabVida's main certificate programme modules	240
C11.1	Annual breakdown of schools, teachers, and students engaged in ABD learning	254

BOXES

1.1	Soils for life	5
1.2	'Growing for the community, by the community, to be enjoyed by the community' – Donegal pupils work the school plot	6
1.3	Philippines ISNM	8
1.4	Centre for ecoliteracy	9
1.5	Peoples garden school programme	10
1.6	What is a crop museum?	12
1.7	School gardens in the East coast – Australia	13
1.8	Edible Schoolyards Leith, Scotland	14
1.9	The Edible Schoolyard	17
1.10	Tohono O'odham Community Action	19
1.11	School gardens and women's empowerment	20
1.12	International Green Academy	21
2.1		34
2.2		36
2.3		38
6.1	Schools offer a platform for practical action, a case study from Machakos County Kenya	96
6.2	Establishing location-specific food tree and crop portfolios in school gardens for targeting food harvest and nutrient gaps	98
7.1	Moringa trees to improve diets and environmental awareness in Brazil	107
7.2	School gardens and conservation of important fruit tree genetic resources in Central Asia	111
9.1	The school garden as a learning garden	129
9.2	The school garden as an inspirational pocket landscape	129

C1.1	In conversation with Driver Primary School	165
C2.1		175
C6.1	The potential of ALVs in Africa	210
C7.1	Plant and seed selection	218
C7.2	Food AID in Lebanese refugee camps	219
C11.1	Changing perspectives of students	251
C11.2	Local skills transferred from elders to youth	252
C11.3	Behaviour changes	253
C12.1	The Learning Garden Program	260
C13.1	The potential of wild edible species	268
C13.2	Wild edibles to enhance agrobiodiversity in Lebanon	271
C13.3	Wild edible species in Turkey	271
C13.4	Testimonials from the Turkish beneficiaries	273

ACKNOWLEDGEMENTS

The editors would like to thank the many individuals who took the time and effort to submit the chapters and case studies that have contributed to the rich diversity of experiences highlighted in this publication. The editors would also like to extend our sincere thanks to Amy Johnston and Hannah Ferguson, and other staff at Earthscan from Routledge for their guidance during the preparation of the publication.

Nyhria, Blesilda, and Bessie would like to acknowledge the support of Dr Gil C. Saguiguit, former director of The Southeast Asian Regional Center for Graduate Study and Research in Agriculture-Southeast Asian Ministers of Education Organization (SEAMEO-SEARCA); Dr Fernando C. Sanchez, Jr., chancellor of University of the Philippines Los Baños (UPLB); and Dr Josilyn S. Solana, school division superintendent, The Department of Education Region 4-A for their methodical guidance of the School-Plus-Home Gardens Project and the ensuing conference *International Conference on School Gardens: Leveraging the Multi-functionality of School Gardens*, from which papers served as valuable inputs to this publication.

Julian and Emily would like to acknowledge the contribution of Dr Annie Wesley of International Development Research Centre (IDRC) Canada; George Sycip; the Department of Education, especially undersecretary Alain Pascua, Dr Rizalino Rosales, Dr Maria C Dumlao, and the School Health Division of Bureau of Learner Support Services; George Aranas of the Department of Agriculture; Dr Mario V. Capanzana and Dr Imelda Agdepa of the Food and Nutrition Research Institute; and IIRR's Food Security and Nutrition team.

Danny and Nina would like to thank colleagues Bessie, Blesilda, Emily, Julian, and Nyhria for their friendship, creativity, and support.

The publication of this book was made possible through support from the Global Environment Facility, UN Environment, and the Food and Agriculture

Organization of the United Nations within the framework of the global project 'Mainstreaming Biodiversity Conservation and Sustainable Use for Human Nutrition and Well-being'.

To the best of our knowledge, materials presented in this manual have been accurately referenced and sourced. Every effort has been made to ensure that the original source of copyright materials has been provided within the text. If any errors or omissions are noted, we would be pleased to rectify them.

CONTRIBUTORS

Editors

Bessie Burgos (Southeast Asian Regional Center for Graduate Study and Research in Agriculture (SEARCA)) was Program Head for Research & Development of SEARCA from 2010 to 2018. She earned her PhD degree in Science and Technology Studies from the University of Wollongong, New South Wales, Australia, and her Master of Management degree in Agricultural Business from the University of the Philippines Los Baños (UPLB). She was Overall Coordinator of the School-Plus-Home Gardens Project of SEARCA, UPLB, and the Department of Education – Laguna in 2016–2017. As Overall Coordinator, she provided oversight, guidance, and direction to the project and established linkages with various national and international organizations.

Blesilda Calub (University of the Philippines Los Baños), a university researcher, serves as Program Leader of the Organic Agriculture Program and Chair of the Interdisciplinary Studies Center on Organic Agriculture at the University of the Philippines Los Baños. Dr Calub leads programmes towards science-based and people-oriented sustainable organic agriculture through research, extension, teaching, public service, information material production, and technical support to various national and international agricultural community development institutions. As Project Leader of the School-Plus-Home Gardens Project she facilitated participatory capacity- and knowledge-building activities that enabled stakeholders to be actively committed to sustaining and scaling up the education and nutrition of schoolchildren.

Julian Gonsalves (International Institute of Rural Reconstruction) is Senior Advisor at the International Institute of Rural Reconstruction, Philippines. He works in a range of areas related to food security, nutrition, and climate change. His work on regenerative agriculture for small holder agriculture and biointensive systems for schools and urban poor spans nearly four decades, mostly in Asia. He has been awarded the Global 500 award for Environmental Achievement by United Nations Environment Programme (UNEP). He has a strong interest in relating science to solving problems of the poor, and he currently spends half his time travelling in rural areas in order to be on the front lines.

Danny Hunter (Bioversity International) is Senior Scientist in the Healthy Diets from Sustainable Food Systems initiative at Bioversity International. He has more than 25 years of experience working in over 30 countries, covering most regions of the world, specializing in the conservation and sustainable use of crop and tree genetic resources and their role in linking sustainable agriculture, environment, health, and nutrition. He is the Agrobiodiversity Research Theme Leader for the Plant and AgroBiosciences Centre (PABC) at National University of Ireland Galway (NUIG) and Series Editor of Issues in Agricultural Biodiversity, a series of books published by Earthscan from Routledge in association with Bioversity International.

Nina Lauridsen (Bioversity International; https://orcid.org/0000-0001-7208-7262) works as a research fellow for the Biodiversity for Food and Nutrition project at Bioversity International. She has previously been engaged with work on neglected and underutilized species, and forest genetic resources. Nina has a master's in agricultural development from the University of Copenhagen and did her thesis studying the impact of deforestation on forest communities in Cambodia.

Emilita Monville-Oro (International Institute of Rural Reconstruction) has spent two decades as a development worker at IIRR, a global research, development, and training institute, which has been developing innovative and practical solutions to alleviate poverty. She holds an MA in public health from James P. Grant School of Public Health, BRAC University in Bangladesh, under a full scholarship. Emily is a primary investigator of two evidence-based projects on integrated approaches to nutrition for school-age children, which is now being scaled up nationwide in the Philippines. She is a staunch advocate of farmer innovations and nutrition-sensitive programming to scale up nutrition.

Carmen Nyhria Rogel (Southeast Asian Regional Center for Graduate Study and Research in Agriculture (SEARCA); https://orcid.org/0000-0002-6844-6557) coordinates the development of projects, provides technical support and oversight, and monitors research projects and activities while also managing the centre's programme for the provision of research grants in Southeast Asia. She is a team member in the research initiatives of the centre towards influencing policy directions, building research capacities, and promoting research activities in the region with a focus on inclusive and sustainable agricultural and rural development (ISARD). She is currently working with the team on developing an online courseware on school gardens and scaling out the School + Home Gardens Project (S+HGP) to other parts of the Philippines and to other countries in Southeast Asia.

Contributors

Neşe Adanacioğlu (Aegean Agricultural Research Institute; https://orcid.org/0000-0001-9009-8635), received her MSc in 2002 with the thesis 'Investigations on the cultivation of *Lentinula edodes* on bag culture without using laminar air flow hood' as well as her PhD in 2011 with the thesis 'Researches on the cultivation techniques of *Agaricus brasiliensis* (Syn. A. blazei Murrill.) mushroom' – both from Ege University, Faculty of Agriculture, where she also worked at as a research assistant between 2006 and 2010. Since 2010 she has been working as a researcher at Department of Biodiversity and Genetic Resources of Aegean Agricultural Research Institute, Izmir, Turkey.

Leila S. Africa (University of the Philippines Los Baños) is an associate professor and current director of the Institute of Human Nutrition and Food, College of Human Ecology, University of the Philippines Los Baños (UPLB). She has a doctorate in Nutrition and has been teaching community nutrition undergraduate and graduate courses since 2002 at UPLB. She served as Study Leader for Nutrition in the School-Plus-Home Gardens Project. She led the impact study of the project and organized nutrition training for teachers and vegetable cooking contests for mother and student teams. She produced a nutrition-based cookbook with standardized formulation for use in schools.

Imelda Angeles-Agdeppa (Food and Nutrition Research Institute) is the chief science research specialist of the Nutrition Management and Monitoring Division of the Department of Science and Technology – Food and Nutrition Research Institute. This division is in charge of conducting national nutrition surveys, modelling nutrition interventions, and developing policy recommendations. She was conferred Scientist II in 2018. She has authored numerous articles in peer-reviewed international and local journals, and is a recipient of the Alberto G. Romualdez, Jr. Outstanding Health Research Award and Outstanding Oral Presentation Award by the Society of International Endocrinology and Metabolism, Seoul, South Korea.

Manivanh Aliyavong (The Agro-Biodiversity Initiative) is currently Project Management Coordinator for the Swiss-funded Agro-Biodiversity Initiative (TABI). Previously she was a Contract Management and Monitoring Officer. She worked for Nam Theun 2 Power Company (NTPC) as Administrative and Program Assistant under the Social and Environment Division, and for Nam Et Phou Loei Integrated Conservation and Development as Project Finance and Admin Assistant.

Contributors **xxiii**

Irish P. Baguilat (International Institute of Rural Reconstruction (IIRR)) is currently the Applied Learning Program Manager at IIRR. As a former Food and Nutrition Program Manager, she led the implementation of several research projects. She co-managed the 'Integrated Approach to Address Food and Nutrition Security in the Philippines' project that developed a school nutrition model. She also served as the project manager for the 'Improving Food and Nutrition Security in the Philippines Using Schools as Platforms' project that scaled up an integrated school nutrition. Irish received her BSc in Agriculture from the University of the Philippines and is currently pursuing her master's in Community Development.

Malek Batal (World Health Organization (WHO); Collaborating Centre on Nutrition Changes and Development (TRANSNUT); https://orcid.org/0000-0001-5672-0371) is professor of Public Health Nutrition at the Nutrition Department of the Université de Montréal's Faculty of Medicine and Director of TRANSNUT. His research focusses on the nutrition transition; the double burden of malnutrition; food security; and the environmental, social, economic, and cultural determinants of food choices, and their relationship to the health of individuals and the ecosystem. He works with many populations, including Indigenous peoples in Canada and South America, and rural populations in the Middle East, South America, and the Caribbean.

Daniela Moura De Oliveira Beltrame (Biodiversity for Food and Nutrition (BFN) project, Brazil) holds an MSc and a PhD in nutrition (food science) from the University of São Paulo. As the national coordinator of the Biodiversity for Food and Nutrition (BFN) project in Brazil, Daniela led the implementation of activities in the country and collaborated with universities and national research agencies to carry out work such as determining the nutrition composition of and developing an online database with 70 underutilized fruit species native to Brazil as well as liaising with partner ministries for the inclusion of food biodiversity in public policies and programmes, such as nutrition education, food procurement, and school feeding.

Dhruba Raj Bhattarai (Nepal Agricultural Research Council) is Chief and Senior Scientist at the Outreach Research Division of the Nepal Agricultural Research Council. He has more than 15 years of experience in the field of food security and vegetable science, with a particular interest in research projects that promote integrated approaches for improving nutrition in Nepal. He has published 5 books and over 100 papers. He holds a BSc in Agriculture from Chaudhary Charan Singh University (CCS) India; an MSc in horticulture from Institute of Agriculture and Animal Sciences, Tribhuvan University; and a PhD in vegetable science from Dr. Y. S. Parmar University of Horticulture & Forestry, India.

Samuel Bikajle (Republic of the Marshall Islands Public School System) is the Learning Garden Program Coordinator for the Republic of the Marshall Islands

Public School System. He is passionate about composting as he believes his country can build up soil to combat what land is lost to sea level rise.

Neio Lúcio De Oliveira Campos (University of Brasília) is an associate professor in the Department of Geography and the Center for Excellence in Tourism at the University of Brasilia, where he is currently also the director. He holds a PhD in urban and regional planning, and his research focusses on socio-spatial dynamics, tourism planning for sustainable development, and research methodologies applied to geography and tourism. He has been a board member on several decision committees, such as the Federal District Tourism Development Council. He is also an ad hoc consultant at Brazilian Higher Education Council – CAPES.

Mario V. Capanzana (Department of Science and Technology Food and Nutrition Research Institute (DOST-FNRI)) is the Director of the DOST-FNRI. He is actively involved in the field of food and nutrition as a researcher and an educator, and in community development and extension. His research interests are on food fortification, functional foods, technology transfer, food quality and safety, and food product development. He has contributed significantly to the crafting of the Food Fortification Law in the Philippines and holds several patents and utility models as an inventor. He is the 2016 Presidential Lingkod Bayan Award awardee for being a key player in addressing malnutrition in the country.

Natalie Ching (Bioversity International and The American University of Rome) was born in Hong Kong but is also a native of Seattle, Washington. She received her BSc in public health from the University of Washington, where she became interested in food- and nutrition-related issues. Currently, she is pursuing an MA in food studies at The American University of Rome and completing her dissertation on urban agriculture.

Elizabeth Cole (The Kohala Center), EdD, is a founding member of The Kohala Center, an institute for research, conservation, and education, turning research and ancestral knowledge into action so that communities can thrive – ecologically, economically, culturally, and socially. Elizabeth has created programmes for community-based food system development, incorporating a public seed initiative, farm-to-school programmes, farmer training, technical assistance, and capitalization for rural enterprises. She supported Nancy Redfeather's leadership in the Hawaii Island School Garden Network and the Hawai'i Farm to School Hui, and was an initial partner in the 'Aina Pono initiative to provide locally produced fresh food to Hawai'i's public school students.

Lidio Coradin (Biodiversity for Food and Nutrition (BFN) project, Brazil) is the National Project Director of the BFN project in Brazil. He is a former employee of the Brazilian Agriculture Research Corporation – Embrapa, where he acted as Research Director of the Genetic Resources and Biotechnology Research Centre and was also in charge of the Species Conservation Division at the Ministry of the Environment. Lidio is responsible for the establishment of the Plants for the Future Initiative in Brazil. He also acted as negotiator during meetings of the Convention on Biological Diversity and Food and Agriculture Organization of the United Nations' (FAO's) International Treaty on Plant Genetic Resources for Food and Agriculture.

Pommelien Da Silva Cosme (Global Diversity Foundation) has a bachelor's degree in Arabic and Islamic Studies, and a master's degree in Business Communications from K.U. Leuven, Belgium. She is based in Marrakech (Morocco), where she has been working for the Global Diversity Foundation since 2017. In her role as Mediterranean Programme and Communications Coordinator, she contributes to the successful implementation of the High Atlas Cultural Landscapes Programme through the delivery of creative and engaging communications, and co-leads on grant management and donor relations.

Peter Dawe (Royal Botanic Gardens) has been the Youth Community Greening Coordinator for the Royal Botanic Gardens for the last four years and has been delivering environmental education to students and communities for the last 30 years. This experience, combined with a Master of Environmental Management, Bachelor of Education, and Diploma of Sustainability, provides him with the expertise, knowledge, and passion to deliver such an important message and programme.

Lesley Drake (Partnership for Child Development, Imperial College London) is the Executive Director of the Partnership for Child Development (PCD), Imperial College London. PCD is recognized internationally for its focus on quality science and building the evidence base around effective, sustainable, and scalable school health and nutrition interventions in low- and middle-income countries. Her work has influenced both UN strategy and government plans to establish schools as scalable and sustainable platforms for the delivery of simple health services to children and to the wider community. She was instrumental in developing the principles of good practice: Focusing Resources on Effective School Health (FRESH) launched at Education for All (EFA) 2000.

Kaia Engesveen (WHO Department of Nutrition for Health and Development) is a technical officer at the Unit for Nutrition Policy and Scientific Advice in the WHO Department of Nutrition for Health and Development, where she supports the monitoring, development, and implementation of national nutrition policies, including the Nutrition-Friendly Schools Initiative (NFSI). Kaia holds an MSc in public health nutrition from the University of Oslo, where her research focussed on a human rights-based role and capacity analysis for breastfeeding. Before joining WHO, she worked at the UN Standing Committee on Nutrition (SCN), the World Food Programme in Afghanistan, and The United Nations Children's Fund (UNICEF) in the Republic of Maldives.

Anthea Fawcett (Remote Indigenous Gardens Network, The EduGrow School Garden Awards and Foodswell Limited) has worked in sustainable design, policy advocacy, social innovation, and research roles for over 25 years. A farmer's daughter, she believes in building resilience and co-designed solutions, and supporting everyone's right to food security and sovereignty. She possesses academic qualifications in history and critical theory; is a member of Al Gore's Climate Reality Leaders programme; and currently works with Vast Solar, an Australian renewable energy technology company. She is the founder of the Remote Indigenous Gardens Network, The EduGrow School Garden Awards, and Foodswell Limited.

Bruce G. Ferguson (Departamento de Agricultura, Sociedad y Ambiente, El Colegio de la Frontera Sur, Mexico; http://orcid.org/0000-0003-3963-2024) (MS, PhD, University of Michigan) is researcher and professor in the Agriculture, Society and the Environment Department at El Colegio de la Frontera Sur in San Cristóbal de Las Casas, Chiapas, Mexico. His current research and teaching explore agroecology, food systems, and critical pedagogy. Together with Helda Morales, he coordinates *Laboratorios para la Vida*, a programme that trains educators in garden- and food system-based education. He is also part of a research group focussed on scaling out agroecology for more just and sustainable food systems. He is associate editor of *Agroecology and Sustainable Food Systems*.

Agnes Gachuiri (World Agroforestry (ICRAF)) holds an MSC in ecology and environmental science, and works with World Agroforestry (ICRAF), Nairobi, Kenya, as research technician. Her research interest is in agricultural biodiversity, tree domestication, sustainable agriculture, and rural development. She undertakes both participatory research and adaptive research with various projects and partners.

Andrea Polo Galante (Food and Agriculture Organization of the United Nations (FAO)) is a senior nutrition consultant for FAO in the Nutrition and Food Systems Division, engaged in providing advice and expertise on mainstreaming nutrition, specifically in food value chains and home-grown school feeding programmes. Previously, she was the President of the Brazilian Nutrition Association and worked closely with the biggest initiative to date by the Brazilian government to combat hunger. She has over 25 years of research consulting and management experience, particularly in the areas of policy and knowledge dissemination. She holds a master's and a PhD in nutrition sciences from University of Sao Paulo Brazil.

Hala Ghattas (American university of Beirut) has focussed in her research on the biological, social, and structural determinants of maternal and child health and nutrition in low-resource settings and marginalized populations. Her research includes mixed-methods studies of food insecurity experience, barriers to appropriate infant feeding, and barriers to antenatal care access as well as survey research on food security, nutrition, and health status of refugees. Her work responds to the challenges identified by designing, implementing, and evaluating public health interventions to address these. One example is a community-based intervention to empower marginalized women through the establishment of social enterprises that cater healthy food to refugee schoolchildren.

Alessandra Grasso (Vrije Universiteit Amsterdam; https://orcid.org/0000-0002-2962-9502) is a PhD student in sustainable nutrition at the Vrije Universiteit Amsterdam, the Netherlands. Her research focusses on the environmental sustainability implications of food intake and food-related behaviour in vulnerable groups in Europe. In 2015, she went to Kenya as a U.S. Borlaug Fellow in Food Security. There she supported the Biodiversity for Food and Nutrition project by documenting knowledge, attitudes, and practices related to locally available fruits and vegetables in Busia County. In the same year she received her MSc in public health from Johns Hopkins Bloomberg School of Public Health.

Francesca Grazioli (Bioversity International) is working as a research officer for the Cacao Genetic Resources Team to implement projects focussed on the challenges of climate change throughout the whole spectrum of the cocoa value chain. She is also involved in the implementation of monitoring and evaluation activities in projects about the impact of biodiversity on improving livelihoods across different countries. Before joining Bioversity International, she worked as an economist for FAO on household food resilience and food security in the sub-Saharan area. Francesca has a background in economics and social sciences, with a focus on development economics and food justice.

Karalyn Hingston (Food Plant Solutions) has over 20 years of experience in the agricultural sector, with a wide range of skills and experience, including production management, freight, administration, human resources, and quality systems. Karalyn joined Food Plant Solutions in October 2012, progressing to the role of Executive Officer. During that time, Karalyn has driven significant growth with Food Plant Solutions. Karalyn's specific achievements include significantly increasing the number of project partners, contracts with major international aid organizations, and international awareness and recognition of Food Plant Solutions' work, and putting structures and systems in place to streamline processes and ensure accountability (both for Food Plant Solutions and its partners).

Ramni Jamnadass (World Agroforestry (ICRAF)), PhD, leads the Trees Theme at World Agroforestry (ICRAF), Nairobi, Kenya. Her research theme promotes tree diversity, domestication, and delivery to promote the use of 'productive' trees in agricultural landscapes and improve food and nutrition security, income, and environmental sustainability. Within the CGIAR Consortium of International Agricultural Research Centers research programme Forests Trees and Agroforestry (FTA), she leads Flagship 1: Tree genetic resources to bridge production gaps and promote resilience. She hosts the African Orphan Crops Consortium; this initiative supports the mainstreaming of 101 crops of nutritional importance to Africans into food systems through the application of new genomic methods.

Aileen R. de Juras (University of the Philippines Los Baños) is an assistant professor at the Institute of Human Nutrition and Food, College of Human Ecology, University of the Philippines Los Baños. She has a BSc in Nutrition and an MSc in applied nutrition from UPLB. Currently, she is working on her doctorate in Public Health at the National Cheng Kung University, Taiwan. Her research and public service involvements include nutrition education, capacity development, and nutrition programme planning and management.

Kevin Kamp (The Agro-Biodiversity Initiative) is currently the Chief Technical Advisor and Team Leader for the Swiss-funded Agro-Biodiversity Initiative, a decade-long investment in agrobiodiversity conservation, development, policy support, and scaling in the Lao People's Democratic Republic. Mr Kamp has held leadership positions in programmes supporting biodiversity conservation, sustainable agriculture, climate smart agriculture, fisheries research, and project formulation in Bangladesh, Cambodia, China, the Lao People's Democratic Republic, and Thailand in the Asia region as well as similar positions in Africa and the Caribbean. He has worked for FAO, Danida, Swiss Agency for Development and Cooperation (SDC), civil society organizations, and other development agencies.

Agnes Katiwa (Feed the Children) is a program officer working with Feed the Children to implement different livelihoods projects in Nairobi, including projects on food trees for diversified diets and improved nutrition. The projects aim at empowering the communities for better and improved livelihoods. Agnes has implemented the World Agroforestry (ICRAF)-led Food Tree/Fruiting Africa projects in Laikipia and Machakos-Mwala counties in Kenya. Agnes is currently finalizing her MA degree in community development at Kenyatta University.

Chris J. Kettle (Bioversity International and Eidgenössische Technische Hochschule (ETH) Zurich; https://orcid.org/0000-0002-9476-013), PhD, is an ecologist and a geneticist. He has 20 years of research experience working in tropical forest landscapes and restoration. Since August 2017, he has been leading Bioversity International's cross-cutting interdisciplinary research team, working on conservation and sustainable use of socio-economically and ecologically important trees, and their genetic diversity. He holds a joint appointment and is Group Leader in the Department of Environmental System Science, ETH Zurich, Switzerland, and an associate scientist in the Department of Plant Science, University of Oxford, UK. Prior to joining Bioversity International, he was a senior lecturer at the ETH Zurich (2007–present).

Aurillia Manjella (University of Nairobi, Kenya) is a PhD student in agricultural and applied economics at the University of Nairobi. Her research focusses on value chains analysis of African leafy vegetables in Busia, Kenya. She holds BSc and MSc degrees in agricultural economics and resource management from Moi University. In 2015 she joined Bioversity International as a research consultant, where she supported research, development, and implementation of programme activities in Busia. She also worked on the Linking Farmers to Market project for 4 years, where she tested and successfully implemented a farmer business school model in Busia.

Reguli Damas Marandu (National Slow Food Gardens Project, Tanzania) has sound experiences in the community development sector with a focus on sustainable agriculture and sustainable livelihoods. Currently, he is a national facilitator for the Slow Food gardens (agroecological gardens) project in Tanzania. He is involved in initiating, planning, designing, and implementing sustainable agriculture and agrobiodiversity projects in the country. He is driven by a commitment to attaining sustainable livelihood through protection of agrobiodiversity, enhancing food sovereignty, and food justice. Reguli holds a post-graduate diploma in International Trade and Development from 'Trade Policy Center in Africa' (Trapca) and a bachelor's degree in Community Development from Tumaini University of Iringa.

Ben Mbaya (Feed the Children), Head of Programs at Feed the Children's (FEED) Kenya Office, oversees FEED programmes in Kenya and ensures quality, rigour, and intended impact. Ben has more than 10 years of experience in participatory development management within a non-profit setting. Ben also has extensive experience in the design and implementation of people-centred community development and innovation programmes which address issues of nutrition security, income generation, education, and preventative health and water, sanitation and hygiene (WASH) in both rural and urban settings.

Stepha McMullin (World Agroforestry (ICRAF)), PhD, is a social scientist working with World Agroforestry (ICRAF) and based in Nairobi, Kenya. She leads research on the contribution of agroforestry and agricultural biodiversity for improved nutrition outcomes (nutritious foods, food seasonality, diversified diets), food security, and livelihood opportunities. She designs, implements, and leads a team undertaking participatory research (quantitative and qualitative) to inform data gaps on food production and consumption as well as quality of diets/dietary gaps in order to identify suitable agroecological recommendations for making local food systems more nutrition sensitive.

Chinda Milayvong (The Agro-Biodiversity Initiative (TABI)) is the Phakhaolao team leader. She has more than 10 years of experience working with community and non-profit organizations as project assistant and on communication; she worked at Village Focus International and led the short film project and Calendar publication on Land Rights and Natural Resources Management. Today, she is engaged in the Phakhaolao- and Story Telling team at TABI. She likes cooking sweet and nutritious Lao recipes for her kids; her main interests are in the area of Lao natural products, especially medicinal plants.

Helda Morales (Departamento de Agricultura, Sociedad y Ambiente, El Colegio de la Frontera Sur, Mexico; http://orcid.org/0000-0001-7583-2125) is researcher and professor in the Agriculture, Society and the Environment Department at El Colegio de la Frontera Sur. She is from Guatemala City and did graduate work at the Tropical Agricultural Research and Higher Education Center (CATIE) in Costa Rica and University of Michigan. Her research has documented the importance of traditional knowledge for sustainable farming and pest prevention. Recently, she has focussed on education and food systems, working with urban and rural growers and farmers markets as well as international organizations. She is a founder and an active member of AMA-AWA, the Alliance of Women in Agroecology, and co-coordinator of *Laboratorios para la Vida*.

Edward Mukiibi (Slow Food International) is Agronomist and Vice President of Slow Food International. He lives and works in Uganda, where he has created agroecological gardens, Slow Food Presidia, Earth Markets, and a huge network of food communities together with a group of passionate young people.

John Kariuki Mwangi (Slow Food Foundation for Biodiversity), Vice President of the Slow Food Foundation for Biodiversity, coordinator of the Slow Food network and projects in Kenya, and councillor for Slow Food representing East, Central, and South Africa. A graduate of the University of Gastronomic Sciences in Pollenzo, John Kariuki has overseen the construction of more than 300 food gardens and the development of the Slow Food Youth Network in his country.

Erick Ngethe (World Agroforestry (ICRAF)) is a project manager working with ICRAF in Nairobi, Kenya. He manages agroforestry for nutrition projects, including food trees for diversified diets, improved nutrition, and better livelihoods for smallholders in East Africa, and agrobiodiversity and land restoration for the food and nutrition security of smallholder farmers in Eastern Africa. Erick holds an MA degree in development studies from Murdoch University, Australia. His research focus and interests relate to identifying best approaches for designing, implementing, and managing sustainable agricultural programmes for poverty alleviation, food and nutrition security, and improved livelihoods in Eastern Africa.

Samson Kiiru Ngugi (National Slow Food Gardens Project, Kenya) is the national coordinator in the Slow Food Kenya Association. He graduated from the University of Gastronomic Sciences in 2014 and is currently the main collaboration partner of John Mwangi. He also has a role in coordinating the initiatives of Slow Food in Kenya, especially in the region of Nakuru.

Ken Njogu (World Agroforestry (ICRAF)) is a Statistician based in the Trees Theme of ICRAF, Nairobi, Kenya. Ken assists teams in research design, development, and implementation: specifically, through research tool development; supporting quality data collection by training enumerators and electronic data collection and management; and performing statistical data analysis, including report writing.

Melari Shisha Nongrum (North East Slow Food and Agrobiodiversity Society (NESFAS)) is currently the Executive Director of NESFAS, based in Meghalaya, India. Her work involves using traditional knowledge of food systems to transform health and nutrition among indigenous communities. She has also been a faculty of the Martin Luther Christian University for 10 years and has been involved in creating a curriculum that links social work to public health with a focus on incorporating traditional knowledge systems to attain the well-being of communities.

Nádia Lúcia Almeida Nunes (University of Brasília) is a nutritionist, specializing in geriatrics and gerontology. She holds a master's in tourism and has professional experience in public health, food and nutrition education, school feeding, food safety, gastronomy, and environment. She was also an instructor and teacher of professional courses and workshops about these subjects. As a researcher, she collaborated with several studies, including the 'Use of regional products and recipes in school food menus' research in the Center of Excellence in Tourism at University of Brasilia, Brazil. She was Executive Coordinator of the 'Educating with School Gardens and Gastronomy' (PEHEG) project from 2010 to 2016.

Stineke Oenema (UN System Standing Committee on Nutrition) has been the coordinator of the UN System Standing Committee on Nutrition since 2016. She previously worked for civil society and chaired the Netherlands Working Group on Nutrition, a working group of NGOs, the private sector groups, and knowledge institutes. She was member of the Coordinating Committee of the Civil Society Mechanism for the Committee on World Food Security and the editorial board of the Right to Food and Nutrition Watch. She also supported the development of the Global Nutrition Report during its initial years. Between 1995 and 2002 she worked for UNICEF and FAO in Ghana, Vietnam, and Chile.

Camila Neves Soares Oliveira (Department of Species Conservation and Management, Ministry of Environment, Brazil) is an Environmental Analyst in the Department of Species Conservation and Management of the Brazilian Ministry of Environment. She acted as the national project manager of the Biodiversity for Food and Nutrition Project in Brazil. She is a Forest Engineer graduate at the University of Brasília, Brazil, and participated in the Managing Global Government Programme, an initiative of the German Ministry for Economic Cooperation and Development (BMZ), implemented by the German Development Institute (DIE), in 2013.

Mamounata Sandaogo Ouedraogo (Ministry of National Education and Literacy, Burkina Faso) is Inspector for Primary Education at the General Directorate of Basic Education, Ministry of National Education and Literacy in Burkina Faso. She was also Country Project Manager for the Vegetables Go to School Project, funded by the Swiss Agency for Development and Cooperation (SDC) from 2013–2017.

Bal Bdr Rai (Ministry of Agriculture & Forests, Bhutan) is National Coordinator of the School Agriculture Programme at the Department of Agriculture, Ministry of Agriculture and Forests, Royal Government of Bhutan. He plans, supports, and monitors the green vegetable and small livestock farming in schools as part of vocational education. He holds a BSc in Agriculture and an MA in public administration from the University of Canberra. He was also Country Project Manager for the Vegetables Go to School Project, funded by the Swiss Agency for Development and Cooperation (SDC) from 2013–2017. He has vast knowledge on the sustainable farming systems in hilly regions.

Nancy Redfeather (The Kohala Center) is an educator and an avid home gardener who has worked in Hawai'i for the past 25 years to create school learning garden programmes statewide. She helped found the state's Farm to School Program and to bring together the collaborative partners in the State Farm to School Hui, and to create the Hawai'i School Garden Teacher Training and Certification Program (Ku 'Aina Pa) and the Hawai'i School Garden Curriculum Map. She also founded the Hawai'i Public Seed Initiative and the Hawai'i Seed Growers Network. Today she gardens at the Kawanui Farm with her husband Gerry Herbert in Kona, Hawai'i.

Nick Roskruge (Tahuri Whenua, the National Maori Horticultural Collective in New Zealand) (Te Atiawa and Ngati Tama Tribes) is the chairman of Tahuri Whenua, the National Maori Horticultural Collective in New Zealand, and an ethnobotanist involved in a wide range of projects aligned with traditional crops and establishing germplasm collections for the benefit of the indigenous communities involved. He is the author of several books on traditional Maori foods and Maori horticulture, and an associate professor at Massey University, lecturing and supervising in horticulture and Maori/Pacific agribusiness, and working in the Pacific in farmer development programmes sponsored by the NZ Foreign Affairs aid programme.

David Ryckembusch (World Food Programme (WFP)) is the Chief of the Technical Assistance, Digital Innovation, and Private Sector Partnership within the

School Feeding Division of the UN World Food Programme and a champion of home-grown school feeding in partnership with FAO, IFAD, and Bioversity. He joined WFP in 2011 after 15 years of Supply Chain Management with private sector companies such as Solvay and Royal DSM in Europe. He has a master's degree in engineering and graduated with two global executive MBAs. He has also published in collaboration with the World Bank (http://dcp-3.org/school-feeding), International Food Policy Research Institute (IFPRI), The State of Food Security and Nutrition, and several universities.

Ana Rosa Domingues dos Santos (University of Brasília) is assistant professor in the Center for Excellence in Tourism at the University of Brasilia, Brazil, where she has coordinated several research projects related to gastronomy and tourism, with a special focus on regional cuisines, food heritages, and sustainability. She is currently completing a PhD in 'Food Heritage: Cultures and Identities' at the University of Coimbra in Portugal, and her current research focusses on senses, uses, values, and materialities of food heritage. She was the general manager of the 'Educating with School Gardens and Gastronomy' (Projeto Educando com a Horta Escolar e a Gastronomia) project from 2010–2016.

Alessandra Santos dos Santos (University College of Brasília (UniCEUB) and at the CEUMA University College (UNIEURO)) is currently a professor at the UniCEUB and at the UNIEURO in Brazil. Her research focusses on gastronomy, rural tourism, ecotourism, and food and sustainable development. She was the founder and President of the NGO 'Araucária – Integrated Sustainable Development Organization', and her expertise is in planning, designing, and executing projects in tourism for governmental and private sector organizations. She took part in the 'Educating with school gardens and gastronomy' (Projeto Educando com a Horta Escolar e a Gastronomia – PEHEG) project, responsible for environment content and technical assistance for the participants.

Pepijn Schreinemachers (World Vegetable Center; http://orcid.org/0000-0003-1596-3179) is Flagship Program Leader for Enabling Impact at the World Vegetable Center. He coordinates the center's work on scaling approaches, monitoring tools, knowledge management, and impact evaluation. He has conducted studies on the impact of improved vegetable varieties, off-season production methods, farmer training in good agricultural practices, and home and school gardens. Pepijn holds a PhD in agricultural economics from the Center for Development Research, Germany, and an MSc in development studies from Wageningen University, the Netherlands.

Barbara Stadlmayr (ICRAF and University of Natural Resources and Life Sciences, Austria) holds an MSc in nutrition and is based at the Centre for Development Research (CDR) at the University of Natural Resources and Life Sciences, Vienna. She is involved in projects with World Agroforestry (ICRAF) in Nairobi on food trees for diversified diets and improved nutrition. With the Food and Agriculture Organization of the United Nations (FAO) she is co-coordinating an international working group on food composition issues. Her research interests include the link between agriculture and food systems for better nutrition, and the potential of underutilized crops to improve diet quality.

Stephanie Alexander Kitchen Garden Foundation provides professional development, educational resources, and support for schools and early learning centres to deliver pleasurable food education through a kitchen garden programme. The model teaches students how to grow, harvest, prepare, and share fresh, seasonal, delicious food, establishing positive food habits for life. It is an integrated approach that meets a range of health and well-being, education, and community objectives.

Luana Swensson (Food and Agriculture Organization of the United Nations (FAO)) is a legal specialist and serves as an international consultant in the Nutrition and Food Systems Division of FAO. With 8 years of experience in the development field, her work focusses on multidisciplinary policy-oriented research and technical support for the design and implementation of projects related to sustainable public food procurement and home-grown school feeding programmes. Before joining FAO in 2013 she was a post-doctoral researcher at the European University Institute and managed an international research project funded by the Inter-American Development Bank. She is also a lawyer and has a PhD in economics and business law.

Maria Theresa M. Talavera (University of the Philippines Los Baños) is an associate professor at the Institute of Human Nutrition and Food, College of Human Ecology, University of the Philippines Los Baños. She has a Bachelor of Science degree in Nutrition from UPLB and finished her MSc in public health and her Doctor of Public Health (major in nutrition) at the University of the Philippines Manila. She completed a postgraduate diploma at the University of Otago, New Zealand. Her research work is focussed on infant and young child feeding, nutrition in emergencies, school nutrition education, and nutrition programme planning and management.

Salma Talhouk (American University of Beirut; https://orcid.org/0000-0002-4797-4342) is currently interested in the promotion of community stewardship of natural resources. She is leading a participatory digital mapping project that encourages residents to identify and document natural and cultural landmarks in their towns. She is also conducting urban greening research, investigating the use of native and ecologically adapted plants for roofs and green walls. Her more recent focus is a project that explores the links between nature and culture by defining nature and natural resources as objects of cultural concern providing nonmaterial services, such as recreation, aesthetic experiences, healing, and spiritual enrichment.

Ayfer Tan (Biodiversity for Food and Nutrition Project, Turkey; https://orcid.org/0000-0003-4843-2104) has a PhD on genetics from Aegean University Faculty of Agriculture, Turkey. Until her retirement in 2014, she was the Head of Biodiversity and Plant Genetic Resources Department and managed the National Genebank as well as the National Biodiversity and Plant Genetic Resources Programme. In addition, she led various ex situ, in situ (GEF, Project), on-farm (Global Project, Coordinated by Bioversity International), and ecosystem conservation projects (Life Program of EU). Today, she coordinates the regional part of the GEF project, Biodiversity for Food and Nutrition and continues to voluntarily study with local initiatives and NGOs.

Florence Tartanac (Food and Agriculture Organization of the United Nations (FAO)) is Senior Officer in the Nutrition and Food Systems Division and Group Leader of the Market Linkages and Value Chain Group at FAO. Her areas of expertise include sustainable value chain development and inclusive business models, voluntary standards and geographical indications, institutional procurement, and small and medium food enterprise development. Before joining FAO in 2001 she worked 10 years in Guatemala for the French Cooperation INCAP (Institute of Nutrition for Central America and Panama) and UNIDO (United Nations Industrial Development Organization). She is a food engineer and has a PhD in economical geography from Paris University.

Saadet Tuğrul Ay (Batı Akdeniz Agricultural Research Institute; https://orcid.org/0000-0002-1261-593X) graduated in 1991 from Faculty of Agriculture, Aegen University, in Turkey. She started to work at Department of Field Crops, Akdeniz University, as an assistant in 1993 and received her MSc on dye plants three years later. In 2005 she earned her PhD on medicinal and aromatic plants from Akdeniz University Department of Field Crops. Today, she works at the Batı Akdeniz Agricultural Research Institute, where she leads and consults various national, EU, and international projects. Over the years she has attended several international meetings, congresses, and conferences, and has contributed to more than 70 publications.

Muhabbat Turdieva (Bioversity International) has an MSc in forestry and horticulture. Since 1999, she has worked as Regional Project Coordinator for Bioversity International office for Central Asia located in Tashkent, Uzbekistan. Her research areas include study, conservation, and sustainable use of temperate fruit and nut trees originating in Central Asia for improving the livelihoods of local people and the environment, including restoration of degraded lands through the use of specific and intra-specific diversity of indigenous fruit and nut tree species. Her job experience also includes work as a Senior Scientist at Uzbek Research Institute of Forestry and Engineer of Forestry at Khorezm Forestry Farm in Uzbekistan.

Victor Wasike (Genetic Resources Research Centre, Kenya) was the National Project Coordinator of the Biodiversity for Food and Nutrition Project in Kenya (2012–2019). In collaboration with the County Government of Busia, he developed the first County Biodiversity Conservation policy in Kenya. Earlier, he was the Project Agronomist for the German Technical Cooperation Agency (GTZ) Soybean Kenya project that undertook pioneering soybean promotion work that led to the release of the current soybean varieties under cultivation in Kenya. He holds a PhD in soil microbiology from Egerton University and an MSc in soil science from the University of Nebraska, United States. He is currently the Centre Director for the Genetic Resources Research Centre.

Torres Webb (Centre for Relational Learning and Indigibee), a proud Erubam man from Darnley Island in the Torres Strait, is a passionate parent and community engagement advocate, and a traditional gardener and horticulturalist, working to improve the well-being and life chances of all children and youth by focussing on 'what's strong within our communities rather than what's wrong'. He has worked with Youth Challenge Australia in Vanuatu, Asia Pacific Indigenous Youth Network in Philippines, Queensland Youth Parliament, and Oxfam International Youth Partnerships in India. Recently he has been supporting school communities to embed traditional Indigenous Science Knowledges and Wisdoms within the schooling curriculum and education system.

Koh Ming Wei (Center for Getting Things Started and Jitdam Kapeel Ippan Doon) is affiliated with the Center for Getting Things Started and Jitdam Kapeel Ippan Doon (JiKID) – seeking knowledge and wisdom together. Ming Wei, who has a PhD in Sustainability Education, is a gardener, educator, independent researcher and consultant, curriculum developer, and programme evaluator. Her research includes how the school learning garden experience is a context conducive to teaching core subjects, science, technology, engineering, and mathematics (STEM), and foundational life skills, and she created the Pedagogy of Food to frame the kind of education she believes in and shares.

Brendah Wekesa (World Agroforestry (ICRAF)) holds an MSc in food, nutrition, and dietetics, and works as a nutrition consultant at World Agroforestry (ICRAF), Nairobi, Kenya. She works on research on food and nutrition security of individuals/smallholder households and communities, designs and implements appropriate nutrition interventions, and assesses the impact. The goal is to promote nutrition-sensitive agriculture and create awareness on consumption of adequate nutritious diets for improved nutrition and health outcomes.

Ray-yu Yang (World Vegetable Center; http://orcid.org/0000-0002-6136-3943) heads the nutrition group of the World Vegetable Center in Taiwan. She specializes in laboratory methods to characterize nutritional and functional properties of vegetables. She works with multidisciplinary teams and develops programmes linking agriculture and nutrition to improve diets and health. She received her PhD in food and nutrition from the Institute of Tropical Agriculture and International Cooperation at Ping-Tung University, Taiwan.

ABBREVIATIONS

ABD	Agrobiodiversity
ACIAR	Australian Centre for International Agricultural Research
AFA	Asian Farmers' Association for Sustainable Rural Development
ALV	African leafy vegetables
AMA-AWA	Alliance of Women in Agroecology
ASEAN	Association of Southeast Asian Nations
AWESOME	Active, well-nourished, and smart
BFN	Biodiversity for Food and Nutrition
BIG	Bio-intensive garden
BMI	Body mass index
CaLaBaRZon	Cavite, Laguna, Batangas, Rizal, and Quezon (five provinces in the Philippines)
CARD	Council of Agriculture and Rural Development
CAPES	Brazilian Higher Education Council
CATIE	Tropical Agricultural Research and Higher Education Center
CCS	Chaudhary Charan Singh University
CDR	Centre for Development Research
CESCR	Committee on Economic, Social and Cultural Rights
CET-UnB	Centre for Excellence in Tourism of the University of Brasilia
CISU	Civil Society in Development
CRC	Committee on the Rights of the Child
CTA	Technical Centre for Agricultural and Rural Co-operation
DA	Department of Agriculture
DA-BPI	DA-Bureau of Plant Industry
DepEd	Department of Education
DFC	Drivers of Food Choice
DFID	UK Government's Department for International Development

Abbreviations **xxxix**

DOLISA	Department of Labour, Invalids, and Social Affairs
DOST-FNRI	Department of Science and Technology Food and Nutrition Research Institute
DSWD	Department of Social Welfare and Development
EBSCO	Elton B. Stephens Co.
EC	European Commission
EENT	Eyes, ears, nose, and throat
EFA	Education for All
ENNS	Expanded National Nutrition Survey
EPP	Edukasyong Pantahanan at Pangkabuhayan
EsP	Edukasyon sa Pagpapakatao
ETH	Eidgenössische Technische Hochschule
EU	European Union
FAO	Food and Agriculture Organization of the United Nations
FAO-RAP	FAO Regional Office for Asia and the Pacific
FEED	Feed the Children
FNDE	Fundo Nacional para o Desenvolvimento da Educação (National Fund for the Development of Education)
FNE	Food and nutrition education
FNRI	Food and Nutrition Research Institute
FNRI-DOST	FNRI of the Department of Science and Technology
FTA	Forests Trees and Agroforestry
FRESH	Focusing Resources on Effective School Health
GarNESupp	Gardening, nutrition education, and supplementary feeding
GDF	Global Diversity Foundation
GDP	Gross domestic product
GEF	Global Environment Facility
GLOPAN	Global Panel on Agriculture and Food Systems for Nutrition
GoV	Government of Vietnam
GPP	Gulayan sa Paaralan Program
GROW	Growing to Renew Our World
GSFP	Ghana School Feeding Programme
GTZ	German Technical Cooperation Agency
HGSF	Home-grown school feeding
HISGN	Hawai'i Island School Gardening Network
HKI	Helen Keller International
HLPE	High Level Panel of Experts on Food Security and Nutrition
ICN	International Nutrition Conference
ICRAF	World Agroforestry
IDRC	International Development Research Centre
IFAD	International Fund for Agricultural Development
IFPRI	International Food Policy Research Institute
IFS	Indigenous Food System
IIRR	International Institute of Rural Reconstruction

IMEIGEP	Action Plan for Strengthening the Link between Education and Employment
INCAP	Institute of Nutrition for Central America and Panama
INFOODS	International Network of Food Data Systems
IPBES	Intergovernmental Science-Policy Platform on Biodiversity and Ecosystem Services
IPC-IG	International Policy Centre for Inclusive Growth
IPES	International Panel of Experts on Sustainable Food Systems
IRSP	Regional Institute of Public Health
ISARD	Inclusive and sustainable agricultural and rural development
ISNM	Integrated School Nutrition Model
JES	Julugan Elementary School
JiKID	Jitdam Kapeel Ippan Doon
KAP	Kū āina Pā (Standing Firmly in Knowledge Upon the Land)
LabVida	Laboratorios para la Vida
Lao PDR	Lao People's Democratic Republic
LGU	Local government unit
LS	Lighthouse school
MAO	Municipal Agriculture Office
MAPEH	Music, Arts, Physical Education and Health
MBLA	Moroccan Biodiversity and Livelihoods Association
MNAO	Municipal Nutrition Action Office
MoE	Ministry of Education
MOES	Ministry of Education and Sports
MoU	Memorandum of Understanding
MSWDO	Municipal Social Welfare and Development Office
NARC	Nepal Agricultural Research Council
NCD	Non-communicable diseases
NCP	Nutrition Center of the Philippines
NESFAS	North East Slow Food and Agrobiodiversity Society
NFSI	Nutrition-Friendly Schools Initiative
NGO	Non-governmental organization
NGTS	Nutrition Goes to School
NHOPI	Native Hawaiian and Other Pacific Islanders
NNC	National Nutrition Council
NPSW	National Parks and Wildlife Service
NSMP	National School Meals Programme
NTFP	Non-timber forest product
NTPC	Nam Theun 2 Power Company
NUI Galway	National University of Ireland Galway
OFSP	Orange-fleshed sweet potato
PAA Africa	Africans for Africa
PABC	Plant and AgroBiosciences Centre

PARRFI	Philippine Agriculture and Resources Research Foundation, Inc.
PCD	Partnership for Child Development
PEHEG	Projeto Educando com a Horta Escolar e a Gastronomia (Educating with School Gardens and Gastronomy)
PIDS	Philippine Institute for Development Studies
PNAE	Programa Nacional de Alimentação Escolar (National School Feeding Program)
POES	Provincial Office of Education and Sports
PPAN	Philippine Plan of Action for Nutrition
PSS	Public school system
PTA	Parent-teacher associations
PTC	Parent-teacher conference
R&D	Research and Development
RACCC	Reiby Aboriginal Community Consultative Committee
RCHE	Red Chiapaneca de Huertos Educativos
RDA	Recommended dietary allowance
RIHE	Red Internacional de Huertos Educativos
RMI	Republic of the Marshall Islands
RMI Map	RMI Jikin kallib ilo jikuul Curriculum Map
RWJF	Robert Wood Johnson Foundation
S+HGP	School + Home Gardens Project
SAKGF	Stephanie Alexander Kitchen Garden Foundation
SBES	Sunny Brooke Elementary School
SBFP	School-based supplementary feeding programme
SDAID	Sawa for Development and Aid
SDC	Swiss Agency for Development and Cooperation
SDG	Sustainable Development Goal
SEAMEO	Southeast Asian Ministers of Education Organization
SEAMEO INNOTECH	SEAMEO Center for Educational Innovation and Technology
SEAMEO RECFON	SEAMEO Regional Centre for Food and Nutrition
SEAMEO–SEARCA	SEAMEO Southeast Asian Regional Center for Graduate Study and Research in Agriculture
SEARCA	Southeast Asian Regional Center for Graduate Study and Research in Agriculture
SFP	School feeding programme
SGP	School Gardens Project
SHN	School health and nutrition
SINGI	Sustainable Income Generating Investment Group (Kenya)

STEM	Science, technology, engineering, and mathematics
SUPW	Socially Useful Productive Work
SW	Severely wasted
TABI	The Agro-Biodiversity Initiative (Lao PDR)
TCP	Teacher-child-parent
TES	Tinabunan Elementary School
TOCA	Tohono O'odham Community Action
ToT	Training of Trainers
TRANSNUT	Collaborating Centre on Nutrition Changes and Development
Trapca	Trade Policy Center in Africa
TREES	Trees for the Future
TVET	Technical and Vocational Education and Training
UN	United Nations
UNEP	United Nations Environment Programme
UNESCO	United Nations Educational, Scientific and Cultural Organization
UNHCR	United Nations Refugee Agency
UNICEF	United Nations Children's Fund
UNIDO	United Nations Industrial Development Organization
UNIEURO	CEUMA University College
UniCEUB	University College of Brasília
UNSCN	United Nations System Standing Committee on Nutrition
UPLB	University of the Philippines Los Baños
USAID	United States Agency for International Development
USD	US dollars
USDA	U.S. Department of Agriculture
VGtS	Vegetables Go to School
VND	Vietnamese Dong
VTAH	Vocational and Technical College
W	Wasted
WASH	Safe water, sanitation and hygiene
WB	World Bank
WFP	World Food Programme
WHO	World Health Organization
WHO WPRO	World Health Organization Western Pacific Regional Office
WMO	World Meteorological Organization
YCG	Youth Community Greening

1
SCHOOL GARDENS
Multiple functions and multiple outcomes

Julian Gonsalves, Danny Hunter, and Nina Lauridsen

Introduction

School garden programmes have been a popular development intervention for many decades. The objectives for school gardens have, however, differed greatly, determined by the purpose, the targeted audiences, and the proponent. In the developing world, these have included teaching improved farming skills, supporting community food production, raising funds, and demonstrating exemplary agricultural practices to the communities surrounding the schools. In the industrialized world (and increasingly in the global South), school gardens have served a broader education function, helping children understand science, nature, and the environment. Increasingly a case is also made for reconnecting rapidly urbanizing school communities with the realities of rural areas, local food culture, local food biodiversity, and farm tourism. There is now a wider recognition of the role of school gardens in environmental and nature education, in local food biodiversity and conservation, food and ecoliteracy, diets, nutrition and health, and agricultural education. The current concerns about environmental degradation and the disconnect of young people with nature and agriculture have resulted in school gardens receiving unprecedented attention.

However, with donors and government, the nutrition agenda is also driving the current interest in supporting school garden programmes. This is a major focus of many of the chapters and case studies in this book, highlighting the importance of school gardens as a tool for improving food and nutrition education – especially through the better incorporation of local agrobiodiversity and enhanced awareness of its nutritional value – to improve healthy eating habits and dietary diversity. Governments are embarrassed and challenged by the growing prevalence of malnutrition among school-aged children. Evidence from nutrition surveys has drawn attention to school-aged malnutrition. In the global South, funding for school nutrition activities including gardens and associated feeding programmes is sourced from health and nutrition sectors resulting in mainstreaming and institutionalization efforts and policy support. In an increasing number of countries, frameworks are being developed to support universal school feeding programmes. This wider attention to the nutrition agenda in schools, a parallel effort to find ways to leverage the nutrition contributions of agriculture through what is now referred to as nutrition-sensitive agriculture, with the engagement of a diverse range of sectors and players (not just agriculture), has brought school gardens back to the development agenda. The increasing appreciation of the wider multiple benefits and multi-functionality of school gardens is indeed the driver of this growing interest in school gardens, irrespective of geography (Figure 1.1).

This chapter provides a brief history of school gardens and an overview of their multiple benefits. These benefits include: a better understanding of the agriculture and nutrition sectors; enhancement of farming and livelihood skills; behavioural and attitudinal changes towards food, including a wider awareness of healthy eating and diets; the conservation of agrobiodiversity; understanding climate change impacts on agriculture and food production; enhancing academic skills and performance; empowerment of girls and women; reconnecting indigenous children with their foods and culture; and using these as a potential space to address mental health and well-being in schoolchildren. The chapter concludes with the identification of some key issues for the future of school gardens and a brief outline of the structure of the book including an overview of the chapters and case studies.

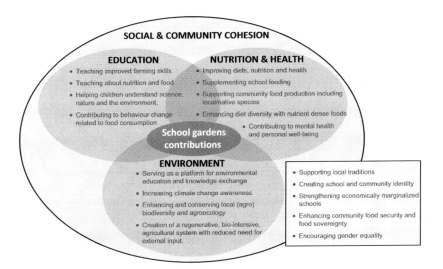

FIGURE 1.1 The multiple benefits of school gardens.

School gardens: a short history[1]

In the last century, in Europe and the United States, school gardens have featured as a hunger intervention. Some of the earliest gardening efforts (George Putnam School in Massachusetts) remain useful reminders of the importance of school gardens and the role they played in hunger mitigation (e.g. the Victory Gardens in the two World Wars and the introduction of 'U.S. Garden Armies' by the Federal Bureau of Education). By the end of 1906, the U.S. Department of Agriculture (USDA) estimated that there were 75,000 school gardens mostly referred to as relief gardening. School gardens were considered a national phenomenon, but they were also considered a part of U.S. culture from the 1890s to 1920s (Wills, 2019). In the 1970s the growing environmental movement helped revive interest in school gardens, resulting in another period of intense growth in the 1990s (Hayden-Smith, 2015). In recent years, the FoodCorps[2] movement has grown, supporting school and community garden efforts. Learning about gardening, the environment, nature, and sustainable diets characterizes current school gardening efforts in Europe, Australia, and the United States.

In the developing world, in the mid-sixties and seventies, school gardens have featured primarily as food security interventions which help encourage children to appreciate agriculture and to learn how food is produced. School gardens are largely featured as part of efforts to address hunger and malnutrition among schoolchildren and occasionally to supplement school feeding programmes. Linking school gardens with school feeding and nutrition education is emerging as a new area to converge the efforts of the agriculture, health, and nutrition sectors in school platforms. Linking schools with communities has brought in an added interest in home gardens and their role in supporting household nutrition. The role of school gardens in behavioural modification in relation to healthy food, sustainable diets, and environmental stewardship is also receiving prominent attention. In the global South, education for vocational agricultural training or agricultural education has been an important focus for school gardens. Some have been used for food production, often with the intention that they might help to augment the ingredient requirements of school meal programmes. In some cases such initiatives have been unsustainable because of the lack of resources, motivation, or expertise, though some countries, such as Costa Rica, with suitable policies and enabling environments are the exception (FAO, 2010). In many instances, though, when the donor support has stopped, so too has the school garden programme. In the Philippines, the Department of Education and the Department of Agriculture have allocated funds to schools to support both gardens and feeding programmes: policy and recent legislation have helped improve the sustainability of such programmes.

School garden programmes in the global South have sometimes had a troubled past often due to poor clarity on the objectives and relevance of school garden interventions to the wider educational role of schools and often further complicated by a lack of vision and creativity, resulting in the perception of school gardens as drudgery and efforts to integrate them into schools as 'ruralisation' of the curriculum (FAO, 2010). This has often led to negative perceptions of school gardens, such as that school garden work can be used as a form of punishment; that school garden activities do not help to pass exams; that gardening is dirty and tiring work; that our children are being exploited; and that the food from school gardens, especially if promoting indigenous crops, was the food of the poor, only eaten in hard times (FAO, 2010). There is also a need to consider the burden school teachers already have with school-based activities. Well-intentioned ideas about promoting school gardens and linking schools with communities and homes have to factor in the increased commitments of human and financial resources. The good intentions of 'outsiders' to link schools with a host of other activities (income generation, community outreach, home gardens of parents, reforestation, and small livestock) must be screened carefully to ensure that teachers and students are not unduly burdened. For community outreach efforts the already burdened teachers should be provided additional human and financial resources, otherwise once again sustainability and quality are sacrificed. More individuals and organizations are realizing the huge potential of school gardens to transform how children learn and understand the world in which they live and act accordingly. There is an increased appreciation that school gardens can be suitable learning spaces to address the complexity of challenges we face by promoting interdisciplinary and holistic approaches. That school gardens not only serve the pupils but also the wider community and society itself by realizing the multiple benefits they can deliver (Figure 1.1).

The multiple benefits of school gardens

Development of agricultural and livelihood skills including knowledge of sustainable food systems

Traditionally school gardens have played an important role, and continue to do so, in teaching agricultural and horticultural skills and associated learning and capacity building. This often covers the full spectrum of the growing cycle from the design of the garden, selection of planting material and agricultural biodiversity, growing and management through harvesting, and preparation for consumption as well as processing for longer-term storage (Figure 1.2). Such activities allow children to learn how to grow and maintain a variety of foods, not just crops and plants but sometimes to raise small livestock and even fish (FAO, 2010). Such learning often also includes enhancing knowledge and skills for the sustainable management of natural resources especially soils (Box 1.1) and water, including recycling or circular economy approaches such as minimizing waste and composting and its addition to soil to enhance soil health, fertility, and water retention. Environment-friendly approaches to managing pests and diseases, and the importance of beneficial insects, including pollinators, are also often taught, including the enhancement of biodiversity in school gardens combined with cultural approaches, such as cover crops, mulching, companion planting, and hand collection of damaging pests. All of this raises awareness and capacity of students in regenerative agriculture including its contribution to a more sustainable food system.

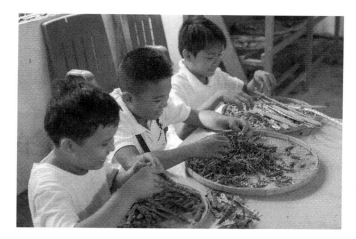

FIGURE 1.2 Sustainability is enhanced with seed saving practices, which are now a special feature of the Philippine government's school garden programme.
Source: IIRR.

BOX 1.1: SOILS FOR LIFE

Soils for Life, an Australian non-profit organization, dedicates its mission to promoting regenerative management practices in farming, also known as regenerative agriculture. Maintaining healthy soils is fundamental to the work of Soils for Life, who believe that regenerative management practices are key to restoring soil quality. Regenerative agriculture not only promotes agrobiodiversity and output productivity but also the overall resilience and sustainability of the system. Through identifying successful regenerative management practices and innovations and disseminating this knowledge through peer-to-peer exchange programmes, through which experienced land managers are partnered with farmer mentors in a 12-month-long dynamic process, Soils for Life works to encourage and support the adoption of regenerative agriculture. Besides promoting regenerative management practices with farmers and land managers, Soils for Life also aims to share its knowledge with other members in the community. One avenue through which Soils for Life works to achieve this is through their school garden programme, which partners with primary schools to establish an educational garden where children can learn about the crucial role soil plays in a healthy ecosystem. The organization believes that children should have an understanding about not only how their food is grown but also the importance of healthy soil to their food. Soils for Life has been advocating and promoting a national school garden policy for Australia, as an engaging medium whereby students can learn biological concepts, such as photosynthesis, as well as environmental issues, such as carbon sequestration.

Source: www.soilsforlife.org.au/program/school-gardens.html

Linked to this is the role of school gardens and associated activities in fostering livelihood and business skills among pupils in the area of market gardening and value adding especially in agriculture-dependent economies where it might be particularly important to focus on developing the horticultural and entrepreneurship skills of older students (FAO, 2010). However, such skills are certainly not exclusive to economies where agriculture dominates. The growing global interest in local food and healthy eating continues to provide increasing opportunities to students with skills in gardening and food irrespective of geography (Box 1.2).

BOX 1.2: 'GROWING FOR THE COMMUNITY, BY THE COMMUNITY, TO BE ENJOYED BY THE COMMUNITY' – DONEGAL PUPILS WORK THE SCHOOL PLOT

Employing the school's instructional outdoor classroom polytunnel, entrepreneurial students at Moville Community College in County Donegal, Ireland have been growing vegetables, which they now supply to the local hotel and restaurant trade. The students began studying horticulture as part of their transition year. When the summer came around, they volunteered to keep working on their plot so that it could benefit from the summer growing season. A local chef who had already spotted the work going on at the school's polytunnel suggested the students link up with the hospitality industry in the area. The owner of the Foyle Hotel, on Moville's main street, says he is proud to list the school on his menus as one of his suppliers. *'The students deliver their produce once a week – they put it in boxes and walk down from the school to the hotel. Their carrots and cabbage were on our Sunday lunch menu last weekend'*. The students did not have much experience of horticulture, though they admit to becoming quite protective of their produce. *'It's not like in class, when you might just be watching'*, says one of the students. *'You're the one doing the planting and the harvesting, so they're your plants'*. The initiative has also led to requests by the restaurant for new crops and plants, which has led to the students testing and evaluating options to see what grows well. From the teachers' point of view, it is a practical way of building interest and skills among their students. *'There's often a fear around growing your own food as adults'*, said one horticulture teacher, *'but they've seen that it takes very little, and that's learning they'll take with them for life'*. The students and wider school community also get to see vegetables they might never have encountered before, and taste them, and know they can grow local produce. It also has a wider relevance. The school is part of the United Nations' Global Schools Programme, which is committed to education around the sustainable development goals including responsible consumption and production and climate action. *'It's about changing the mindset of students in schools'*, explained the home economics teacher. *'They are learning habits which they*

> *then bring home to their community'*. The students also supply another local restaurant, Inish Fusion; its owner is a very satisfied customer. *'The quality is as good as anything else out there, it's hard to beat it, and it's so fresh. You couldn't ask for anything more local than this'*.
> Source: www.irishtimes.com/news/environment/we-couldn-t-stop-the-lettuce-growing-donegal-pupils-work-the-school-plot-1.3997850

Nutrition and the role of school gardens in complementing school feeding

The number of undernourished people has increased to 821 million (FAO et al., 2019), signalling a rise in world hunger and a reversal of trends following a prolonged decline. Child stunting remains unacceptably high with approximately 151 million children affected and 51 million children wasted. About 2 billion people lack the key micronutrients they need for physical and mental development such as iron and vitamin A. More than one in eight adults are obese – over 672 million people worldwide – while three out of four deaths are caused by non-communicable, diet-related diseases (e.g. diabetes, hypertension), particularly in emerging economies and in low- to middle-income countries.

Clearly, current agriculture and food systems are failing to deliver on positive nutrition (and environmental) outcomes, and the agriculture sector is increasingly under pressure to better deliver on nutrition objectives. A small part of that debate on nutrition-sensitive agriculture mentions the role of bio-fortification, which involves breeding new varieties of crops. Others promote diversification of agriculture and the need to ensure that nutrition outcomes accrue in all agriculture programmes through the deliberate inclusion of nutrition outcomes in the impact pathways and value chains for agriculture. It is believed that new ways of approaching agriculture, including biodiverse and agroecological approaches to gardening, smallholder diversification, and agroforestry can provide the level of dietary diversity needed to reduce malnutrition, by promoting a more diverse range of crops, tree species, and protein (livestock, legumes) options. The permaculture movement, the agroecology, and bio-intensive garden (BIG) movements have supported more permanent, structured, and diverse forms of agriculture. School gardens have also proven to be an excellent mechanism to promote nutrition-sensitive agriculture when integrated with nutrition education (Chapter 3) and especially if agroecological approaches are used for ensuring safe food, free of residues.

School feeding programmes receive considerably more attention as mechanisms to address childhood level malnutrition. A recent analysis by the World Bank (WB), World Food Programme (WFP), and the Partnership for Child Development identified that, today, most countries are seeking to provide food, in some way and on some scale, to its schoolchildren (Bundy et al., 2009). School gardening has often not been explicitly mentioned as an intervention but is increasingly being recognized as having a supporting role (Chapter 2). School health and nutrition (SHN) provides a useful platform for the inclusion of school gardens and for eventual convergence with the health and nutrition sectors.

School gardens are usually not linked with school feeding programmes, which is primarily the result of structural problems associated with the fact that school gardens are considered the mandate for Department of Agriculture with feeding being relegated to Department of Education and the rest of the services a responsibility of the health sectors. Increasingly, convergence efforts are being advocated which look at these different initiatives to seek complementarities and synergies such as using the school garden as a platform for more practical nutrition education as well as production of specific nutrient-rich foods that might supplement school meals (Chapter 4). The Department of Education in the Philippines has successfully led the Integrated School Nutrition Model (ISNM), which is currently being institutionalized and mainstreamed throughout the country (Box 1.3 and Chapter 4).[3]

More holistic and integrated school garden approaches including links to school meals and healthy eating are also receiving increasing attention in the industrialized world (Box 1.4).

BOX 1.3: PHILIPPINES ISNM

The Philippines ISNM was an action research project undertaken in the Philippines with the Department of Education, developed and tested with the support of the International Development Research Centre (IDRC), Canada. The ISNM consisted of 3 components: a bio-intensive school garden; nutrition education for children and parents; and supplementary school feeding with indigenous nutrient-rich vegetables from the school garden as well as iron-fortified rice. Fifteen menus with indigenous vegetables were developed, lab-tested, and used in the school feeding programme. Serving vegetables produced in the school garden resulted in better nutrition while lowering feeding costs. Results also highlighted improvements on nutrition knowledge, attitudes, and practices among children and parents. Overall, the ISNM resulted in:

- Enhanced garden productivity and functionality
- Improved year-round availability of a diverse range of nutrient-rich indigenous vegetables with less reliance on inputs and easier day-to-day maintenance
- Improved nutritional status of schoolchildren through the use of standardized recipes using indigenous vegetables and iron-fortified rice in school feeding
- Conservation and management and dissemination of indigenous vegetables
- Improved knowledge and attitude towards nutrition and gardening through education.

Source: International Institute of Rural Reconstruction

BOX 1.4: CENTRE FOR ECOLITERACY

The Centre for Ecoliteracy, a non-profit organization, was established in 1995 by a group of committed people who wanted to change how we normally understand education and transform it into having social and sustainable impact. The centre is dedicated to nourishing education for sustainable living and creates learning material to further ecological teaching and training including guidelines to classroom discussions, integration of school meals, and development of school garden cookbooks. Systems thinking is an essential part of ecoliteracy, and the centre has created numerous resources to foster community, cultivate networks, and understand the ecological system. Material for establishing school gardens is also developed by the centre including guides demonstrating how to establish gardens on all imaginable levels – from the windowsill to large-scale vegetable, fruit, and flower gardens. According to the centre, school gardens are important for understanding systems because it allows children to interact and react on nature while fostering a deeper understanding of relationships in the nature – relationships between climate, seasons, water, soil, insects, plants, bacteria, and people.

One of the biggest achievements of the centre is their California Thursdays, which is a collaboration with a network of public-school districts in California, serving healthy, freshly prepared school meals made from locally grown food. The network includes 3,195 schools across the state, and meals are served to more than 2,000,000 students. The aim is eventually to turn the Thursday meals into an everyday event, ensuring healthy foods to pupils all week.

Source: www.ecoliteracy.org

Promotion of healthy diets and healthy eating habits by influencing behaviours

The increasing prevalence of malnutrition among school-aged children, including the growing obesity challenge and other issues around unhealthy food and diets, and unsustainable food systems, is contributing to increasing advocacy for sustainable diets. Gardens and nutrition education can help foster school environments which promote healthy diets and eating behaviours (FAO, 2010; FAO 2015), which can have a positive influence on children's health and well-being (Box 1.5). Behavioural change communication is increasingly viewed as an effective tool in bringing about desirable change. Gardens in schools can serve as a powerful mechanism to educate students, teachers, and parents alike. FAO in their guidance for school gardens acknowledges that the school might be torn between the practical and educational objectives of school gardens. Gardening and nutrition education are considered a winning combination. We are also reminded that 'Children cannot learn how to grow food without actually growing food' (FAO, 2010). In fact, FAO suggests prioritizing the educational aspects in children's gardening activities.

Behavioural changes are expected with such approaches. A 2017 evaluation of FoodCorps school gardens by the Tisch Center for Food Education and Policy

---

BOX 1.5: PEOPLES GARDEN SCHOOL PROGRAMME

Between 2011 and 2013, four universities across the United States worked together to examine the influence of school gardens on children's health and well-being. Washington State University served as the lead institution in collaboration with Cornell University, Iowa State University, and the University of Arkansas to develop the People's Garden School Pilot Project. These universities were chosen because the states they are in offer a wide variety in climate, seasonality, and local food preferences. The research project was primarily funded by the USDA's People's Garden *Healthy Gardens, Healthy Youth* project and by the Robert Wood Johnson Foundation (RWJF), through its *Active Living Research* programme.

The objective of the project was to increase fruit and vegetable consumption, empower youth in their communities, contribute towards a sustainable environment and food system, and build a national network. Community-based cooperative extension systems were used to develop and implement school community gardens in 47 elementary schools. The gardens were designed to offer students at high-poverty schools an opportunity for improved access to nutritious food through learning about nutrition and agriculture production. Each class in the schools received a raised bed or container garden kit and got access to an educational toolkit, specifically developed for the project, containing a garden implementation guide, lessons, activities, and recipes. The toolkit was put together by experts in nutrition, youth development, and horticulture from the participating universities.

Children's health and well-being in third, fifth, and sixth grade was assessed before and after the garden intervention. Assessment indicators included nutritional knowledge, fruit and vegetable consumption, and physical activity. Schools that had been through the garden intervention were compared to control schools that had not. Though not being statistically significant, the results showed an increase in physical activity and consumption of fruits and vegetables in the schools with the intervention compared to the schools without it. The garden intervention also had a significant influence on children's nutrition and plant science knowledge.

Source: http://peoplesgarden.wsu.edu/research-outcomes/ and http://wellslab.human.cornell.edu/research/

(Teachers College, Columbia University) found that schools that provide frequent high-quality opportunities for hands-on nutrition learning for students do have an impact on eating habits: students eat up to 3 times more fruits and vegetables (Laurie M. Tisch Center for Food, Education & Policy, 2017). A recent randomized study by Nancy Wells at Cornell University showed that children whose schools provide regular school garden lessons had more access to low-fat vegetables than children without that curriculum did. The study suggests that it does, however, take 35 to 50 hours of nutrition education per year to change children's preferences over the long term (Wells et al., 2018).

Other studies have also stressed the role of gardens in influencing the food habits of children. Children who grow their own food are more likely to eat fruits and vegetables and to show higher levels of knowledge about nutrition. They are more likely to continue healthy eating habits throughout their lives. Eating fruits and vegetables in childhood has been shown to be an important predictor of higher fruit and vegetable consumption in adulthood, which can prevent or delay chronic disease conditions over a lifetime (Blair, 2009). A Harvard study suggests that school gardens 'provide students with a real time look at how food is grown', suggesting that gardens can help shift children's perception of food enhancing access to health needs. The same study indicates that a long-lasting benefit can accrue on health and wellness of students who might choose healthful eating of nutritious foods. Gardens can serve as a counterweight to poor nutrition and serve as a respite for children (Shafer, 2018).

Conservation and sustainable use of local agrobiodiversity

With a growing recognition of the value of local and indigenous vegetables in diets, an effort to revive food culture and foster recipe development which features such crops represents a new window of opportunity that has arisen for using school gardens as a platform for the conservation of agrobiodiversity (Chapter 4), including indigenous tree species (Chapters 6 and 7). The BIG initiative within the national school systems in the Philippines is relatively unique in its advocacy for the conservation of climate resilient agrobiodiversity of nutritional and local food culture relevance (it advocates for two-thirds of the crops used in school gardens to be locally adapted crops and varieties, featuring intra-species and inter-species diversity).

Local agrobiodiversity of vegetables is now difficult to conserve on-farm but could be effectively conserved in school gardens where they can continue to evolve adapting to changes in the environment. The Crop Museum Initiative (Box 1.6) in schools of the Philippine government Department of Education recommends conserving, multiplying, and sharing this diversity of locally adapted genetic resources through annual sharing events (DepEd et al., 2017). A total of 520 crop museums have been set up by the Department of Education across the country.

BOX 1.6: WHAT IS A CROP MUSEUM?

Crop museums in schools serve as a focal point for safeguarding crop diversity through saving crop varieties. The crop museum is a garden where teachers, students, and community members can view a diverse range of nutritionally relevant and climate hardy vegetable varieties. It can include trees, shrubs, roots and tuber crops, vines, and short season annual crops. These crop museums serve as focal points for conserving inter-species and intra-species diversity, as propagation centres and seed banks and as platforms of seed exchange fairs. A primary reason for crop museums is to ensure sustainability and outscaling which relies on locally adapted plant materials.

Crop museums serve as nurseries and sources of planting materials that can be distributed and exchanged with surrounding schools and communities (Figure 1.3). Seed banks are maintained in crop museums, and outplanting is done annually. The Philippines was once known for its diverse backyard gardens. However, with modernization and increasing reliance on the commercial import of vegetables, the country is losing this rich diversity of crops and the culinary heritage associated with it. Restoration of local agrobiodiversity is an important new agenda for schools. School gardens and home gardens can be used to restore crop diversity for future generations. Diverse gardens can lead to richer dietary diversity and therefore better nutrition for kids and families.

Source: International Institute of Rural Reconstruction

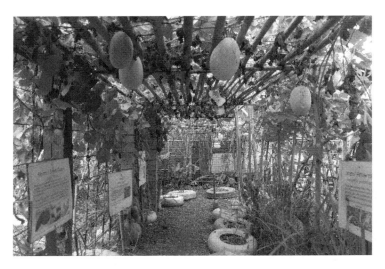

FIGURE 1.3 School gardens across the Philippines now feature crop museums where local agrobiodiversity is demonstrated. School gardens serve as a platform for self-learning for parents, students, and the local community.

Source: IIRR.

Children in urban localities are particularly prone to being disconnected from nature and an understanding of where their food comes from. There are particular challenges facing urban schools in addressing these problems from limited space to grow food to the logistical challenges in visiting rural areas and farms. Trends in greening urban areas and creating move liveable, sustainable cities provide opportunities to address these challenges. While local agrobiodiversity in urban centres may be increasingly difficult to conserve, school gardens can provide appropriate spaces for this to take place, thereby providing an important platform for urban schoolchildren to gain a better understanding of nature and biodiversity and the diversity of foods available and where they come from and their role in healthy eating (Box 1.7).

BOX 1.7: SCHOOL GARDENS IN THE EAST COAST – AUSTRALIA

Although there is a rich body of literature about the impact of school gardens on children's knowledge, preference, and consumption of fruits and vegetables, Guitart, Pickering, and Bryne (2014) identified a research gap with regard to the evaluation of agricultural biodiversity in school gardens. Thus, they conducted a survey of 23 school-based community gardens in the cities of Brisbane and Gold Coast, located in Southeast Queensland in Australia. The state of Queensland has been experiencing rapid urbanization and growth in population, which has impacted the food environment in its cities and the health outcomes of its citizens. More than one-quarter of children in Queensland are overweight or obese, a persistently high rate that has endured since 2007 (Queensland Government, 2016). Moreover, 96% of children in 2016 did not meet the daily-recommended intake for vegetables, and discretionary foods accounted for 41% of total energy intake. School gardens present a valuable opportunity to address these diet-related issues in Queensland, as it is located in a very fertile region in Australia with a favourable agricultural climate.

Through conducting cross-sectional surveys with school garden managers in Brisbane and Gold Coast, 230 different types of plants, encompassing 159 species in 66 families were identified across 23 schools. On average, each garden hosted 63 different plant types (with the most diverse gardens having up to 139 types of plants), 12 different types of fruits, and 26 different types of vegetables. The size or age of the school garden was not found to have an impact on the diversity of plants, nor with the initial motivations of starting the garden. Moreover, Australian native food plants, such as bush tucker, made up 12% of all plants identified in the gardens. The most common fruits and vegetables found in school gardens were then evaluated using a colour code system to quantify food diversity. It was found that school gardens contained highly diverse environments and that over three-quarters of these grew plants that encompassed the total spectrum of seven colours.

(Continued)

Moreover, the project investigated the motivations behind and the utilization of school gardens in the two cities. Education, health of students, and environmental sustainability were the three most commonly reported reasons for establishing school gardens. Many schools also used the produce in cafeterias, utilized the gardens as a learning space, and encouraged students to bring the produce home. Thus, school gardens in these two cities were found to be a powerful strategy to increase consumption of diverse and nutritious foods for children and good spaces for the conservation of agrobiodiversity.

Source: Biodiversity for Food and Nutrition. (n.d.). School Gardens in the East Coast. www.b4fn.org/case-studies/case-studies/school-gardens-in-the-east-coast/

School gardens to increase awareness of climate change

Climate change modelling studies suggest that at the global level, climate change will reduce crop yields and land suitable for agriculture with the greatest impacts in tropical latitudes. Climate change could increase the numbers of malnourished children in the least developed countries. Climate change impacts on food security will spread unevenly, affecting the populations that are currently most at risk. Food prices will increase as a result of climate change, affecting the poor who are likely to eat more carbohydrates and less of the nutrient-dense food. Climate change will also negatively influence the nutritional quality of food produce. School gardens can serve as learning laboratories for understanding the risks and impacts of climate change, and for demonstrating ways to adapt to it (Box 1.8).

BOX 1.8: EDIBLE SCHOOLYARDS LEITH, SCOTLAND

Reduction of carbon emissions, healthier diets, and increased attention to the importance of biodiversity for sustainable food production are a few of the benefits that the Edible Schoolyards in Leith have brought along. It all started with the founder of Edible Schoolyards, Evie Murray's enthusiasm about children's physical and emotional well-being, and concern about climate change, mass extinction, and the role of industrial agriculture. She realized that by creating gardens where children could grow their own fruits and vegetables it was possible to address all these issues at once. Furthermore, by teaching in the garden she experienced how much simpler it was to explain environmental concepts, referencing to plants, pollinating insects, and compost making directly, compared to teaching these themes in the classroom. She also noticed that spending time in the garden was important, especially for children with difficulties in class.

> News about the success of this one school garden quickly spread, and neighbouring schools got keen on establishing their own vegetable gardens. Therefore, supported by the Climate Change Fund, the Edible School Gardens concept was developed and rolled out in one nursery and four schools under the foundation Leith Community Crops in Pots. Today, throughout the year, children learn about soil health, nutrient cycles, pollination, and photosynthesis in the gardens. They experience how to plant fruit trees, sow seeds, harvest vegetables, and plant out seedlings and potatoes, and thus get a much better understanding of the whole producing cycle.
>
> It all started in the backyards of a few schools, but the outreach has moved far beyond. The school gardens today function as a channel to transmit messages about the environment and sustainable living to the broader community. Furthermore, events celebrating the environment, the establishment of a community orchard, and the community growing area known as 'Leith Community Croft' are now all part of this community movement that has led to reduced food waste, more sustainable shopping patterns, more people growing wild flowers for the bees, and more people composting their organic waste in Leith. Through the schools and community gardens, the Edible Schoolyards have reached people that have never grown their own food before and that were not particularly concerned about biodiversity, climate change, and environmental topics before. Moving back to the original purpose of the establishment of the gardens in Leith, the project has also shown clear evidence of a positive correlation between children's engagement in nursing the plants and their general well-being and health.
>
> *Source: https://leith-community-crops-in-pots.org/our-initiatives/edible-schoolyards/*

School gardens in the Philippines have effectively promoted and scaled climate resilient approaches such as water-conserving agrobiodiverse, BIGs across the national school education system (Chapter 4). BIGs are considered Climate Smart Agriculture. Such gardens, advocated by the bio-intensive agriculture movement of the International Institute of Rural Reconstruction in the Philippines, and others feature deep-dug beds that serve to harvest rainwater (including excess rain associated with climate change) and conserve limited water during dry periods (as result of a deeper soil profile rich in organic matter including residues of roots, mulch, and cover crops). Deep beds allow for the close planting of diverse crops which extract both nutrients and moisture from different parts of the soil profile, thus maximizing efficient use of nutrients. At harvest time, plant roots are retained in the ground to regenerate soils and rebuild and enrichen soil life. Biodiversity below the soil is conserved as the result of the combination of deep beds; rich organic matter, above and below ground; and well-conserved moisture (Figure 1.4). Multipurpose trees grown on garden boundaries help sequester

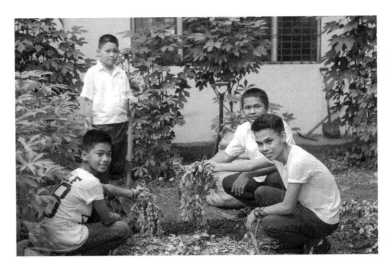

FIGURE 1.4 Green leaf manure (with *Gliricidia*) helps to feed soil microbial life, to regenerate soils, to store moisture, and to store carbon in the soils in school gardens.

Source: IIRR.

carbon, storing it in tree biomass and soils. By advocating that two thirds of the crop selections should feature locally adapted and climate resilient crops/varieties risks are substantially reduced. School gardens have been challenged by sustainability issues associated with a range of factors. Climate change is the new threat to sustainability of gardens and must be dealt with in ways that can be managed with local resources and with the lowest costs. Efficient and regenerative gardening systems with climate resilient practice can contribute to a better understanding of adaptation options by schoolchildren and local communities.

Enhancing academic skills and learning aptitude and academic performance

Research with teachers has shown that they use school gardens to enhance the learning of their students, promote experimental learning, and teach environmental education (DeMarco, 1999; Skelly and Bradley, 2000). Studies have also found that using school gardens to support teaching also does, in fact, improve student learning (Sheffield, 1992) and environmental disposition (Skelly and Bradley, 2007). Studies in industrialized countries have shown that students who are actively engaged in garden projects tend to enjoy learning and show improved attitudes towards education. Third, fourth and fifth grade students who participated in school gardening activities scored significantly higher on science achievement tests than students who did not experience any garden-based learning activities (Klemmer et al., 2005) (Box 1.9).

BOX 1.9: THE EDIBLE SCHOOLYARD

The first Edible Schoolyard was established in 1995 at a public middle school in Berkeley. Here, almost 25 years after, the Edible Schoolyard has provided capacity building to teachers, administrators, nutritionists, food service staff, parents, and community leaders from more than 367 schools worldwide. Moreover, the project facilitates the Edible Schoolyard network including 5,513 school garden programmes located all over the world. Under the concept of Edible Education, the idea is to use food as a tool to teach lessons of the academic curriculum. This is done by involving children in the preparation of soil, compost, cultivation, and harvest, and thereafter cooking the vegetables together in the kitchen. Putting learning into practice is one of the very cornerstones of edible education because it increases children's perception of what is possible. The school garden serves as a rich teaching environment, while the kitchen classroom brings everybody to the table to share thoughts and considerations on what has been learnt. Through the project, values such as nourishment, stewardship, and community are fostered, which is believed to give children a better foundation for healthy eating now and in the future. Parents and other adults are invited to participate and learn as well in certain evening classes. The edible schoolyard has developed an education curriculum for children of all ages, from pre-kindergarten to high schools. Lesson plans are targeted to children of specific grades and in a certain stages of learning progression. For instance, students learn about volume, measurement, and density as well as the concept of species varieties while pressing cider in sixth grade or learn about pH by measuring the soil in different sites in the school garden in eighth grade. All resources are free of charge and can be downloaded from their website.

Source: https://edibleschoolyard.org/

A literature review conducted by Norman and her colleagues concluded that there is 'meaningful evidence that environmentally related education using the best educational practices can increase academic achievement across curriculum subjects'. Studies of natural environments, as the review concluded, can be a significant factor in academic achievement gains. Certain teaching practices and teaching support in environmental education appear to strengthen academic outcomes (Nomann et al., 2006). The potential for gardening as an environmental subject especially in the context of climate change and nutritional awareness has not been maximized in the developing world. Gardens in schools can serve as a powerful mechanism to educate students, teachers, and parents alike.

Other benefits of school gardens

The concept of biodiverse edible schools highlights the important role of school gardens in reconnecting schoolchildren with nature and food production in an urban setting especially through the role of edible wild plants and local urban biodiversity (Fischer et al., 2019; see also Box 1.7). The key elements of the concept of biodiverse edible schools include: a school kitchen supplied with foods from local producers, a school garden actively producing food, a nearby empty wild space as a habitat for wild edible plants, and stakeholder participation and collaboration in planning and implementation. The school link to a neighbouring vacant wild site was particularly important as a site for learning about wild species and foraging for wild edible species. Vegetation surveys of one such site revealed 121 wild species, of which 56 were edible or had edible plant parts. Such foraging connects children with nature, but more importantly, earlier studies have shown that people who learn to collect wild edible species in childhood are more aware of biodiversity issues later in life (Figure 1.5). The topic of schoolchildren foraging for wild edible species is one taken up later in this book in Case study 13, *Where the wild things are*.

School gardens can also play a critical role in reconnecting indigenous children with their traditional foods, food culture, and the ecological knowledge associated with this. Such actions can be important in empowerment of indigenous children, creating a strong sense of pride and biocultural heritage as well as contributing to physical and mental health and personal well-being (Box 1.10). This topic is further explored in Case studies 2, 5, 8, and 9.

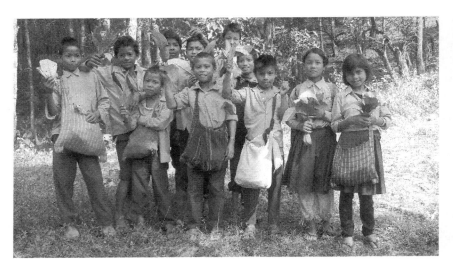

FIGURE 1.5 School garden activity with children from the Khasi community in Mulieh, Jaintia Hills, Meghalaya.

Source: NESFAS.

BOX 1.10: TOHONO O'ODHAM COMMUNITY ACTION

Located in southwestern Arizona in the United States is the Tohono O'odham Nation, the second-largest reservation in the state with 2.8 million acres and more than 28,000 members. In order to address the challenges the community has been facing with diet-related diseases, such as type II diabetes and the decreasing cultivation of traditional indigenous crops (by an astonishing amount from 20,000 acres in 1936 to less than 2 acres in 2000), non-profit organization Tohono O'odham Community Action (TOCA) has been utilizing school gardens to connect multiple objectives. The organization was founded in 1996, and the mission of TOCA is to create a *'healthy, sustainable, and culturally vital community'*. Through establishing community-based projects, TOCA aims to transform the food system in the Tohono O'odham Nation which promotes the health of humans and the environment using traditional methods and practices. TOCA achieves this objective through a variety of programmes, ranging from operating two farms to produce traditional crops such as tepary bean, squash, and O'odham 60-day corn to organizing cultural events to educate about and to celebrate traditional food traditions. TOCA organizes many projects to engage youth through agriculture. One example is Project Oidag, a community garden and mentoring programme, which was established by a group of young people in 2011. Project Oidag is an internship programme for students ranging from 14 to 27 years old to take part in establishing and maintaining school gardens in their community. Project Oidag aims to *'empowering O'odham youth to grow food, be active in their communities, and stand strong in being Oodham'*, and has developed its own educational curriculum GROW (Growing to Renew Our World) in order to engage more youth in agriculture.

Source: www.facebook.com/pg/TOCA-Tohono-Oodham-Community-Action-137202393001616/about/?ref=page_internal

Education and empowerment of girls and women is an equally important dimension of school gardens and related activities (Box 1.11), a topic also taken up in Case study 4, *Preserving local cultural heritage through capacity building for girls in the Moroccan High Atlas* (Figure 1.6). School gardens can enhance the learning and future actions and livelihoods of girls through many of the benefits already highlighted in this chapter including agricultural and livelihood skills, nutrition education and awareness of healthy eating and diets and nutrient-rich foods, their preparation and cooking as well as traditional knowledge and conservation and use of biodiversity. Empowerment is not limited to school-aged girls. Where school gardens are linked to surrounding villages, especially to home gardens, women in these communities can also benefit in similar ways.

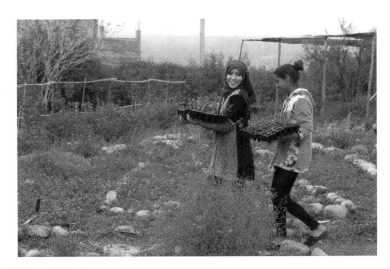

FIGURE 1.6 *Dar Taliba* students in the garden on their way to plant vegetable seedlings which they cultivate.

Source: Pommelien Da Silva.

> **BOX 1.11: SCHOOL GARDENS AND WOMEN'S EMPOWERMENT**
>
> In a village in Burkina Faso, not only are women responsible for subsistence agriculture and growing food for their families, but those with children going to school also contribute to maintaining the school garden to provide vegetables for the canteen. The school garden is highly valued by these women, as it contributes to nutritious school lunches and continuous school attendance. Moreover, the school garden also became an activity that supported the empowerment of women in this community.
>
> The school garden in this village in Burkina Faso initially faced low output and many problems, including bad soil and water quality, infestation of insects and pests, and the overuse of chemical fertilizers and pesticides. After the identification of these challenges, the women worked with a project supported by the Canadian International Development Agency to create and implement more sustainable agricultural production methods and solutions. These strategies included environmental education about chemical contaminants and the gradual reduction in use of chemical inputs; the use of natural sources of fertilizer from goat manure, which was abundant in the community; and the implementation of plant diversification techniques to combat weeds.
>
> After one year of implementing these strategies, the school garden in this community experienced a variety of successes – not only did the school environment improve, which could be observed through healthier-looking vegetables, less pests, and better water retention in the soil, but the year witnessed

the highest number of graduates from the community. Most remarkably, there were more female graduates than there were in previous years, which was attributed to better access to food. Through this process, which included environmental education sessions with women as well as their participation and maintenance of the school garden, women felt empowered as they were able to learn about the impact of chemicals on the health of their community as well as sustainable agricultural production methods, eventually applying them with success. The successful adoption of these methods was attributed to the fact that they did not require the adoption of other activities and thus did not add to the workload the women already experienced. Moreover, the women felt that they were able to contribute directly to the education and success of their children.

Source: Vasseur, L. (2016)

The benefits of school gardens and green spaces in schools for mental health and personal well-being constitute an area receiving increasing attention but still very much under-researched. Schools are often in the front line of mental health yet gardens as spaces of health and mental well-being can be an important tool in addressing mental health issues including using the school garden as a space for therapy and for counselling (Box 1.12).

BOX 1.12: INTERNATIONAL GREEN ACADEMY

The International Green Academy is a unique partnership between the University of Glasgow's School of Geographical and Earth Science, and the University of Arizona's School of Geography and Development. The goal of our team is to construct an international school garden network that bridges distinct urban biomes: Tucson, in the arid Sonoran Desert, and Glasgow, in the temperate Scottish Lowlands. This 'biome bridging' will resource a new generation of urban learners with practical knowledge, ecological awareness, and the skills to build more resilient – and internationally sensitive – urban ecologies. More than this, we are interested in how these green spaces can work to change student and teacher subjectivities. How exactly is pupil mental health and well-being implicated in the practice of outdoor learning and gardening? And how might we be able to design curricula that enhance and empower young people's ecological mindset and confidence? To answer these questions, we are working with school counsellors, teachers, and students of all ages to build therapeutic garden spaces (one potato at a time).

Source: Ian Shaw and Cheryl McGeachan, School of Geographical and Earth Sciences, The University of Glasgow

Key issues for the future of school gardens

Key issues for the future of school garden initiatives include:

1 Schools have distinct features that make them unique platforms for delivering nutritional, agricultural, and environmental education outcomes. School gardens can provide students with a better understanding of the value of healthy diets, lifestyles, and their links with food systems. The multiple benefits of school gardens are now better understood and accepted. With the growth of global nutrition movements, the current emphasis on nutrition sensitive programming and the value of linking nutrition-specific and nutrition sensitive interventions, new spaces have been created for a wider educational role for school gardens. Despite this widening recognition, the reality is that sustainability remains a threat, for example if government does not make significant and continuing financial commitments while also putting in place supportive policies, school garden interventions will continue to be challenged by sustainability. The majority of school nutrition programmes globally are still over-reliant on external donor funding: this is a weak link in efforts to ensure long-term commitment and institutionalization of school garden programmes. Sustainability of school garden programmes have been a persistent and a major issue that proponents of school gardens will continue to have to be conscious of, and to plan for accordingly. This includes avoiding the pitfalls of tokenism, showcasing, and a bias for glamourism.

2 The workload of the schoolteachers is another important consideration. School garden teachers are already burdened with responsibilities aside from their roles in garden education. Poor planning of teacher and school administrator time, and overambitious goals for school gardens and teachers could, in themselves, be determinants of the level of success and chances for scaling and sustainability. Design features and school garden interventions would have to be incremental in nature. As such, programming approaches should feature team and partnership-based approaches, if the complexities of managing, sustaining, scaling, and mainstreaming school gardens are to be effectively managed.

3 Convergence of efforts at local levels is crucial to reduce the diverging atmosphere created by the well-meaning proponents of school garden programmes. Conflict of interests and narrow vested interest might prevail. With the resurgence of nutrition sensitive agriculture programming, the health, agriculture, and education sectors will have to converge, collaborate, and complement each other: this is best done at sub-national and local levels (e.g. municipalities, districts). Harmonization of new efforts arising from the new interest in nutrition sensitive agriculture is likely to be best managed locally. Stakeholder organizations would do well to pick 'niches' for their engagement within such a framework, keeping comparative advantages and complementary contributions in mind.

4 A new agenda for schools in future is likely to be geared towards multiple objectives, which include better nutrition, sustainable lifestyles and behavioural change while also being supportive of a conservation, regenerative agriculture and food systems orientation. A need for evidence to back up claims can be expected as more development partners become engaged, and financing mechanisms are put into place. However, there is little doubt that the best time for engagement in school gardening initiatives is ahead of us.

Book structure

The book is divided into two parts. Part one contains a series of chapters (Chapters 2–10) which look at the role of school gardens in food and nutrition education to improve healthy eating habits, dietary diversity and nutrition, with a number of the chapters focussing on the contribution of nutrient-rich agrobiodiversity, including fruit trees, to these outcomes. Part two is a diverse collection of short case studies from all over the world many of which address improving diets and nutrition using local agrobiodiversity but which also go beyond these goals to look at many of the other benefits school gardens can provide.

In 2018, the United Nations System Standing Committee on Nutrition (UNSCN) published the discussion paper 'Schools as a system to improve nutrition'. Oenema and colleagues, in Chapter 2, provide a summary of that discussion paper, highlighting the role of school gardens in the overall vision of schools as a system to improve nutrition. They argue that the key path to better health and well-being is early adoption of long-lasting, healthy food-related outlooks, practices, and habits. While stressing that school gardens cannot be regarded as bulk sources of school food, they point out there are instances where a school garden can provide limited amounts of locally available and culturally appropriate nutrient-rich leafy or other vegetables to supplement school meals and enhance dietary diversity. School gardens are a critical element in an integrated approach linked to nutrition education, school meals, and wider academic learning and actions. The authors emphasize that school gardens can have an important role in the rediscovery of traditional crops especially if they are nutrient-rich and can play an important role in reconnecting children from indigenous communities with their rich heritage of traditional foods and indigenous food systems. Moreover, school gardens provide a suitable space to engage other stakeholders such as local authorities, parents, and those who have gardens at home, a coupling which is suggested as important in later chapters (Chapters 8 and 9) for longer-term nutritional gains.

Talavera and de Juras, in Chapter 3, take up one of the themes covered in the previous chapter and review strategies and practices aimed at integrating nutrition in the primary school education curriculum and the challenges facing the incorporation of key concepts of school gardening and nutrition in countries in Southeast Asia. They highlight several approaches implemented in nutrition education for schoolchildren: namely, integration of nutrition in the primary school curriculum, school gardening, technology/web-based approaches, parental involvement, and school feeding programmes. They provide a brief description of key school garden activities which have been put in place in some ASEAN countries in recent years, as well as the results of studies on the effectiveness of school gardening on several outcomes such as improvement in consumption of fruits and vegetables, preferences for fruits and vegetables, and willingness to taste fruits and vegetables. They conclude with a summary of the challenges and constraints as well as needs and opportunities facing the better integration of food and nutrition education in the school curriculum.

Monville-Oro and colleagues, in Chapter 4, provide an overview of an ISNM implemented and tested in the Philippines, and highlight good practices and lessons learned. The model features 3 main components: (i) *BIG* featuring climate smart and regenerative agricultural practices to rebuild soil fertility and promote the use of and conservation of local agrobiodiversity; (ii) *Supplementary school feeding of underweight children* using iron-fortified rice and indigenous vegetables from school gardens; and (iii) *Nutrition education* for students, parents/care providers/guardians, and teachers to promote the importance of nutrient-dense food and good eating habits. Testing of the integrated model in 27 pilot schools generated data on its effectiveness, resulting in improved nutritional status of children. The adoption of the BIG standards and practices contributed to sustained school gardens and innovative crop museums helped conserve locally important crop cultivars while improving year-round availability of a diverse range of climate resilient, locally adapted, and nutritionally important vegetables. Furthermore, nutrition education brought about increased knowledge, attitude, and good practices on nutrition.

The *Vegetables Go to School* project, funded by the Swiss Agency for Development and Cooperation, was designed to address malnutrition by establishing comprehensive school vegetable garden programmes in selected countries in Africa and in Asia. Bhattarai and Schreinemachers, in Chapter 5, describe the implementation of this project in Nepal and provide details of how the school garden programme was designed, piloted in two districts, and subsequently scaled at a national level. The project was piloted in ten schools per year over a three-year period in two districts in the mid-hills of Nepal. While the pilot study found a significant increase in children's awareness about fruit and vegetables, their knowledge about agriculture and nutrition, and their stated preferences for eating fruit and vegetables, it did not find a significant effect on vegetable consumption. The authors suggest that this might be due to food items such as fruit and vegetables being insufficiently available within children's households and children being unable to make food choices independently as their parents largely decided what they ate and the food behaviour of parents was perhaps insufficiently affected by the intervention (see Chapters 8 and 9). An ongoing pilot project is currently testing these hypotheses.

For the most part, school gardens focus on annual vegetables and fruits. The potential of neglected indigenous fruit trees, which have an important role in providing vital minerals and micronutrients to growing children, is something rarely considered. This is a topic explored in Chapter 6 by McMullin and colleagues, who highlight the considerable diversity of indigenous fruit trees in Africa and their nutritional value and contribution to micronutrient and wider dietary needs. Such diversity also has an important role to play in addressing seasonality and hunger periods facing many rural communities by ensuring the availability of nutritious fruits for a healthy diet year-round. The authors highlight the 'Portfolio Approach' – for addressing seasonal and nutrient-specific gaps in local diets. Schools also offer a platform for wider community engagement by promoting practical learning and engagement of parents and local farmers.

The topic of trees is explored further by Grazioli and colleagues, in Chapter 7, who examine the role of school gardens as conservation networks for underutilized and threatened tree genetic resources. In addition to linking children to the nutritional benefits of a diverse diet, school gardens offer a huge opportunity to engage children in the wider context of plant identification, conservation and sustainable use of plant genetic resources for sustainable development. This chapter discusses the role that schools and children can play in documenting the diversity of socioeconomically important tree species around their school and community, the role that trees can play in their diet and the multiple co-benefits of trees for delivery of sustainable food systems. In particular, the chapter highlights the critical role schools can play in establishment in ex situ conservation of genetic resources through school arboreta, seed orchards, and school nurseries. Engaging children and youth through school gardens offers a unique educational opportunity to introduce restoration and plant diversity as a solution to multiple environmental and social challenges.

Chapter 8 revisits the *Vegetables Go to School* project, described earlier in Chapter 5, and synthesizes the results of three recent impact evaluations, using cluster randomized controlled trials, of school garden programmes in Bhutan, Nepal, and Burkina Faso. The results showed that while school garden interventions significantly improved children's knowledge about food and agriculture and showed improvements in children's awareness of fruit and vegetables and their stated preferences for eating them, in none of the countries did these improvements translate into an increase in the frequency of fruit and vegetable consumption, nor in the number of different fruits and vegetables consumed. These findings suggest that for school garden programmes to contribute to healthier food choices a more holistic intervention design may be needed that addresses the household-level supply of healthy foods and which influences the food choices of parents.

The lack of availability of healthy foods in students' homes highlighted above is a constraint further examined in Chapter 9, by Calub and colleagues, which describes the School-Plus-Home Gardens Project (S+HGP) in the Philippines. The S+HGP attempts to couple school gardens to home garden and emphasizes greater parent engagement to establish home gardens and to involve them more effectively in school gardening as a way of sustaining nutritional gains. Results demonstrate increased dietary diversity and improved nutrition of students. Additional activities included values strengthening so that parents improved their sense of responsibility in ensuring year-round availability of diverse, nutritious food for their children. Factors that contributed to the success in engaging parents included, regular joint parent-teacher consultations, participatory development approach, training, seminars, parent-child tandem cooking contests using vegetables harvested from the school gardens and close collaboration with the local government units in providing garden inputs and services.

The final chapter in the book, by Monville-Oro and colleagues, revisits the ISNM described in Chapter 4 and shares some experiences and lessons learned in efforts to expand the model from one province (Cavite) to an entire region comprising five provinces of the Philippines. In order to facilitate this, fifty-eight light house schools, which serve as focal points for research, learning, and scaling, are now influencing at varying levels, 2,732 public elementary schools benefitting a total student population of 1,839,445. Through capacity building, multi-stakeholder engagement and partnerships, the ISNM is being scaled up in schools across the country, via institutionalization and increased investments by the government and private sector. The Department of Education, recognizing the value of the model, has pursued a capacity building programme to establish 273 light house schools all over the Philippines.

The first case study in the book comes from the Stephanie Alexander Kitchen Garden Foundation (SAKGF) in Australia. Formally established in 2004 in response to the growing childhood obesity crisis in Australia, SAKGP is driven by a belief that involving children in the food production process in their school environment, ensuring their experience is pleasurable, fun, and delicious, can help change behaviours and attitudes to fresh food and provide them with the skills and understanding to last a lifetime. SAKGF now works with a growing number of over 2000 early childhood services and schools to run programmes and deliver pleasurable food education with children developing key life skills, self-confidence, and a positive relationship with food through practical learning. Evaluations have highlighted multiple outcomes for the schoolchildren, teachers, and parents involved in the programme, including health, well-being, education, and community benefits. As one of the school principals involved highlights, it's the best thing he has seen in 30 years of teaching.

The experiences of the Hawai'i Island School Gardening Network (HISGN), established by the Kohala Center, to promote school gardens as an initiative to build a strong local food economy and improve diets and nutrition of youth is highlighted in Case Study 2. Like most Pacific islands, Hawai'i is increasingly dependent on imported, processed foods; is known for its low consumption of fruits and vegetables; and has disproportionately high rates of obesity and related chronic diseases among native Hawaiian and Pacific Islanders. To address this challenge, HISGN places an emphasis on native Hawaiian plants and practices, and assists garden leaders, school faculty, and administrators in the creation and implementation of gardening and agricultural programmes. The HISGN through the Hawai'i Farm to School and School Garden Hui now supports more than 217 school gardens on five islands and is actively working to change institutional procurement policies to increase the purchase and preparation of fresh, locally produced food, as well as to provide resources for school gardening programmes.

Case study 3 comes from Vietnam and describes the efforts of a partnership between a local non-profit organization (AOG World Relief Vietnam) and an Australian-based Rotarian Action Group (Food Plant Solutions) to improve the nutritional status of children and their communities in Dai Hung and Tam Phu where access to nutritious foods is often impeded by the lack of nutrition information and education. Many farming families and households are unaware of the nutritional value of the diversity of locally available plants. To address this, AOG World Relief Vietnam and Food Plant Solutions implement school garden programmes focussing on promotion of nutrient-rich *rau muong* or water spinach (*Ipomoea aquatica*), Malabar spinach (*Basella alba*), *rau den* (*Amaranthus tricolor*), and *bi dao* or winter melon (*Benincasa hispida*) which have contributed to improvements in health outcomes for the students.

Improving empowerment and capacity of schoolgirls through links to school gardens and local ethnobotanical knowledge is highlighted in Case study 4 from the High Atlas, Morocco. *Dar Taliba*, which in Arabic means 'house of the female student', is an innovative boarding school system in Morocco, enabling girls to pursue their secondary education and overcome challenges such as distance and lack of public transport that all too often limit participation. Through a collaborative ethnobotanical school garden project at a *Dar Taliba* in Ourika, the Global Diversity Foundation supports girls' education beyond primary school while educating students about traditional plant knowledge and the conservation of endemic, threatened, and valuable plant species. The project is not only supporting girls' access to further education but providing healthy outdoor activities, livelihood skills, and nutritious food for the students in residence while offering opportunities to learn about traditional agriculture, local agrobiodiversity, and wild plant use. So far, 700 Moroccan girls have benefited from the school garden training programme.

As Australia increasingly reflects upon the legacies of over two centuries of European settlement, a growing number of people are taking action to address food sovereignty, food security and food justice to help build healthier, more equitable, more diverse, and resilient food systems. In this context, Case study 5 shares the story of three approaches that utilise food gardens, traditional knowledge and strengths-based learning to engage indigenous youth and older generations in learning together to foster better health, nutrition, and emotional well-being. The stories shared in this case study offer additional perspectives on potential well-being benefits that garden based activities may offer indigenous youth and communities. The case study cautions that as attention turns to the potential of cultivating indigenous plant species as food crops, it is important to not again appropriate indigenous knowledge and practices for the benefit of others rather than Aboriginal people. Multiple benefits are being realized by taking a strengths-based approach that focusses on *what's strong rather than what's wrong*.

In certain instances, school gardens can supply or complement school feeding programmes by using local food biodiversity and improving dietary diversity in schoolchildren, as described in Case study 5 from Kenya. School gardening has been practised as part of education in Kenya for many years, especially in rural areas where it goes back to colonial times. While the crops that are commonly grown in the school gardens are healthy and important, they do not cover all the necessary vitamin and mineral intake necessary for a balanced, healthy diet. Locally available and generally more highly nutritious and biodiverse foods are simply not finding their way to the plates of Kenyan students in schools. In Busia County in western Kenya, the Biodiversity for Food and Nutrition (BFN) project has tried to change this by encouraging the cultivation of nutrient-rich African leafy vegetables (ALVs) in school gardens and, where feasible, linking this produce to school meals programmes.

What can be done where there are few schools, or the land available and accessible for gardens is very limited, or those you are trying to educate live a precarious life in limbo? This is very much the everyday experience of refugees and those working with them face and is a context taken up in Case study 7. Due to the conflict in Syria, Lebanon is home to one of the largest refugee populations in the world. Despite the support provided and recent improvements in school and training enrolment, Syrian refugees in the region are becoming increasingly vulnerable, and more than half of displaced Syrian children are still out of school. Working with Syrian communities displaced as refugees in Lebanon, the organization Zaher implement learning gardens as a means to support and engage marginalized youth by creating a network of partners that connects local permaculture experts with education facilities for Syrian children in order to transform unused patches of land into functioning learning gardens. It is hoped learning gardens can make a major contribution to ensuring the continuation of traditional agricultural knowledge and practices and improve employment prospects for Syrian youth through skills-based training and provide them with the necessary skills to rebuild their country if and when they return.

The rapid urbanization of Māori following the Second World War has contributed to limited opportunities for successive generations of young Māori to experience growing their own foods, or learning with their parents and elders how to interact and gain from working their own whenua or land. Addressing this challenge is the subject of Case study 8 where intergenerational activities are being applied to introduce younger generations of Māori to growing and utilizing foods through a variety of approaches. This case study shares the 'Spud in a Bucket' project promoted to schools through the National Māori Horticultural Collective known as *Tahuri Whenua*. From a Māori perspective, *māra* or gardens are not just about growing food products but are important contributors to providing an experience that contributes to the well-being of those involved, children and adults alike. The project has helped to restore and enhance *Mana*, that unique cultural value which recognizes the contribution to the status of Māori within society.

The efforts of the North East Slow Food and Agrobiodiversity Society (NESFAS) to raise awareness among indigenous children of the value of traditional foods by promoting school gardens in Meghalaya, India is shared in Case study 9. The purpose of the school gardens is to enhance the connection of indigenous children to farming, to enhance intergenerational transfer of knowledge and to increase dietary diversity in mid-day meals. Nestled in the hills and biodiversity of Meghalaya are three matriarchal indigenous communities, Khasi, Jaintia, and Garo communities. Though a large proportion of the communities live amidst a high diversity of micronutrient-rich species, dietary diversity levels are low with corresponding high rates of anemia and vitamin A deficiency. NESFAS focusses on planting the missing food groups using local edible species in the school gardens and training the mid-day meal cooks on their inclusion into school meals through cooking demonstrations.

Case study 10 represents a slight departure and focusses on targeting educators within a school garden programme as a way to scale agroecology approaches and more sustainable food systems. The *Laboratorios para la Vida* (LabVida) action research team in Chiapas, Mexico trains educators to use school gardens and local food systems as venues for experiential learning while stimulating conversation and promoting agroecology, and conscientious eating based on regional agrobiodiversity. Chiapas is a biodiversity region with traditional farming systems rich in crop diversity; however, mainstream education and agriculture typically disregard this diversity, hastening its erosion. Faced with these challenges, and inspired by California's Life Lab programme, LabVida has promoted school gardens and local agrofood systems as teaching-learning environments and are extending these networks to other regions and countries.

Case study 11 shares the experiences of the Swiss Agency for Development and Cooperation-funded Agro-Biodiversity Initiative (TABI) to support the inclusion of agrobiodiversity knowledge in school curricula, in Naxaithong Village, Khoun District, in Xiengkhouang Province, Laos, to ensure the transfer of indigenous knowledge and appreciation for agrobiodiversity to future generations, especially the importance of agrobiodiversity for local livelihoods. The case study highlights the many successes of the programme as well as opportunities for future expansion.

Case study 12 ventures into the Pacific Ocean again, to the challenging atoll conditions of the Marshall Islands where the impacts of climate change are increasingly manifested and the tyranny of distance can constrain the implementation and impact of even the best thought-out efforts to improve lives. The Marshallese once had access to a wide diversity of foods and a balanced diet of traditional root crops, fruits, vegetables, and seafood. This diet has been disrupted since the First World War and the events that followed, from atomic fallout to mass migration from outer atolls to urban areas to a shift to a cash economy, so much so that the country now sees most residents reliant on imported convenience foods, such as canned goods, white rice, white flour, ramen noodles, white sugar, salt, and fat, leading to severe malnutrition problems. In an effort to address these negative trends *Jikin kallib ilo jikuul*, the School Learning Garden Programme, has put together activities consisting of school garden teacher training and curriculum integration, co-development of learning garden curriculum maps, and a train the trainers capacity building initiative, including expansion of the programme to outer islands/atolls. While progress is being made, the multiple unique challenges faced illustrate the difficulties of working in an atoll environment.

Where the wild things are, the title of Case study 13, takes the reader away from the school garden to explore ways to engage schoolchildren and students in consumption and foraging for wild edible plants and to create a sense of awareness and appreciation of their nutritional value. As the authors suggest, 'imagine removing the limitation of the school garden and letting the nature around the school – the wider school garden – form the extension of the classroom and the wild plants growing there serve as a basis for heathy and ecological learning and other benefits'. In Turkey and Lebanon, wild edible plants are still common in local cuisine, yet traditional dishes are increasingly unpopular or 'less prestigious' with younger generations who prefer more Western-style foods. The two projects described in this case study promote the revival of awareness of the value and importance of wild edible species. In the Lebanon, the focus is on the incorporation of wild edible species as a cheap option to boosting school meals by providing a mid-morning snack based on traditional recipes optimized to contain wild edibles with high nutrient levels. In contrast, the project in Turkey worked closely with young chefs attending vocational colleges to encourage them to forage and integrate wild species into their learning, cooking, and recipes.

In 2011, Slow Food launched the 1,000 Gardens in Africa project, the topic of Case study 14. The original objective of the initiative was to create a thousand gardens in schools, villages, and urban areas to ensure that communities had access to high-quality, healthy, and sustainable food. Having surpassed this target it has now been scaled up to 10,000 gardens.

Among the purposes of school gardens are promoting a positive perspective on food, agriculture, and the environment to young people, raising awareness of the threats to their food sovereignty and empowering them to question increasing corporate control of the African food system. With school gardens, Slow Food is promoting an idea of agriculture based on knowledge of the landscape and respect for the biodiversity and local cultures. To date, 1623 school gardens in 35 countries have been established involving over 300,000 students, parents, and teachers. These gardens are positively changing children's perception of farming as a profession. Students have gained new knowledge on local agrobiodiversity and on how to safeguard it. In some instances, school gardens are supplying this agrobiodiversity to supplement school meals with nutrient-rich species.

The final case study comes from Brazil and shares the experiences of efforts to promote awareness of native food biodiversity and its integration into school curricula through the use of school gardens and gastronomy. As highlighted by the authors, 'Brazil is a country of superlatives in almost every way' especially when it comes to biodiversity being one of the richest in the world. Brazil also represents a great paradox in its food system, largely dominated by industrial agriculture and based on exotic crops and animals with the vast majority of native food biodiversity relegated to a minor role, a situation mirrored in the national school meals programme in Brazil, the second-largest national school feeding programme in the world. The Brazil case study describes projects and related initiatives that have used school gardens and gastronomy as vehicles for pedagogical practices to develop actions on healthy and sustainable habits towards the environment, diets, and local food cultures, including greater awareness of the value of native food biodiversity. These actions have prompted significant debates on the importance of organic and agroecological production, biodiverse production systems, regional foods and habits, and traditional and unconventional vegetables. The inclusion of Brazilian food biodiversity in school feeding and school curricula represents a cultural appreciation of local resources and food practices, raising awareness and recognition of traditional knowledge and practices, and encouraging students and communities to promote the necessary transformations to build a more sustainable society.

Acknowledgement

Special acknowledgement is given to Natalie Ching, who has assisted putting together the boxes, exemplifying a wide variety of school gardens.

Notes

1 Adapted from Hayden-Smith, R. (2015). A History of School Gardens…and how the model is getting a boost today from FoodCorps. UCFood Observer. http://ucfoodobserver.com/2015/05/06/a-history-of-school-gardens-and-how-the-model-is-getting-a-boost-today-from-food-corps/.
2 FoodCorps, Inc. website: https://foodcorps.org/about/.
3 Integrated School Nutrition Program website: https://schoolnutritionphils.wordpress.com/.

References

Blair, D. (2009) 'The child in the garden: An evaluative review of the benefits of school gardening' *The Journal of Environmental Education* 40(2).
Bundy, D., Burbano, C., Grosh, M., Gelli, A., Jukes, M. and Drake, L. (2009) 'Rethinking School Feeding: social safety nets, child development, and the education sector', World Bank, Washington D.C., ISBN 978-0-8213-7974-5.
DeMarco, L. (1999) 'The factors affecting elementary school teachers' integration of school gardening into the curriculum', Doctoral dissertation, Virginia Tech University, Blacksburg.
DepEd, DA BPI, DA and IIRR (2017) 'Crop Museums in Schools: Conserving agrobiodiversity of nutritional importance. A primer for school teachers in public elementary and secondary schools', Department of Education, Department of Agriculture - Bureau of Plant Industry, Department of Agriculture, International Institute of Rural Reconstruction https://schoolnutritionphils.files.wordpress.com/2017/04/crop-museum-primer.pdf, accessed 5 Sept 2019.

FAO (2010) 'A New Deal for School Gardens', Food and Agriculture Organization of United Nations, www.fao.org/3/i1689e/i1689e00.pdf, accessed 5 Sept 2019.

FAO, IFAD, UNICEF, WFP and WHO (2019) 'The State of Food Security and Nutrition in the World 2019- Safeguarding against economic slowdowns and downturns', Rome, FAO.

Fisher, L., Brinkmeyer, D., Karle, S., Cremer, K., Huttner, E., Seebauer, M., Nowikow, U., Schütze, B., Voigt, P., Völker, S. and Kowarik, I. (2019) 'Biodiverse edible schools: Linking healthy food, school gardens and local urban biodiversity', *Urban Forestry and Urban Greening*, doi:10.1016/j.ufug.2018.02.015.

Guitart, D.A., Pickering, C.M. and Byrne, J.A. (2014) 'Color me healthy: Food diversity in school community gardens in two rapidly urbanising Australian cities', *Health & place*, 26, 110–117.

Hayden-Smith, R. (2015) 'A history of school gardens… and how the model is getting a boost today from FoodCorps', UCFood Observer, 6 May 2015, http://ucfoodobserver.com/2015/05/06/a-history-of-school-gardens-and-how-the-model-is-getting-a-boost-today-from-food-corps/, accessed 5 Sept 2019.

Klemmer, C.D., Waliczek, T.M. and Zajicek, J.M. (2015) 'Growing Minds: The effect of school gardening program on the science achievement of elementary students', *Horticulture Technology*, 15(3), 448–452.

Laurie M. Tisch Center for Food, Education & Policy (2017) 'FoodCorps: Creating Healthy School Environments – Tisch report', Teachers College, Columbia University, New York, www.tc.columbia.edu/media/centers/tisch/FoodCorps-Report-FINAL-08-30-17-v5.pdf, accessed 5 Sept 2019.

Nomann, N., Jennings, A. and Wahi, L. (2006) 'The impacts of environmentally related education on academic achievement. A literature survey', *Community Resources for Science*.

Queensland Government (2016) 'The Health of Queenslanders 2016- Report of the Chief Health Officer Queensland', www.health.qld.gov.au/__data/assets/pdf_file/0036/651879/child-overweight-and-obesity-key-facts.pdf, accessed 5 Sept 2019.

Shafer, L. (2018) 'Let it grow', Usable Knowledge, Harvard Graduate School of Education, www.gse.harvard.edu/news/uk/18/07/let-it-grow, accessed 5 Sept 2019.

Sheffield, B.K. (1992) 'The affective and cognitive effects of an interdisciplinary garden-based curriculum on underachieving elementary students', Unpublished doctoral dissertation, University of South Carolina, Columbia.

Skelly, S. and Bradley, J. (2000) 'The importance of school gardens as perceived by Florida elementary school teachers', *Horticulture Technology*, 10(1), 1–3.

Skelly, S. and Bradley, J. (2007) 'The growing phenomenon of school garden: measuring their variation and their effect on students' sense of responsibility and attitudes towards science and the environment', Cornell Plantations and Department of Horticulture, Cornell University, Ithaca, NY, USA, doi:10.1080/15330150701319438.

Vasseur, L. (2016) 'Burkina Faso–Diversifying the garden: a way to ensure food security and women's empowerment', in A.J. Fletcher and W. Kubik (eds) 'Women in Agriculture Worldwide' (pp. 117–129), Routledge.

Wells, N.M., Myers, B.M., Todd, L.E., Henderson, C.R., Barale, K., Gaolach, B., Ferenz, G., Aitken, M, Tse, C.C., Pattison, K.O., Hendrix, L., Carson, J.B., Taylor, J.B. and Franz, N.K. (2018) 'The carry-over effects of school gardens on fruit and vegetable availability at home: A randomized controlled trial with low-income elementary schools', *Preventive Medicine*, 112, 152–159.

Wills, M. (2019) 'The first school gardens', JSTOR Daily, https://daily.jstor.org/the-first-school-gardens/, accessed 5 Sept 2019.

2
SCHOOLS AS A SYSTEM TO IMPROVE NUTRITION

Stineke Oenema, Lesley Drake, Kaia Engesveen, Andrea Polo Galante, Danny Hunter, David Ryckembusch, Luana Swensson, and Florence Tartanac

In 2018 the United Nations System Standing Committee on Nutrition (UNSCN) finalised the discussion paper "Schools as a system to improve nutrition" (UNSCN, 2018), with the invaluable support of several partners: FAO, WFP, UNICEF, WHO, IAEA as well as PCD, WB, BMGF, Bioversity International and IFPRI. This chapter is a summary of that discussion paper and highlights the role of school gardens in the overall vision of schools as a system to improve nutrition. In addition, it sketches a few recent developments that are of interest for both school-based nutrition programs and School Health and Nutrition (SHN) interventions as well as more specifically in the area of school gardens.

Introduction

This chapter states the multiple benefits of school-based nutrition interventions that span far beyond having an impact on education through school retention (specifically in low- and middle-income countries) and dietary and nutritional outcomes. Social, health, economic, and ethical arguments coalesce in and around schools. The potential benefits of SHN interventions are maximized when they are designed as multi-sectoral interventions and integrated into broader national social protection systems, leveraging existing and potential synergies with other social protection and development programmes.

The year 2020 sees the 20th anniversary of the FRESH Initiative (Focussing Resources on Effective School Health), that was jointly launched by a number of UN agencies. FRESH provides an evidence-based framework to guide countries in the development of comprehensive SHN programmes. With so many governments and partners now involved, it is recognized as an essential tool in SHN policy and implementation development. The UN is currently 'Refreshing' FRESH to reflect the learnings and experiences of contemporary SHN (Box 2.1).

> **BOX 2.1**
>
> Governments and international development partners are increasingly interested in school gardens. These have traditionally been used for science education, agricultural training or generating school income. Today, given the urgent need for increased food security, environmental protection, more secure livelihoods and better nutrition, perceptions of the potential of school gardens are changing. Some roles which are gaining prominence are the promotion of good diet, the development of livelihood skills, and environmental awareness. The belief is that school gardens can become a seed ground for a nation's health and security; this idea is increasingly backed up by experience and research (FAO, 2010).

The publication of Disease Control Priorities 3rd Edition in 2017, that was used as an important reference in the aforementioned UNSCN publication, clearly states that food and nutrition education (FNE) was critical at all stages and school gardens play a critical role in developing awareness and understanding on nutrition, not only for the school-age child but for the community more generally (Bundy et al., 2017).

Food and nutrition education (FNE) in the school setting aims to facilitate the voluntary adoption of long-lasting, healthy food-related outlooks, practices and habits conducive to better health and well-being. School gardens form a relevant school food and nutrition tool to be used as a platform for learning. It should not be regarded as bulk sources of food or income. Though a school garden can provide limited amounts of locally available and culturally appropriate nutrient-rich leafy or other vegetables to sometimes supplement school meals, its key path is to better nutrition and education.

SHN programmes offer the opportunity to connect with and improve local agriculture and local economy, for example through home-grown school meal programmes. SHN programmes also offer opportunities for lifestyle changes when children, through the meals they are served at school, get to acknowledge and appreciate nutritious crops as part of a healthy diet. This can have lifelong benefits and even span beyond current generations. School meals can contribute to dietary diversity by serving a variety of food products. When these products are part of local culture, for example because of their origin – indigenous crops – this may help to protect cultural diversity as well as agrobiodiversity. SHN programmes can also address the school environment and influence to what extent, diverse and healthy and fresh products are available. School garden programmes have proven to be very beneficial in most of the aforementioned areas: education and agronomic knowledge, local economies, and food security globally. When done properly, it helps to stimulate the interest of young children to pursue careers in agriculture and related areas, a deeper understanding of the nutritional value of a balanced diet primarily composed of local foods and, overall can promote long-term food security. These benefits and outcomes are clearly articulated in many of the case studies that make up the second part of this book. On the other hand, if not properly handled, school gardens can become an unpleasant chore or punishment and can easily undermine the potential or interest from the children. It is therefore important that as learners, children are inspired to enjoy their time in the garden whilst learning, and those involved in planning and coordination of school garden activities give this serious attention.

Recognition is now given to SHN programmes as significant investments in human capital and consequentially an investment in the wealth of nations. We are now at a critical juncture in developing contextually appropriate policies and programmes that can be sustainably financed and taken to scale. This chapter focusses upon the critical role that schools – and school gardens – can play in increasing the understanding of good nutrition and healthy diets.

The following paragraphs highlight the several chapters of the recent UNSCN discussion chapter:

Human rights: rights of the child, right to adequate food, and right to health. Steps towards a healthy school environment

Schools can play an important role contributing to the realization of rights for children. The Committee on the Rights of the Child, in interpreting and operationalizing Article 24, states in General Comment 15 that

> School feeding is desirable to ensure all pupils have access to a full meal every day, which can also enhance children's attention for learning and increase school enrolment. The Committee recommends that this be combined with nutrition and health education, **including setting up school gardens** and training teachers to improve children's nutrition and healthy eating habits.
>
> *(CRC, 2013, emphasis added)*

The Committee further highlights the need to limit exposure to '*"fast foods" that are high in fat, sugar or salt, energy-dense and micronutrient-poor, and drinks containing high levels of caffeine or other potentially harmful substances*', typically the opposite to the kinds of foods grown in a school garden.

The Committee on Economic, Social and Cultural Rights (e.g. rights to food and to health) identifies three levels of obligation for states to realize such rights: namely, to 'respect', 'protect', and 'fulfil' (through facilitation or provision) (CESCR, 1999). In the context of school nutrition, this means that the duty bearers – the government, teachers, and other school personnel – must respect the rights of children to good nutrition, and respect local food cultures that are conducive to healthy diets. School gardens can be used to grow fruits and vegetables that might be traditionally important as part of local food culture. In many countries such foods for a variety of reasons have been forgotten or neglected and school gardens can have an important role in their rediscovery especially if they are nutrient rich. Second, protecting the right to adequate food and the highest attainable standard of health means ensuring that children are not confronted with an unhealthy or unsafe school food environment, or are subject to abuse by third parties, including misleading marketing of unhealthy foods and beverages. The third level of obligation, to 'fulfil', implies duty bearers should act to fulfil children's rights through facilitation (e.g. school food standards, school gardens, nutrition education, training of staff, parent involvement) or provision (e.g. school meals).

Specific attention should be paid to marginalized groups, including girls, indigenous peoples, and ethnic minorities. In many communities, girls' right to education is violated; they are often less likely to enter secondary education and more likely to drop out for economic and socio-cultural reasons (see Case Study 4). This has severe consequences for the realization of their other rights, including the right to adequate food. Health- and nutrition-related interventions have shown to be effective in keeping girls at school. The importance of providing culturally appropriate food in school meals is paramount among indigenous communities, whose cultural concerns often go unaddressed by school administrations. School gardens can play an important role in reconnecting children from indigenous communities with their rich heritage of traditional foods and indigenous food systems (see Case studies 2, 5, 8, and 9).

In short, the school environment needs to be conducive to promoting the health and nutritional wellbeing of children. It should promote healthy diets, using diverse approaches, by ensuring the availability of a variety of foods, including plenty of fruits, vegetables, and legumes, and regulate the promotion, marketing, and sale of foods and beverages that are high in fats, sodium/salt, and sugars (WHO, 2015). One step being taken by several countries is to promote drinking water, as well as a ban on the sale or serving of sugar-sweetened beverages in cafeterias, kiosks, and/or vending machines, as well as in shops and stores around schools (WHO WPRO, 2016). Having a school policy or guidelines on school meals or foods to be brought from home would also help to develop an enabling school environment for the promotion of healthy diets (Box 2.2). Not only will school gardens provide hands on learning for children about how fruits and vegetables can be grown, but their produce may also be used to supplement school meals with fresh fruits and vegetables. In addition, it may create opportunities for children to learn about local food culture and to reinforce messages about healthy diets and sustainable environment (see Case Study 15), this may be of specific importance for children of indigenous peoples. School gardening, can also be used as a tool to teach students about food, the environment, health and hygiene. Moreover, it has engaged other stakeholders such as local authorities, parents and those who have gardens at home (FAO, 2019).

The school environment also presents an important opportunity to foster various health-promoting behaviours that can impact nutrition, by ensuring that clean

> **BOX 2.2**
>
> In the Philippines, for example, the Philippines Department of Education (DepEd) set out new regulatory standards for foods served, sold, and marketed in schools through its Policy and Guidelines on Healthy Food and Beverage Choices in Schools and in DepEd Offices. The policy uses a specially designed national nutrient profile model to categorize foods as 'green' to be served frequently (e.g. fruits and vegetables with little to no processing and lean meats), 'yellow' to be served only occasionally and avoided in large quantities (e.g. juice and biscuits), and 'red' to not be served at all (e.g. foods containing high amounts of saturated fats, sugars, or salt).

drinking water, hand-washing facilities, appropriate sanitation infrastructure, such as sanitary latrines, and areas for physical activity are easily accessible to schoolchildren throughout the school day and regularly maintained. School gardens can serve to show and teach where/what products can be grown and are nutritious.

Other examples are provided through the World Health Organization's (WHO) Nutrition-Friendly Schools Initiative (NFSI): In selected cities in Benin and Burkina Faso, the World Health Organization, Helen Keller International (HKI), the Regional Institute of Public Health (IRSP) and the University of Montreal launched the NFSI in 2006 to combat the double burden of malnutrition. In both countries, street vendors received training to improve hygiene and the nutritional value of the food sold to schoolchildren. In addition to integrating nutrition into the school curriculum, activities included special school-based nutrition events and sanitation measures, gardening and the raising of poultry. About 6,500 children were involved in the project. Evaluations found that vitamin A deficiency and anaemia had declined more significantly in intervention than control schools, although rates remained high (>25%), however consumption of unhealthy diets was on the rise in these urban areas and requires sustained efforts.

School meals and social protection

School meals programmes have the potential to directly address nutrition by improving the quality of student diets, including those of pre-school, primary, and secondary school-aged children. According to the WHO *Healthy Diets Factsheet*, a healthy diet contains an adequate intake of fruit, vegetables, and foods high in fibre, such as wholegrains, and limits the intake of fats, free sugars, and sodium (WHO, 2015). School meals should be based on national food-based dietary guidelines, which are, in turn, often based on international standards, to ensure they are diverse, likely to meet nutrient needs, and aligned with local food availability and preferences. Many countries have national school-meal policies that provide guidance on limiting the consumption of highly processed foods, or guidelines that set out the percentage of total nutrient or caloric needs that school meals should contribute (see example in Box 2.3). In addressing nutrient needs, schools can help prevent and manage micronutrient deficiencies in schoolchildren, considering that many children already start school with a micronutrient deficiency. Among preschoolers, the global prevalence of vitamin A deficiency in low- and middle-income countries is estimated at 33% (though it is 45% in Africa and Southeast Asia) (WHO, 2009), while the prevalence of anaemia is estimated at 47.4% (WHO, 2008). The nutrient requirements shall be informed by age, sex, and local food cultures, as well as the special needs of vulnerable groups, such as those impacted by infectious diseases or malnutrition.

BOX 2.3

In Slovenia, several laws have been adopted on school nutrition, the first in 1953. The Slovenian School Meals Act of 2010, amended in 2013 (Uradni, 2010), and the National Dietary Guidelines for Healthy Nutrition in Kindergartens (Gabrijelčič Blenkuš et al., 2005), defined in the Act, set the standards for the National School Meals Programme (NSMP) through which schools must provide at least one nutritionally balanced meal a day for all pupils. The meals, typically consisting of a mid-morning snack or lunch, must comply with the requirements for energy and nutrient content as well as a specific list of recommended and non-recommended food groups. The Act requires schools to determine the content, amount, education, and training activities related to meals and encourage a healthy food culture in their annual operational plan. Thus, the school plays a significant role in developing knowledge about healthy food, healthy eating habits, and food culture, and in teaching students how to develop a responsible attitude towards themselves and their health. In addition to ensuring nutritionally balanced meals, the programme is also linked to complementary initiatives, such as a weekly fruit and vegetable scheme, which currently covers 90.5% of students in basic education. The scheme largely offers fresh fruits and vegetables; dried or canned products are only included occasionally (<10%). Complementary activities include nutritional education, cooking-skills classes, tasting sessions, school gardening, visits to farms, and the promotion of local food procurement (Uradni, 2010).

Evaluations (Gregorič et al., 2015; WHO, 2016) showed that compliance of school lunches with dietary guidelines and meal quality varied between schools across regions in a pattern that mirrored availability of resources and capacity: schools with more students and in areas of higher socioeconomic status more often complied with dietary guidelines. The evaluation recommended measures to support a healthier food selection and preparation by food-service managers, through actions such as nutrition education and training.

Beyond their immediate benefits for children, school meals, when linked to local smallholder farming and agricultural development, can also shorten supply chains and ensure the diversification of food procurement, increasing the use of traditional, neglected and underutilized foods, while enhancing biodiversity conservation and environmental sustainability (Case Study 15; UNSCN, 2018). Such initiatives can also be linked to the establishment of gardens in schools as awareness raising and nutrition education tools, such as the introduction of African leafy vegetables to school gardens in the Kenya case study referred to in this book (Case study 6). They also have the potential to promote dietary diversification from local sources and local dietary habits, as well as local economic development and smallholder farmers' integration into markets (Morgan et al., 2007; Bundy et al., 2009; Espejo et al., 2009; Gelli et al., 2010; FAO and WFP, 2014). Further, such programmes can contribute to enhanced food biodiversity on farms and agricultural landscapes, and increase the resilience of households and communities (Valencia et al., 2019). Strategies for diversifying diets using local procurement should identify situations in which local foods may not be sufficient to meet nutrient requirements. In such scenarios, school meals may need to incorporate fortified foods or other nutritional supplements to address these shortfalls.

The 2016 Global Panel Foresight Report (GLOPAN, 2016) draws attention to the need to 'institutionalize high-quality diets through public sector purchasing power', including food provided in schools, which should be of the highest nutritional benefit. When school meals programmes are thoughtfully planned and supported by an appropriate institutional, political, and legal environment, and implemented with strong cross-sectoral coordination, they can act as an investment, producing benefits across multiple sectors and be integrated into broader national social-protection systems. School meals programmes are ideally placed to form part of comprehensive government plans to address multiple social needs and be integrated into national strategies to fight hunger, poverty, and malnutrition, and improve health-seeking behaviour and health outcomes.

Home-grown school feeding

School meal programmes can bolster local economies and create job opportunities when they forge ties between the provision of safe, diverse, and nutritious food and sourcing from local producers. Programmes linking local food production, purchasing, and delivery, such as home-grown school feeding programmes have the potential to create a more sustainable, inclusive local food system in their community. When a school meals programme is designed to provide children in school with safe, diverse, and nutritious food, sourced locally from smallholders, it is called home-grown school feeding (HGSF) (WFP et al., 2018). Among the multiples benefits of HGSF are the improvement of the economic lives of local farmers, facilitation of access to markets, as well as to productive inputs and credit, and increasing income and opportunities for growth

(Drake et al., 2016). Shifts in purchasing to support small- and medium-sized enterprises, such as small-scale food processing businesses, can also have an impact on social equity, as many such businesses are managed by women, and foster other job opportunities.

As institutional markets, schools can also promote the sourcing of healthy food, the development of short supply chains and the creation of alternative retail infrastructures, as well as support sustainable agroecological approaches to agriculture (IPES-Food, 2016). This approach has the potential to shape the norms around foods that contribute to high-quality diets, which could incentivize those involved in the supply chain to align their value chains accordingly (Tartanac et al., 2018). Demand from schools for a diversified food basket can also stimulate agricultural diversification and overall agricultural production, increase biodiversity and the use of traditional, neglected and/or underutilized foods (Niebylski et al., 2014; IPES-Food, 2016; Bioversity International, 2016; HLPE, 2017; Tartanac et al., 2018).

Recent experiences in countries such as Brazil, Ghana, and Ethiopia as well as from the Africans for Africa (PAA Africa) programme in Malawi suggest the potential for significant and multiple positive benefits from HGSF programmes, including the potential and opportunities of school gardens, as shown in some of the examples below.

In Brazil, family farming has benefited from the requirement that at least 30% of food used in school meals be bought from family farms and rural family entrepreneurs. Beltrame et al. (2016) in the context of the Biodiversity for Food and Nutrition (BFN) Project note how these public food-procurement requirements in Brazil can be strategically targeted to increase the use of nutritious, native foods in schools and to diversify public food procurement for school meals, while supporting family farming. Activities of the project include Partnership with the Educating through School Gardens and Gastronomy (PEHEG) initiative to diversify school curriculums using school gardens and gastronomy as educational tools to promote healthy eating habits; an appreciation of regional ingredients and recipes; the learning of cooking techniques; and the experience of flavours, food textures, and aromas of native biodiversity (see Case Study 15). While investment in native biodiverse products remains small compared with overall food purchases, BFN project initiatives have been able to include native biodiversity in the diets of their beneficiaries, thus becoming strategic tools in promoting the conservation and sustainable use of diverse foods.

The Purchase from Africans for Africa (PAA Africa) project – developed jointly by the Food and Agriculture Organization (FAO) and the World Food Programme (WFP) with the support of Brazil and the United Kingdom – shows similar results. The programme had a twofold objective: improve the income security of smallholder farmers and improve the nutritional status of children in food-insecure areas (FAO and WFP, 2014; Gyoeri et al., 2016). Data from the implementation in Malawi show that PAA Africa has contributed to community diet diversification and food security. Through the programme's production support, smallholder output has become more diversified and producers have been able to meet schools' demand for a wide range of local foods, including cereals, pulses, vegetables, tubers, fruits, and meat. This has not only contributed to dietary diversification at school but also to the regular consumption of diverse and nutritional foods at home. School committees have received training in nutrition and have begun to reproduce school menus at home, incorporating new foods into their diet (FAO, WFP and IPC-IG, 2016; Gyoeri et al., 2016).

More recently, in Ethiopia, an increase in the diversification of commodities being planted and offered locally was already assessed as a result of an HGSF initiative (WFP et al., 2016; WFP, 2018). A study of the HGSF Pilot Program in the Southern Nations Nationalities and People's Region – developed through a partnership among the Ministry of Education (MoE) and technical partners, including the WFP and the FAO – demonstrates that this increase was led by the substantial demand from schools, which served as a guarantee for farmers who would otherwise be reluctant to plant new crop types (WFP, 2018). Considering that local agricultural production and dietary consumption are closely coupled in this country context, this may directly contribute to dietary diversity of the population, which is still considerably low (IFPRI, 2018; Swensson, 2019). Ethiopia is one of the countries currently supported by the FAO Project on 'Policy Support on Public Food Procurement for Government-led HGSF initiatives'.

In **Ghana** preliminary evidence from the national HGSF also suggest multiple positive impacts of the programme, including those on education, health, nutrition, and agriculture. Regarding the latest, data collected by Gelli et al. (2016) indicates that individual dietary diversity improved among school feeding communities and that children receiving school feeding were more likely to consume nutritious foods, like green leafy vegetables and other types of vegetables; roots; and, in the case of 5- to 10-year-olds, meat and fish. Regarding the agriculture, farming activity increased 15% in communities receiving school feeding relative to communities without school feeding and farmers in HGSF communities saw an increase of 5% in household income (Gelli et al., 2016). This programme was the first to use the 'School Meals Planning' tool (Fernandes et al., 2016). This utilizes the WHO guidelines on RDA, FAO food consumption tables and government internal policy to identify locally sourced food (and local farmers to produce the food) to develop nutritionally balanced meals for each school day. It has now been adopted and adapted in multiple countries as a planning tool to ensure that the supply chain (from farmer to child) is strengthened. It is also now used as an FNE tool in the schools and in the development of school gardens. The school garden initiative was introduced in Ghana in 2012 by 4-H Ghana, through the Enterprise School Garden Innovation Project. This was first piloted in the Eastern Region involving 120 schools (primary, junior high and senior high schools) in 12 districts in the Eastern region. The project now reaches over 65,000 (31,150 girls and 33,850 boys) youth in 750 schools, in 25 districts, in 6 regions (Ashanti, Eastern, Volta, Greater Accra, Northern, and Central) in Ghana, concentrating mainly on improved crop varieties such as orange-fleshed sweet potato (OFSP), hybrid corn, and cowpeas.

School garden clubs with over 3,750 members have also been formed and are being provided with sets of garden tools, small animals such as rabbit and grass cutter, and a broad variety of vegetable and grain seeds to enable the practice of crop rotation. Training kits and other manuals are also made available to clubs to facilitate and boost their interest. In addition, over 1,500 school teachers with science and agriculture backgrounds, have been trained as experiential educators/advisors to instruct the school garden programme in schools.

The national school feeding program (GSFP) and 4H Ghana are currently collaborating to effect full integration of the school garden initiative into the GSFP to achieve holistic implementation as well as its educational benefits for the learner.

Food and nutrition education in schools

Food and nutrition education (FNE) in the school setting aims to facilitate the voluntary adoption of long-lasting, healthy food-related outlooks, practices and habits conducive to better health and well-being. FNE may comprise a combination of evidence-based and behaviourally focussed educational strategies, which involve the active participation of all relevant actors (schoolchildren, parents, school staff, community leaders, etc.) and are reinforced by an enabling school environment. FNE actions should be based on the local situation; be developmentally and culturally appropriate; and have an adequate duration and intensity, and a practical focus (Pérez-Rodrigo and Aranceta, 2003; FAO, 2018).

School gardens form a relevant school food and nutrition tool to be used as a platform for learning. It should not be regarded as bulk sources of food or income, though a school can provide limited amounts of nutrient-rich leafy or other vegetables, but rather as a path to better nutrition and education. Students can learn how to grow, tend, harvest, and prepare nutritious seasonal produce in the educational settings of the classroom, the garden, the kitchen, the school cafeteria, and the home. The experience promotes the environmental, social, and physical wellbeing of the school community and fosters a better understanding of how the natural world sustains us. Links with home gardens reinforce the concept and pave the way for an exchange of knowledge and experience between the school and the community (FAO, 2010; FAO and Swensson, 2015).

It is fundamental to explore synergies between *food and nutrition education strategies* and *school meals programmes,* using the participatory approach to promote the full development of children's capacities and motivation for healthier food-related practices. Effective food and nutrition education involves providing children, school staff, teachers, cooks, canteen staff, communities, families, and local smallholder farmers with hands-on learning experiences tailored to facilitate the voluntary adoption of healthy eating and other positive nutrition-related behaviours. Smallholder farmers can also understand the importance of producing local safe and diversified food for school meals programmes. In many communities, schools are the only place where children can learn such basic life skills. Linking classroom learning to practical activities that are reinforced by a nutrition- and health-friendly school environment and involve the participation of families and the school community, provides a wide range of practical, community-based learning opportunities aimed at creating positive attitudes, skills, and behaviours (Psaki, 2014; Lobstein et al., 2015).

Agents of change

To realize the full potential of school-based food and nutrition interventions, it is important to highlight the importance of capable, trained agents of change. Teachers, school staff, students, parents, caterers, food vendors, and farmers all have an important role to play in helping promote positive nutritional behaviour. Developing capacity for these actors and equipping them with the necessary knowledge and skills on nutrition, food hygiene, healthy diets, and lifestyle is paramount. Teachers, in particular, will require more formal training and capacity development, as they can be among the most important promoters of positive nutritional behaviour among the youth. They have the opportunity not only to influence eating habits through food and nutritional education but also to address other issues, including the nutritional needs of adolescent girls and pregnant women, and maternal and infant care.

Benefits and costs of school-based nutrition interventions

As argued above school-based food and nutrition interventions can underpin nutrition and health services, including nutrition education and other health promoting behaviours as well as contribute to social protection and local economic development. Growth monitoring and/or regular screening can help detect children with various forms of malnutrition and health problems. School-based food and nutrition intervention comes at a **cost**, but because of the multiple objectives and benefits involved, any narrowly defined cost-benefit analysis will underestimate the full impact of school-based nutrition measures. One key outcome is to increase regular school attendance by both girls and boys. This serves as a basis for educational achievement, leading to better economic productivity and, consequently, a greater contribution to national GDP. While this outcome is still relevant in some low- and middle-income countries, it has become less central as school participation has increased. Thus, the total value of school-based food and nutrition interventions increasingly is based on their contribution to learning as well as in social protection and sustainable development.

Finding sustained sources of funding for school-based intervention, including school gardens, can pose a challenge for many lower- to middle-income countries. However, school-based interventions should:

- Be part of the national budget;
- Plan a clear transition period from donor support to sustainable domestic budgetary support, rather than resort to abrupt programme termination; and
- Be supported by UN agencies and other partners, in close coordination with governments and local stakeholders, to ensure that programmes become part of long-term, sustainable social-protection and local development strategies led by countries, both in the global North and South.

Concluding remarks

Schools offer an extremely important entry point to improve health and nutrition to children in a sustainable way. As described above, SHN interventions, when implemented in an integrated way, have huge potential to improve the nutritional status of schoolchildren and at the same time shape their health-seeking behaviour for the rest of their lives. School gardens can be an important element of SHN interventions as many of the benefits and outcomes highlighted throughout this book reinforces. School gardening, can also be used as a tool to teach students about food, the environment, health, and hygiene. Moreover, it provides a suitable space to engage other stakeholders, such as local authorities, parents, and those who have gardens at home (FAO, 2019).

Specific benefits are expected when school gardens grow a variety of indigenous crops, thus contributing to pupils' knowledge, understanding, and appreciation of the importance of a diverse production system that underpins healthy and sustainable diets.

Home-grown school feeding can also have an important spin off effect on local economic development in instances where local farmers and caterers are involved in the supply and preparation of safe and diversified foods and nutritious meals. Despite the many countries and projects experiences, it is important to note that there is still considerable opportunity to further improve the understanding of the role of school meals programmes on job creation for low-skilled and/or rural women, youths and farmers, as well as of the enabling institutional, policy and legal enabling environment that may inform the sustainability of the programme and its benefits. In this respect it is interesting to know if school gardens can help prompt students to opt for employment in agriculture.

To conclude, it is possible to affirm that when school meals programmes are thoughtfully planned, supported by an appropriate institutional, political, and legal environment, and implemented with strong cross-sectoral coordination, they can act as an investment, producing benefits across multiple sectors (Morgan and Sonnino, 2008; Espejo et al., 2009; Gelli et al., 2010; Sumberg and Sabates-Wheeler, 2011; Drake et al., 2016; Tartanac et al., 2018; WFP et al., 2018).

They also provide the opportunity to involve a multitude of community actors, including civil society, farmer organizations, and the private sector. Consequently, schools, especially those with HGSF programmes and linked to food and nutrition education activities, have the potential to create a more sustainable, inclusive local food system (HLPE, 2017) in their community and also to contribute to healthier and more sustainable diets.

References

Beltrame, D.M., Oliveira, C.N.S., Borelli, T., de Andrade Cardoso Santiago, Monego, E.T., Vera de Rosso, V., Coradin, L. and Hunter, D. (2016) 'Diversifying institutional food procurement – opportunities and barriers for integrating biodiversity for food and nutrition in Brazil', *Revista Raízes*, 36 (2), 55–69.

Bioversity International (2016) 'Mainstreaming agrobiodiversity in sustainable food systems: scientific foundations for an agrobiodiversity index', Bioversity International, Rome.

Bundy, D., Burbano, C., Grosh, M., Gelli, A., Jukes, M. and Drake, L. (2009) 'Rethinking school feeding: social safety nets, child development and the education sector', World Bank, Washington DC.

Bundy, D., Schultz, L., Sarr, B., Banham, L., Colenso, P. and Drake, L (2017). 'The school as a platform for addressing health in middle childhood and adolescence', in: D. Bundy, N. de Silva, S. Horton, D.T. Jamison and G.C. Patton (eds) 'Disease control priorities in developing countries', Third edition, Vol 8: *Child & Adolescent Health Development*, World Bank: Washington, DC.

Committee on Economic, Social and Cultural Rights (CESCR) (1999) 'Substantive issues arising in the implementation of the international covenant on economic, social and cultural rights: General comment 12 (Twentieth session, 1999), The right to adequate food (art. 11)', ECOSOC, Geneva.

Committee on the Rights of the Child (CRC) (2013) 'General comment No. 15 (2013) on the right of the child to the enjoyment of the highest attainable standard of health (art. 24)'.

Drake, L., Woolnough, A., Burbano, C. and Bundy, D. (eds) (2016) 'Global school feeding sourcebook: Lessons from 14 countries', Imperial College Press, New Jersey.

Espejo, F., Burbano, C. and Galliano, E. (2009) 'Home grown school feeding: A framework to link school feeding with local agricultural production', World Food Programme, Rome.

Fernandes, M., Galloway, R., Gelli, A., Mumuni, D., Hamdani, S., Kiamba, J., Quarshie, K., Bhatia, R., Aurino, E., Peel, F. and Drake, L. (2016) 'Enhancing linkages between healthy diets, local agriculture, and sustainable food systems: The school meals planner package in Ghana', *Food Nutrition Bulletin*, 37(4), pp. 571–584.

Food and Agriculture Organization of the United Nations (FAO) (2010) 'A new deal for school gardens', FAO, Rome.

FAO (2018) 'Regional overview of national school food and nutrition programmes in Africa', FAO, Rome, accessible from www.fao.org/3/I8063EN/i8063en.PDF.

FAO (2019) 'FAO school food and nutrition framework', FAO, Rome, accessible from www.fao.org/3/ca4091en/ca4091en.pdf.

FAO and Swensson, L.F.J. (2015) 'Institutional procurement of food from smallholder farmers: The case of Brazil', FAO, Rome, accessible from www.fao.org/3/a-bc569e.pdf.

FAO and World Food Program (WFP) (2014) 'Promoting local food assistance in the African continent: Purchase from Africans for Africa', FAO and WFP, Rome.

FAO, WFP and International Policy Centre for Inclusive Growth (IPC-IG) (2016) 'PAA Africa program midterm monitoring report: Malawi', FAO, WFP and IPC-IG, Rome and Brasilia.

Gabrijelčič Blenkuš, M., Pograjc, L., Gregorič, M., et al. (2005) 'Smernice zdravega prehranjevanja v vzgojno izobraževalnih ustanovah: od prvega leta starosti naprej' (National Dietary Guidelines for Healthy Nutrition in Kindergartens and Schools), Ljubljana: Ministrstvo za zdravje RS.

Gelli, A., Masset, E., Folson, G., Kusi, A., Arhinful, D.K., Asante, F. et al. (2016) 'Evaluation of alternate school feeding models on nutrition, education, agriculture and other social outcomes in Ghana: Rationale, randomised design and baseline data', *Trials*, 17, 37.

Gelli, A., Nesse, K. and Drake, L. (2010) 'Home grown school feeding: Linking smallholder agriculture to school food provision', Working paper 212, Partnership for Child Development (PCD), London.

Global Panel on Agriculture and Food Systems for Nutrition (GLOPAN) (2016) 'Food systems and diets: Facing the challenges of the 21st century', GLOPAN, London.

Gyoeri, M., Miranda, A.C. and Soares, F. (2016) 'Linking vulnerable smallholder farmers to school feeding programs: The experience of PAA Africa', *Policy in Focus*, vol 13, no 2. IPC-IG and the United Nations Development Program (UNDP), Brasilia.

High Level Panel of Experts on Food Security and Nutrition (HLPE) (2017) 'Nutrition and food systems. A report by the High Level Panel of Experts on Food Security and Nutrition of the Committee on World Food Security', Report 12, FAO, Rome.

International Food Policy Research Institute (IFPRI) (2018) 'Food systems for healthier diets in Ethiopia: Toward a research agenda', IFPRI, Washington DC.

International Panel of Experts on Sustainable Food Systems (IPES-Food) (2016) 'From uniformity to diversity: A paradigm shift from industrial agriculture to diversified agroecological systems', IPES-Food, Brussels.

Lobstein, T., Jackson-Leach, R., Moodie, M.L., Hall, K.D., Gortmaker, S.L., Swinburn, B.A., James, W.P.T., Wang, Y. and McPherson, K. (2015) 'Child and adolescent obesity: Part of a bigger picture', *The Lancet*, 385(9986), 2510–2520.

Morgan, K., Bastia, T. and Kanemasu, Y. (2007) 'Home grown: The new era of school feeding, Project report, World Food Programme (WFP), Rome.

Morgan, K. and Sonnino, R. (2008) 'The school food revolution: Public food and the challenge of sustainable development', Earthscan Publications, London, Washington DC.

Niebylski, M.L., Lu, T., Campbell, N.R.C., Arcand, J., Schermel, A., Hua, D., Yeates, K.E., Tobe, S.W., Twohig, P.A., L'Abbé, M.R. and Liu, P.P. (2014) 'Healthy food procurement policies and their impact', *International Journal of Environmental Research and Public Health*, 11, 2608–2627.

Pérez-Rodrigo, R. and Aranceta, J. (2003) 'Nutrition education in schools: Experiences and challenges', *European Journal of Clinical Nutrition*, 57(suppl 1), 82–85.

Psaki, S.R. (2014) 'Addressing early marriage and adolescent pregnancy as a barrier to gender parity and equality in education', Background paper for the 2015 UNESCO Education for All Global Monitoring Report, Population Council, New York.

Sumberg, J. and Sabates-Wheeler, R. (2011) 'Linking agricultural development to school feeding in sub-Saharan Africa: Theoretical perspectives', *Food Policy*, 36, 341–349.

Swensson, L.F.J. (2019) 'Aligning public procurement rules and practices to support the implementation of home-grown school feeding (HGSF) initiatives: The case of Ethiopia', FAO, Rome, accessible from www.fao.org/3/CA3614EN/ca3614en.pdf.

Tartanac, F., Swensson, L.F.J., Galante, A.P. and Hunter, D. (2018) 'Institutional food procurement for promoting sustainable diets', in B. Burlingame and S. Dernini (eds) *Sustainable Diets: The Transdisciplinary Imperative*, CABI, Wallingford.

United Nations System Standing Committee on Nutrition (UNSCN) (2018) 'School as a system to improve nutrition', UNSCN, Rome.

Uradni (2010) Zakon o šolski prehrani (ZŠolPre) 'Ljubljana: Uradni list 43' accessible from www.uradni-list.si/1/content?id=98032.

Valencia, V., Wittman, W. and Blesh, J. (2019) 'Structuring markets for resilient farming systems', *Agronomy for Sustainable Development*, 39, 25.

World Food Program (WFP) (2018) 'Ethiopia school feeding programme', WFP, Rome.

WFP, FAO, IFAD, NEPAD, GCNF and PCD (2018) 'Home-grown school feeding: Resource framework', Technical document, FAO and WFP, Rome, accessible from www1.wfp.org/publications/home-grown-school-feeding-resource-framework.

WFP, PCD and Dubai Cares (2016) 'Home Grown School Feeding (HGSF) Pilot Programme in Southern Nations Nationalities and Peoples Region, Ethiopia: Programme Evaluation', World Food Programme, Partnership for Child Development and Dubai Cares, Ethiopia.

World Health Organization (WHO) (2008) 'Global anaemia prevalence and number of individuals affected', WHO, Geneva.

WHO (2009) 'Global prevalence of vitamin A deficiency in populations at risk 1995–2005', WHO Global database on vitamin A deficiency, WHO, Geneva.

WHO (2015) 'Healthy diets factsheet. no. 394', (updated September 2015), accessible from www.who.int/en/news-room/fact-sheets/detail/healthy-diet.

WHO (2016) 'Evaluating implementation of the resolution on the Slovenian food and nutrition action plan 2005–2010 – Upgraded evaluation, 2016', Regional office for Europe, Copenhagen.

WHO Western Pacific Regional Office (WHO WPRO) (2016) 'Be smart drink water: A guide for school principals in restricting the sale and marketing of sugaring drinks and around schools', WHO and WPRO, Manila.

3

STRATEGIES FOR INTEGRATING FOOD AND NUTRITION IN THE PRIMARY SCHOOL CURRICULUM

Maria Theresa M. Talavera and Aileen R. de Juras

Introduction

Every child has a right to food, nutrition, health, and education. However, millions of children around the world are suffering from malnutrition, diseases, and poor education. Based on the *Education for all - Global monitoring report*, around 58 million children are out of school globally and around 100 million children do not complete primary education (UNESCO, 2015). UNESCO has identified barriers to inclusive education categorized as follows: child (homelessness and the need to work, illness and hunger, birth registration, violence, pregnancy), family (poverty, conflict, inadequate caregiving, HIV/AIDS); community (gender discrimination, cultural differences and local tradition, negative attitudes); and school (costs, location, scheduling, facilities, preparedness, class sizes, resources, and teachers' workload).

Malnutrition continues to affect millions of children globally (FAO et al., 2017) and in the Association of Southeast Asian Nations (ASEAN) countries (ASEAN/UNICEF/WHO, 2016). However, the nutrition situation of schoolchildren is not as well measured as that of pre-school children. In Asia and the Pacific, there is a dearth of information on the nutritional status of schoolchildren (SEAMEO INNOTECH, 2016). Understanding malnutrition is important as it affects populations throughout the life cycle, from conception through childhood into adolescence, adulthood, and older age (IFPRI, 2016). Among schoolchildren, under-nutrition has been linked with poor school achievement and performance, reduced school attendance, and diminished income-earning capacity in adulthood (ASEAN/UNICEF/WHO, 2016).

The school has been recognized as a setting for advancing nutrition in a large group of young people, school staff, families, and community members

(Perez-Rodrigo and Aranceta, 2003; FAO, 2005). Nutrition education is identified as one of the key interventions addressing malnutrition and in promoting lifelong healthy eating and exercise behaviours (Center for Disease Control and Prevention, 1996; McNulty, 2013). According to Perez-Rodrigo and Aranceta (2003), school-based nutrition education should (a) address the needs and interests of the students, teachers, and school; (b) be relevant to programme goals; (c) take into account what children already know and can do; (d) be culturally appropriate; and (e) be delivered in a way children can understand and teach the skills and knowledge required to improve or strengthen healthy eating habits.

Methodology

This chapter aims to review current strategies on how food and nutrition education is integrated in the primary school curriculum focussed on countries in Southeast Asia. The interventions were identified using Elton B. Stephens Co. (EBSCO) research database, information searches on Google Scholar, and targeted internet searching of key organization websites. The search keywords used were "food and nutrition education" AND "integrated" AND "school curriculum" AND English language; and "food and nutrition education" AND "school feeding program" AND English language. Additional search was done using the keyword "school gardens", "school meals", and "school feeding". Search results were refined to include full text copies of peer-reviewed journals published from 2005 onwards.

Main Findings

Health and nutrition problems among schoolchildren

Nutrition and health problems affect many schoolchildren in Southeast Asian countries though there are some variations from country to country. Based on the study of SEAMEO INNOTECH (2016), the most common school health and nutrition problems in the countries are underweight and dental problems, followed by overweight, and then EENT (eyes, ears, nose, and throat) problems and water- and sanitation-related illnesses (see Table 3.1). In terms of diet, SEAMEO RECFON (2018) has documented the nutritional practices of schoolchildren, including not eating breakfast regularly; not bringing food from home; poor consumption of fruits and vegetables; and high consumption of sweet drinks and processed food high in sugar, salt, and oil or fat. Said practices were reported to be a reflection of situations in countries in the region which contribute to nourishment-related problems among schoolchildren such as stunting, being underweight or overweight, anaemia, and obesity.

TABLE 3.1 Most common SHCN problems by country

Country	School health and nutrition problems					
	Underweight	Overweight	EENT Problems	WASH related illnesses	Skin disorders	Dental problems
Brunei Darussalam		✓	✓			✓
Cambodia	✓			✓		✓
Indonesia	✓	✓				✓
The Lao PDR	✓		✓	✓		
Malaysia	✓	✓			✓	
The Philippines	✓			✓		✓
Thailand		✓	✓			✓

Source: SEAMEO INNOTECH (2016).

Strategies in nutrition education

The governments of Southeast Asian countries have formulated and implemented policies and programmes addressing the problems identified among schoolchildren. Nutrition education is one of the interventions implemented to protect and promote the health and well-being of schoolchildren. Recently, there are several initiatives that have been implemented such as training of trainers on integrating nutrition in primary education curriculum by FAO in 2016 (FAO-RAP, 2016), development of comprehensive documents on school food and nutrition education by FAO that started in 2017 (FAO and United Arab Emirates University, 2019), and SEAMEO-RECFON has introduced the Nutrition Goes to School (NGTS) programme first in Indonesia and then to be expanded to other ASEAN countries (SEAMEO RECFON, 2018). This programme aims to produce active, well-nourished, and smart (AWESOME) schoolchildren using three approaches: 1) active (students perform physical activities); 2) well-nourished (students have a body mass index (BMI) that falls within the normal range; and 3) smart (students reduce their number of absences due to sickness and show improved academic performance).

While there are efforts to step up school-based food and nutrition education, several strategies have been implemented in nutrition education for schoolchildren: namely, (1) integration of nutrition in primary school curriculum, (2) school gardening, (3) technology/web-based, (4) parental involvement, and (5) school feeding programmes. In this chapter, the curriculum approach is defined as nutrition education programmes delivered by teachers or specialists and cross-curricular when nutrition education programmes are delivered across two or more traditional primary school subjects. The technology/web-based approach is defined as students interacting with website(s) via the internet to enhance their knowledge of healthy eating or internet-based resources or feedback mechanisms that could be accessed by students at home or school. Parental involvement is defined as parents playing a role in the delivery of messages in the classroom and/or reinforcement of messages at home or programmes requiring active participation or assistance from a parent within or outside the school environment. School feeding programmes are defined as providing meals to schoolchildren. According to FAO (2019), integrating food and nutrition education with school meal helps establish meal times as learning opportunities and, at the same time, enhances effects on food practices.

Curriculum approach

Primary schools have been identified as a suitable place for nutrition education because of its systematic environment. They reach a large proportion of children and can influence schoolchildren at a critical stage when eating habits and attitudes are being established (FAO, 2005). One of the interventions to incorporate nutrition education in the school curriculum is through activities and/or lessons in a specific subject or programme related to healthy eating. With the narrow strategy currently employed in Southeast Asian countries, a 'tripartite curriculum' on school-based nutrition education developed by the FAO is put forward wherein the classroom curriculum is linked with the family, community, and school environment.

Integration is an act of bringing together small components (subjects) into a single system (a particular grade curriculum) that functions as one (specific knowledge domain + nutrition education). The goal is to develop a curriculum that can help learners to recognize the links between food, health and the environment and the causes and consequences of hunger, malnutrition and food insecurity, and (where possible) to act on this understanding. The expected output is a seamless integration of learning knowledge, skills/behaviour domains as specified in the school curricula and proper nutrition. The question has been why integrate concepts of nutrition in primary education. The answer is basically because it offers a unique venue for inculcating proper nutrition behaviour and healthy lifestyles at an important stage in a person's lifelong learning and total development and can provide the important multiplier effect when families and communities are engaged.

When integrating food and nutrition concepts, several factors have to be considered such as country context (food and nutrition issues in the country and focus on the most urgent), content (select curriculum content that will contribute to the objectives of nutrition education, i.e. healthy eating and nutrition literacy), development (structure learning so that it is age group appropriate and develops systematically though the school years), relevance (learning is relevant to local practices, beliefs, and attitudes, and makes direct connections to children's daily lives), and framework (spread nutrition education and school gardening through the primary school curriculum while at the same time maintaining its coherence and impact).

In deciding the level of integration, several questions have to be answered such as how much nutrition is already taught, what subjects are already taught and how are they grouped, which subjects are examinable, how much time is available, how much competition for time exists, whether the current system favours cross cutting subjects, and whether schools are used to project work, team teaching. There are several ways by which nutrition can be integrated, namely, nutrition education as a separate subject (considered as most ideal, raises profile of nutrition, and easier to develop appropriate teaching materials), infusion into subjects such as science, social sciences, literature and math, themes and projects with a nutrition focus such as Nutrition Month in the Philippines, World Food Day, and a combination of the strategies. The types of learning needed include food-based knowledge rather than information on basic nutrition science and nutrient-based; procedural knowledge, with emphasis on developing self-efficacy, skills and practices (food preparation/cooking, label reading, the habit of breakfast, food gardening); application of learning to the food environment (school, home, community, and the food system) and involving families.

If you take a look at the topics included in the curriculum, the most common ones are nutrients, functions, and/or nutritional value of foods; food safety, hygiene, and/or sanitation; and relationship between diet and health and disease. On the other hand, the least common topics are producing and growing diversified and nutritious foods, procuring/shopping for good food value, planning and preparing healthy meals, and trying out new foods or new food practices. New topics have to be included in the context of changing food systems, such as increasing dependence on mass-produced convenience and fast foods; the fact that it is not only women who need to understand and practice healthy eating and lifestyles; climate change; food culture; right to food; and household practices: for example, who does what in the home and why, and how long it takes.

Results of the literature search revealed that Cambodia, Indonesia, the Lao People's Democratic Republic (the Lao PDR), Malaysia, Myanmar, Philippines, Singapore, and Thailand integrate food and nutrition education by using the curriculum and cross-curricular approaches. Nutrition knowledge and principles are covered in Science, Health Education, and Home Economics subjects. Topics discussed are food groups, nutrients, eating a variety of foods, meal preparation, and proper hygiene. Moreover, the curriculum in some countries was designed using developmentally appropriate and learner-centred approaches.

Within the Asian countries, there is an integration process taking place where different educational levels are being revisited and improved. This is because of the recognition of the need to integrate nutrition and use of school gardens as a platform for acquiring lifelong skills and positive nutrition behaviours. In 2016, a FAO Regional Training of Trainers on Integrating Nutrition in Primary Education Curriculum was conducted. Representatives from countries of Bangladesh, the Lao PDR, Myanmar, Timor Leste, Nepal, Cambodia, and Thailand were represented (FAO-RAP, 2016). The aims were to develop regional capacity and national capacity on how to integrate nutrition and related key concepts on nutrition in the curriculum and promote the use of school garden-based learning as a more sustainable strategy for promoting and acquiring lifelong skills and positive nutrition behaviours that translate to improved food and nutrition security. The experiences among the said countries revealed that primary or elementary curriculum varies among countries. In addition, primary education has incorporated nutrition mostly in science, health, physical education, and life skills subjects. The quality of teaching nutrition needs to be addressed due to lack of knowledge of schoolteachers and lack of teaching materials. Many of the countries have also implemented school garden learning but it is not widely promoted (Myanmar, the Lao PDR, Bangladesh, and Timor Leste) and linking school gardens with nutrition and with curriculum are not well established.

School gardening

There are many studies on the use of school gardens as an effective experiential learning strategy. Garden-based learning is an educational strategy that utilizes school gardens to supplement instruction in a variety of disciplines. It provides an atmosphere that incorporates hands-on activities and strengthens academic, personal, and social skills. In addition, school gardens allow children to develop life skills in areas such as nutrition, leadership, and decision-making.

School gardening programmes have been implemented in both developed and developing countries. In Cambodia, the FAO and Council of Agriculture and Rural Development (CARD) initiated the implementation of garden-based learning using the farm to table food path as a framework. Children are taught to produce, prepare, and consume food through the school feeding programme or at home where they bring the harvested food. In the Philippines, both government and private agencies are involved in implementing school feeding programmes. The Southeast Asian Regional Center for Agriculture (SEARCA) recently implemented school and home gardens as learning sites and as sources of nutritious food and income. Furthermore, the International Institute for Rural Reconstruction (IIRR) also implemented school gardening projects in selected schools using the bio-intensive gardening (BIG) method (see Chapter 4). The project has developed a model which integrates school gardening, supplementary feeding, and nutrition education. An evaluation of the project showed that supplementary feeding of malnourished schoolchildren using iron-fortified rice and indigenous nutrient-rich vegetables from school gardens significantly improved their nutritional status. Likewise, parents were reported to have enhanced knowledge, attitude, and practices on gardening and nutrition. The project also used climate resilient, locally adapted, and nutritionally important vegetables. The Philippine Department of Education is one of the government agencies implementing school gardening through the *Gulayan sa Paaralan* (School Vegetable Garden). *Gulayan sa Paaralan* employs different models, that is, Model A or Patch Gardening, Model B or Dish or Potted Gardening, Model C or Vertical

Gardening, Model D or Aerial Gardening, Model E or Refrigerator Gardening, and Model F or Pocket Gardening. A preliminary assessment of the programme showed minimum involvement of stakeholders, insufficient landscaping and garden fixtures, and lack of proper arrangement and classification of vegetables according to the specified garden models (Inocian and Nuneza, 2015).

Davis et al. (2015) systematically reviewed the impact of garden-based programmes conducted in school on dietary behaviours in children (kindergarten through 8th grade students). Results showed that garden-based programmes increased vegetable intake and preference for vegetables; improved attitudes towards willingness to taste; and identification of and self-efficacy to prepare/cook fruit and vegetables. The strategies employed by the majority of the programmes included: 'hands on' curriculum, incorporation of a cooking component, instructor-aided classes, parental and stakeholder support, provision of food, and use of garden as focal point for media promotion. Another systematic review by Williams and Dixon (2013) of 48 articles published from 1990 to 2010 evaluated the impact of garden-based learning on academic outcomes among schoolchildren. The results showed a preponderance of positive impacts on direct academic outcomes with the highest positive impact for science followed by math and language arts. Indirect academic outcomes were also measured with social development surfacing most frequently and positively.

Studies on the effectiveness of school gardening were focussed on the measurement of several outcomes such as improvement in consumption of fruits and vegetables, preferences for fruits and vegetables, willingness to taste fruits and vegetables. In the study of Dudley et al. (2015), experiential learning approaches such as school/community gardens, cooking lessons, and food preparation reported on outcomes associated with reducing food consumption and energy intake. The study of Morgan et al. (2010) showed that school gardens can impact positively on primary-school students' willingness to taste vegetables and their vegetable taste ratings but not on vegetable intake which was attributed to the complexity of dietary behaviour change. Another study which determined the effects of garden-based nutrition education on sixth grade adolescents' fruit and vegetable consumption showed that those who participated in the garden-based nutrition intervention increased their servings of fruits and vegetables more than students in the two other groups. There were also significant increases found in vitamin A, vitamin C, and fibre intake (Mcaleese and Rankin, 2007).

Technology/Web-based approach

New technologies such as the Internet provides opportunities for interactive learning experiences since they are popular among schoolchildren (Perez-Rodrigo and Aranceta, 2003). Classroom phones and voice mail, video technology, radio announcements, and school websites to link homes and schools can enhance communication with parents beyond the traditional formats. In the paper of Graham-Clay (2005), the authors showed enhancement in communication between parents and teachers through phones (teachers can contact parents from their classrooms when students are not present); voice mail (daily one-minute voice mail message for parents and students to call at the end of each day, recorded message provided updates on homework assignments, classroom highlights), use of video technology particularly for parents of students who have severe disabilities, school websites are used to convey a broad range of school information and update parents on homework assignments, test schedules, resource links, and student learning plans may be accessed online, enabling goals and progress to be shared with parents.

A systematic review to assess the effectiveness of promoting the consumption of fruits and vegetables among primary schoolchildren showed that computer-based interventions were effective in increasing their intakes (Delgado-Noguera et al., 2011). However, the studies included were conducted in developed countries wherein most schools were noted to have computers. The study of Ahn and Kim (2007) examined the utilization status of the internet, health or nutrition websites, and need for developing nutrition websites and education programmes for Korean children. Results showed that topics on nutrition websites and education programmes should include assessment of obesity or diet, weight control, and special information (e.g. diet for growth). Consideration should also be given to the design and methods of nutrition websites and programmes to induce the interest and involvement of children. In addition, the use of online games was examined. An evaluation on the efficacy and acceptability of an online game called 'ETIOBE Mates' was carried out by Baños et al. in 2012. The study aimed to compare the children's nutritional knowledge using the online game vis-à-vis the traditional paper–pencil mode of information delivery. Results showed that both groups increased their scores on nutritional knowledge but the acquisition of knowledge was superior using the 'ETIOBE Mates'.

Parental involvement

In the Philippines, the teacher–child–parent (TCP) approach was developed by the Nutrition Center of the Philippines (NCP) and institutionalized by the Department of Education. In this approach, the teacher, schoolchild, and parents, through a well-designed guidebook, work on improving knowledge and practices on health and nutrition. Messages were conveyed between the school and the home by the child. It was chosen as one of the innovative components of Educational Technology for Basic Education of the Education for All Program of the Philippines for the decade 1991–2000 (Solon, 2006).

Presently, a number of opportunities are available to improve the communication between teachers and parents such as school-to-home communication books like the TCP, parent conferences (through parent-teacher association), and use of internet technology. In a study which examined the family-school linkage component of a school-based health education programme and its viability, acceptability, and effectiveness, interactive children's books were the mechanism by which students, parents, and teachers received consistent messages at home and school regarding nutrition information. Results showed that the interactive children's books were feasible to implement in the school context. Parents who received the books demonstrated increased knowledge of five servings of fruits and vegetables a day and children were eating additional servings of fruit and vegetables per day compared with children in the control group (Blom-Hoffman et al., 2008). In a more recent study, Baghurst and Eichmann (2014) examined the effectiveness of a child-only (i.e. control) versus a child-plus-parent (i.e. experimental) nutritional education programme in reducing risk factors associated with childhood obesity such as knowledge of nutrition, dietary behaviour, physical activity, behaviour, and sense of self-efficacy. Results showed parental education improved participant self-efficacy where a child's willingness to ask their primary caregivers to buy fruits and vegetables increased significantly.

School feeding programmes

The school feeding programme is another learning strategy with high potential of impact in making children become food and nutrition literate. Providing meals to schoolchildren have been shown to be a valuable opportunity for nutrition education. Bartrina and Perez-Rodrigo (2006) pointed out that school meals should make high-quality foods available and should be part of the educational process, providing a valuable opportunity to practise what children learn in the school, share tasting experiences with their peers and teachers while they learn from them, supported by policies that facilitate a positive school. Available data from school feeding programmes in eight Southeast Asian countries - Cambodia, Indonesia, the Lao PDR, Malaysia, Myanmar, Philippines, Thailand, and Vietnam, showed that school feeding provides social safety nets and promotes education and nutrition outcomes. The Ministry or Department of Education in each country commonly leads the programme. Moreover, geographic targeting is employed in selecting beneficiaries, that is, schools are chosen based on a set of criteria (WFP, 2007). The programme design of school feeding differs across countries in terms of scope and modality; food selection, preparation, and distribution; community involvement; complementary activities; institutional arrangements; and policy or legal frameworks. Food and nutrition education is included as one of the complementary activities wherein teachers discuss simple nutrition lessons about proper hand washing and nutrients in foods. Given the limited integration, school feeding activities can be incorporated in a broader school nutrition programme that includes food and nutrition education; school learning gardens; and local food production and purchase.

In South Korea, free school meals have been implemented since 1953 (Woo, 2015). In addition to ensuring that schoolchildren have nutritious meals while in school, nutrition education materials were developed with the aim of improving the health of students, promoting traditional Korean diet, and extending opportunities for a healthier dietary life. Nutrition education is done through club activities and experiential learning activities such as school gardens, traditional outdoor food storage, and kimchi making. Likewise, Benn and Carlsson (2014) evaluated the effects of free school meals on pupils' learning and on the learning environment in schools. Free lunch was provided to children for 20 weeks. Results showed that the pupils developed knowledge and skills related to novel foods and dishes, and that school meals can contribute to pupils' learning, whether this learning is planned or not.

Challenges

This section summarizes the limitations of integrating food and nutrition education in the school curriculum and other strategies paralleled with the findings. Most countries have a primary school curriculum that outlines the subjects and topics per grade level to be taught to schoolchildren. However, schools have limited capacity to assess the knowledge and skills needed by the schoolchildren to become food- and nutrition-literate. While the curriculum cannot be changed by individual schools, the teachers can be innovative and creative in their teaching strategies. To help the teachers, lesson plans for different subjects and various grade levels have been developed in the Philippines, Cambodia, and the Lao PDR which can be used by teachers as reference.

Teachers need to be trained on the various topics on food, nutrition, and health. They cannot teach the topic when they themselves are not knowledgeable of what nutrition and health are. In addition, they need to be able to assess the nutrition education needs of their students so that they can decide the depth and breadth of the topic on food, nutrition, and health they are going to teach.

The process of integrating nutrition in the curriculum requires the approval of the education department. It is a tedious process that requires the involvement of other sectors such as health and agriculture. Experts are necessary to provide technical assistance in countries who have limited capacity on this activity. Materials for both the schoolchildren (i.e. posters, workbooks) and teachers (e.g. lesson plans, teaching materials), are necessary to be developed.

There are several operational challenges in the school feeding programmes such that the nutrition education component is often overlooked or neglected. In addition, limited planning, monitoring, and evaluation of meals: for example, how much it contributes to meeting the nutritional requirements of the schoolchildren and observance of food safety practices. There are many schools that do not have school kitchens or canteen, toilets, and washing facilities. There is also no paid staff that prepares the food regularly. Schools may rely on teachers, mothers, or volunteers to prepare and cook school meals. They are not trained and supported to prepare nutritious school meals. Children are assigned into groups and are tasked to collect the food for their class from the improvised school kitchens, distribute the food to classmates, and eat on their own with minimal or no supervision from teachers or no nutrition education inputs. Funding that either comes from the government and/or non-governmental organizations (NGOs) is limited, resulting in irregular availability of meals.

Recognizing that not all schools have equal opportunities and resources (manpower, materials, money/funds) for the use of new technologies, the traditional 'chalk and talk', books, film showing, and television/radio programmes are expected to be continually used as learning strategies for children. The advantages include access to free electronic books and lesson plans, readily available and searchable information especially in schools where there is no library or with a small collection of books, and opportunities for sharing of materials and interactions among teachers and schoolchildren. However, several concerns to its full utilization and sustainability have been identified such as absence of electricity especially in geographically isolated and distant areas, high cost of computers, lack of internet access, or if with internet access, high cost of internet connection fees.

The use of the digital communication, that is, Seesaw, Facebook, and Remind, was studied by Bosch et al. (2017) in early elementary and middle school classrooms. The study question focussed on the extent by which each digital tool facilitated parent-teacher communication, quality information sharing, and active parent engagement. Moreover, each tool was found to have distinguishing attributes and limitations for some sorts of communication and interactions. For instance, parents whose first language is not English appreciated Facebook and Remind because of the automatic translation, and parents responded the most to posts with personal information such as pictures, awards, or student work.

The schoolchild's learning environment includes the school, home, and community. However, there are very few activities which ties or links these three avenues of learning or encourages the participation of parents and community. In Cambodia, using the school garden as a learning venue, schoolchildren are taught how to produce food, and volunteer families are organized to take care of the school gardens during the school vacation. The school committee composed of the principal or school head and community leaders also provides support to ensure the continuity of the school gardens. A day of celebration of the food harvested is done with the parents and community. In the Philippines, the Department of Education and Nutrition Center of the Philippines, implemented the teacher-child-parent approach wherein teacher, children, and parents through a well-designed guidebook work together towards attaining better knowledge and practices on health and nutrition. In the past, the workbooks were bought by the Department of Education. To date, the question remains on how children can take ideas and information home when workbooks are scarce or no longer available. Lastly, an enabling environment supportive of school food nutrition and education should be put in place. There are examples such as policies or laws in the Philippines' Republic Act 11037 (Republic of the Philippines, 2018) which provides for the implementation of a national feeding programme for undernourished children and the Lao PDR's National School Lunch Policy (WFP, 2019).

References

Ahn, Y. and Kim, K.-W. (2007) 'Study on utilization status of internet and needs assessment for developing nutrition education programs among elementary school children', *Nutrition Research and Practice*, 1(4), 341–348.

ASEAN/UNICEF/WHO (2016) 'Regional report on nutrition security in ASEAN', Vol 2. Bangkok, UNICEF, accessible from www.asean.org/wp-content/uploads/2016/03/Regional-Report-on-Nutrition-Security-in-ASEAN-Volume-2.pdf.

Baghurst, T. and Eichmann, K. (2014) 'Effectiveness of a child-only and a child-plus-parent nutritional education program', *International Journal of Child Adolescent Health*, 7(3), 229–237.

Baños, R.M., Cebolla, A., Oliver, E., Alcañiz, M. and Botella, C. (2012) 'Efficacy and acceptability of an Internet platform to improve the learning of nutritional knowledge in children: The ETIOBE mates', *Health Education*, 2–15, doi:10.1093/her/cys044.

Bartrina, J.A. and Carmen Perez-Rodrigo, C. (2006) 'Resources for a healthy diet: School meals', *British Journal of Nutrition*, 96(Suppl. 1), S78–S81, doi:10.1079/BJN20061705.

Benn, J. and Carlsson, M. (2014) 'Learning through school meals?' *Appetite*, 78, 23–31, doi:10.1016/j.appet.2014.03.008.

Blom-Hoffman, J., Wilcox, K. R., Dunn, L., Leff, S. S., and Power, T. J. (2008) 'Family involvement in school-based health promotion: Bringing nutrition information home', *School psychology review*, 37(4), 567–577.

Bosch, N., Bosch, S., Cline, K., Hochhalter, S., Rieland, A., Takekawa, E. and Walther, T. (2017) 'The effects of parent-teacher communication using digital tools in early elementary and middle school classrooms', retrieved from Sophia, the St. Catherine University repository website: https://sophia.stkate.edu/maed/23.

Center for Disease Control and Prevention (CDC) (1996) 'Guidelines for school health programs to promote lifelong healthy eating', *MMWR*, 45, 1–33, accessible from www.cdc.gov/mmwr/preview/mmwrhtml/00042446.htm.

Davis, J.N., Spaniol, M.R. and Somerset, S. (2015) 'Sustenance and sustainability: Maximizing the impact of school gardens on health outcomes', *Public Health Nutrition*: 18(13), 2358–2367, doi:10.1017/S1368980015000221.

Delgado-Noguera, M., Tort, S., Martínez-Zapata, M.J. and Bonfill, X. (2011) 'Primary school interventions to promote fruit and vegetable consumption: A systematic review and meta-analysis', *Preventive Medicine*, 53(1–2), 3–9, doi:10.1016/j.ypmed.2011.04.016.

Dudley, D.A., Cotton, W.G. and Peralta, L.R. (2015) 'Teaching approaches and strategies that promote healthy eating in primary school children: A systematic review and meta-analysis', *International Journal of Behavioral Nutrition and Physical Activity*, 12(28), 1–26, accessible from https://ijbnpa.biomedcentral.com/articles/10.1186/s12966-015-0182-8.

FAO (2005) 'Nutrition Education in Primary Schools: Vol. 1: The Reader', Rome, Italy.

FAO (2019) 'Nutrition guidelines and standards for school meals: A report from 33 low and middle-income countries', Rome, 106 pp.

FAO and United Arab Emirates University (2019) 'Stepping up school-based food and nutrition education: Exploring challenges, finding solutions and building partnerships', Rome, 128 pp, accessible from www.fao.org/3/CA3063EN/CA3063EN.pdf.

FAO, IFAD, UNICEF, WFP and WHO (2017) 'The State of Food Security and Nutrition in the World 2017. Building resilience for peace and food security', Rome, FAO.

FAO-RAP (2016) 'FAO-RAP Documentation Report', Regional training of trainers on integrating nutrition in primary education curriculum, 30 Aug–2 Sept 2016, Royal Princess Hotel, Bangkok, Thailand. Accessible from www.fao.org/fileadmin/templates/rap/files/meetings/2016/160830_Final_report.pdf.

Graham-Clay, S. (2005) 'Communicating with parents: Strategies for teachers', *School Community Journal*, 15(1), 117–129, accessible from https://files.eric.ed.gov/fulltext/EJ794819.pdf.

International Food Policy Research Institute (IFPRI) (2016) 'Global Nutrition Report 2016: From Promise to Impact: Ending Malnutrition by 2030', Washington, DC, accessible from https://globalnutritionreport.org/reports/2016-global-nutrition-report/.

Inocian, R.B. and Nuneza, L.M. (2015) 'The "Gulayan sa paaralan" (School vegetable garden) in response to sustainable development', *European Scientific Journal*, 11(8), ISSN 1857-7881.

McAleese, J.D. and Rankin, L.L. (2007) 'Garden-based nutrition education affects fruit and vegetable consumption in sixth-grade adolescents', *Journal of the American Dietetic Association* 107(4), 662–665.

McNulty, J. (2013) 'Challenges and issues in nutrition education', Rome: Nutrition education and consumer awareness group, Food and Agriculture Organization of the United Nations, accessible from www.fao.org/ag/humannutrition/nutritioneducation/en/.

Morgan, P., Warren, J., Lubans, D., Saunders, K., Quick, G. and Collins, C. (2010) 'The impact of nutrition education with and without a school garden on knowledge, vegetable intake and preferences and quality of school life among primary-school students', *Public Health Nutrition*, 13(11), 1931–1940, doi:10.1017/S1368980010000959.

Pérez-Rodrigo, C. and Aranceta, J. (2001) 'School-based nutrition education: Lessons learned and new perspectives', *Public Health Nutrition*, 4(1a), 131–139, doi:10.1079/PHN2000108.

Perez-Rodrigo, C. and Aranceta, J. (2003) 'Nutrition education in schools: Experiences and challenges', *European Journal of Clinical Nutrition*, 57, Suppl 1, S82–S85.

Republic of the Philippines (2018) 'Republic Act 11037' - An act institutionalizing a national feeding program for undernourished children in public day care, kindergarten and elementary schools to combat hunger and undernutrition among Filipino children and appropriating funds therefor.

SEAMEO RECFON (2018) 'Flagship Programme: NTGS Programme', *SEAMEO Education Agenda Magazine*, (6), 43–44, ISSN 1905–4289, accessible from www.seameo-recfon.org/en/news/item/263-seameo-recfon-flagship-program-on-seamag-nutrition-goes-to-school.

SEAMEO INNOTECH (2016) 'School health care and nutrition in primary schools in Southeast Asia: Policies, programs and good practices', Quezon City, Philippines, accessible from www.seameo-innotech.org/wp-content/uploads/2016/10/SHN-Report-2015.pdf.

Solon, F.S. (2006) 'Good governance for nutrition in the Philippines: Elements, experiences, and lessons learned', *Food and Nutrition Bulletin*, 27(4), 343–352, The United Nations University.

UNESCO (2015) 'Education for all 2000–2015: Achievements and challenges', accessible from https://unesdoc.unesco.org/ark:/48223/pf0000232205.

WFP (2007) 'Guidelines for targeting of food for education programmes'.

WFP (2019) 'Lao people's democratic republic annual country report 2018, Country strategic plan 2017–2021, ACR reading guidance', accessible from https://docs.wfp.org/api/documents/WFP-0000104271/download/.

Williams, D.R. and Dixon, P.S. (2013) 'Impact of garden-based learning on academic outcomes in schools: Synthesis of research between 1990 and 2010', *Review of Educational Research*, 83(2), 211–235, doi:10.3102/0034654313475824.

Woo, T. (2015) 'The school meal system and school-based nutrition education in Korea', *Journal of Nutritional Science and Vitaminology (Tokyo)*, 61(Suppl), S23–S24, doi:10.3177/jnsv.61.S23.

4
LINKING SCHOOL GARDENS, SCHOOL FEEDING, AND NUTRITION EDUCATION IN THE PHILIPPINES

Emilita Monville-Oro, Imelda Angeles-Agdeppa, Irish P. Baguilat, Julian Gonsalves, and Mario V. Capanzana

Introduction

School gardening in the Philippines was institutionalized as a programme in 1974 by the Department of Education (DepEd), formerly known as Department of Education Culture and Sports (DepEd, 2017). Today, the school gardening programme is known as *Gulayan sa Paaralan* (Vegetable Gardens in School) and is being implemented to support the school feeding programme (SFP) and agriculture curriculum. An initial assessment done by the International Institute of Rural Reconstruction (IIRR) in 2011 in Cavite province showed that in practice there is very little focus on the link between garden and the SFPs (IIRR, 2011). It is only in recent years that the connection between these two has been made, mostly through various DepEd memoranda. The revival of gardening through the *Gulayan sa Paaralan* programme in 2007 was a response to the growing incidence of hunger and malnutrition and food price hikes in the country. The programme aimed to increase the awareness of the general public especially students, parents, and teachers on the health, nutrition, and economic contributions of gardens (DepEd, 2007).

In 2014, through DepEd Memorandum Order No. 5, s. 2014, the department revitalized the *Gulayan sa Paaralan* as part of the National Greening Program. The National Greening Program within DepEd integrates school gardening with waste management and tree growing and caring. These school-based gardens were intended to ensure food security and help meet the nutritional needs of schoolchildren; strengthen schoolchildren's appreciation and skills in agriculture and the environment; upgrade parents' knowledge in nutrition and agriculture; and improve family livelihood prospects through enhanced knowledge and skills in food production (DepEd, 2014). The programme provided garden tools, certified vegetable seeds, and trainings on food production. In support of this programme, in 2011 former Senator Edgardo Angara launched the nationwide *Oh My Gulay!* (Oh, my vegetable) campaign, with national agencies and the private sector sponsoring school vegetable gardens in public elementary schools. The campaign focussed on encouraging Filipinos to consume vegetables that are packed with vitamins and minerals needed by school-age children. Involvement of children in planting, growing, and harvesting vegetables in school and home gardens are crucial in achieving the increased consumption of vitamin- and mineral-rich crops (Philippine Senate, 2011).

The SFP, on the other hand, an intervention within the Department of Education, was enacted into law in 2018. DepEd implements the SFPs to address under-nutrition and short-term hunger among learners to improve school attendance and to reduce dropouts in schools (DepEd, 2016). The SFPs may be school-initiated or sponsored by individuals, non-governmental organizations (NGOs), and private companies. DepEd's SFP implementation guidelines resulted from the roundtable discussion conducted in July 2012 with government and NGOs.

SFP, complemented by deworming and micronutrient supplementation, has been proven to increase school attendance, cognition, and educational achievement (Bundy et al., 2009). In their analysis of SFPs, Bundy and colleagues found that in many parts of the world, SFPs have been used with the belief that education and learning capacity depend on good nutrition. SFPs also serve as platforms for other human development outcomes (reducing hunger and aiding in the development of children, improvement of nutritional status, and promotion of good health, see chapter 2). Furthermore, SFPs reduce gender and social inequalities by encouraging families to send their children to school (Bundy et al., 2009).

For DepEd, SFPs are considered a sound investment for education and human development. SFPs are also one of the thrusts of public-private partnerships as many private companies see SFPs as effective in providing interventions to schoolchildren in need. In other countries, health and nutrition programmes are lodged under the Department of Health. In the Philippines, there is a health unit under the Department of Education and it is their responsibility to look at the health and nutrition of all school-aged children enrolled in public elementary schools. This is done through the School Health and Nutrition Programmes, which have three components: nutrition support to learners, healthy school environments, and medical/dental health management.

School gardening and school feeding guidelines present each other as complementary programmes. However, these two programmes have been implemented independently of each other to date in the Philippines. Documentation of challenges have identified a wide range of contributing factors including availability of resources, knowledge and skill gaps, unsustainable gardening approaches, and weak monitoring and evaluation of support programmes.

Responding to these challenges, IIRR, Food and Nutrition Research Institute of the Department of Science and Technology (FNRI-DOST), and DepEd implemented a 2-phase action research project. In 2012 to 2015, the integrated school nutrition model was developed and adapted in a single province. In 2016 to 2018, the model was improved and implemented at the sub-national level. Initial outcomes led to its adoption at the national level.

Action research methodology

The integrated school nutrition model that links three related programmes was developed capitalizing on the potential of schools as platforms to address food and nutrition challenges. As part of the model: (i) school gardens were enhanced with agroecological technologies such as bio-intensive gardening (BIG) to improve garden productivity and sustainability; (ii) supplementary feeding with iron-fortified rice and indigenous vegetables from school gardens was provided to identified malnourished (wasted and severely wasted) students. Recipes with indigenous vegetables were also developed and used; and (iii) nutrition education methodologies for children and caregivers were tested and adapted (IIRR, FNRI-DOST, and DepEd, 2018). The model was initially developed through an action research project (Phase 1) implemented in 2012 to 2015 in a single province with the support of the International Development Research Centre (IDRC).

The model builds on existing nutrition interventions of DepEd, such as the school-based supplementary feeding programme (SBFP) and *Gulayan sa Paaralan*. The model emphasizes sustainability and synergy of programmes. Nutrition education was also initially identified as a missing link. The study has revealed the effectiveness of the integrated model in improving the nutritional status of children; improving the knowledge, attitude, and practice of both children and parents; and sustaining the implementation of bio-intensive nutrition gardens and crop museums that aim to retrieve and conserve crop cultivars while improving year-round availability of a diverse range of climate resilient, locally adapted, and nutritionally important vegetables.

Phase 2 was a 28-month action research project, conducted in 2016–2018, that aimed to institutionalize and scale up the integrated school nutrition model to improve nutritional awareness and status of school-age children in the Philippines. The model was improved with emphasis on ways to strengthen all three components. It also tested a scaling up approach. The scaling up relied largely on a critical mass of schools also known as *lighthouse schools* (Figure 4.1) to demonstrate the model on a wider scale whilst also generating data and training of other schools (chapter 10). The research was undertaken in Region IVA of the Philippines with there are 19 school divisions and 2691 elementary schools, with 80,222 children enrolled in the school year 2016–2017. Lighthouse schools are action research sites, expected to influence the rest of the elementary schools in the region that has a total population of around 1,760,000 schoolchildren.

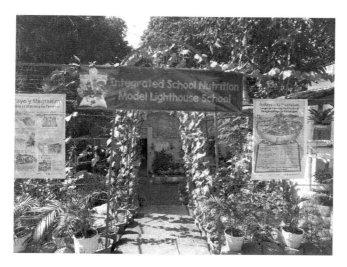

FIGURE 4.1 An example of a lighthouse school.
Source: IIRR.

Three sentinel research schools in Cavite Province were selected through purposive sampling from the wider pool of lighthouse schools. It is within the sentinel research schools that fine-tuning of the model and rigorous data collection were done. Both qualitative and quantitative data were collected in the 3 sentinel schools and 55 lighthouse schools. Survey forms and questionnaires were developed and distributed to teachers at the start and end of the project to support data collection. All schools were required to undertake nutritional assessments of Kinder to Grade 6 children during the first 3 weeks of classes (June). All children enrolled in the schools were weighed and their height measured to determine their nutritional status. This data was used to verify and validate whether they still need to receive the supplementary feeding for the current year. Normally, the basis of DepEd in computing the fund allocation for supplementary feeding per school is the data on weights of children taken before school ends in March. Hence, there is a need for them to update their data during school entry to identify the true feeding beneficiaries. For the study, FNRI-DOST verified the nutritional assessments in three sentinel schools and three lighthouse schools from July to August 2016. Weight was measured using a calibrated digital double window weighing scale (SECA) recorded to the nearest 0.1 kg. Students wore light clothing, their footwear removed, and pockets emptied. Height was measured using a stadiometer (SECA) recorded to the nearest 0.1 cm.

All lighthouse schools went through a series of capacity building programmes, such as training, exchange visits, study programmes, and field-based coaching. Different types of information, education, and communication materials were developed and were given to schoolteachers. Planting materials of indigenous vegetables were produced and distributed as part of the starter kit for school gardens.

The integrated school nutrition model

Bio-intensive Gardening (BIG), characterized as a low-external input approach, was implemented to strengthen school gardens. Supplementary feeding included use of iron-fortified rice (100 g of cooked rice provides 1–2 mg iron) and chemical-free indigenous vegetables from the school gardens. To improve the consumption and acceptance of indigenous vegetables, standardized recipes of indigenous vegetables were developed and used in the feeding programme. Nutrition education was delivered via different modalities to children and caregivers to foster healthy eating habits of children both at school and at home. Different methods to link the various nutrition-related programmes were implemented, resulting in improved nutritional status of children as well as improved knowledge, attitude, and practice of both children and their parents (Figure 4.2).

BIG approach

The BIG approach (Figure 4.3) was adapted to address sustainability challenges faced by schools, nutrition needs, and climate-related challenges. The different practices were translated into school gardening standards to serve as an implementation guide. BIG, a climate- and nutrition-smart garden, is an agroecological approach to gardening that makes the best use of available natural resources and does not rely on external chemical inputs (IIRR, 2017). Deep-dug and raised beds are presented as climate-smart garden beds due to their ability to respond to prolonged drought and anticipated prolonged rainy days. In these types of beds, water is stored for longer periods of time and water drains better during heavy rains. The presence of

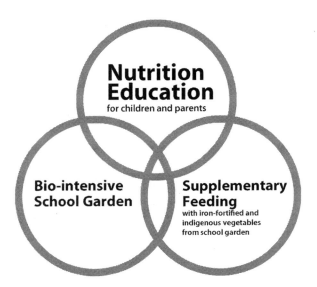

FIGURE 4.2 Integrated school nutrition model.
Source: IIRR, FNRI-DOST and DepEd, 2018.

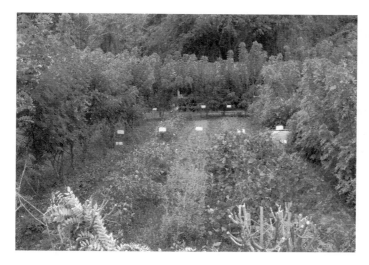

FIGURE 4.3 An example of a bio-intensive garden.
Source: IIRR.

fertilizer trees planted around the garden allows schools to have continuous access to organic material that is crucial in maintaining overall soil health whilst protecting gardens from adverse effects of strong winds brought by typhoons.

With the planting of trees, microclimates are manipulated (i.e. low soil and air temperatures) creating garden ecosystems that are more conducive to crop growth, even with rising temperatures. Cooler garden environments also present a more favourable space to work in for schoolchildren, teachers, and parents. Elaborated through the BIG approach is the role of continuous application of organic matter complemented by soil and water conservation practices such as regular use of green manure, mulching and cover cropping in enriching biological life and in reducing soil temperature. The green manuring practices reduce soil temperature while the deep placement of organic matter reduces its rapid decomposition. The organic matter helps store moisture for dry spells. IIRR also promotes drought tolerant crop varieties through BIG and has undertaken extensive searches for local drought-resistant indigenous materials for use in school gardens. In order to reduce risks of failure due to drought or rain, the BIG guidelines recommend that two thirds of the crops in the school garden should be indigenous.

With prolonged dry seasons being experienced, installation of rainwater harvesting was also encouraged. Intra-species diversity was also encouraged to allow selection of hardy varieties that adapt well within the local context. Liquid fertilizer's contribution to boosting hardiness of seedlings was also supported.

In Phase 1, the approach was translated into BIG standards for schools which outline practices and principles. In phase 2, the garden standard was enhanced by elaborating concepts of climate and nutrient smart gardens, nutrition-sensitive agriculture and its link to school feeding, and the value of school gardens as learning laboratories. A simple crop-planning tool that takes into consideration feeding centre requirements was developed and introduced to schools.

Supplementary feeding with iron-fortified rice and indigenous vegetables

For supplementary feeding, DepEd's implementation guideline was enhanced by integrating concepts and principles learned in Phase 1 of the programme. The promotion of iron-fortified rice and the 15 recipes with indigenous vegetables (Figure 4.4) were supplemented by development of iron-rich recipes for areas or cases where iron-fortified rice is not available (e.g. no delivery because of floods, typhoons, etc.).

Nutrition education for children and their parents

Nutrition education for children includes use of nutrition-sensitive lesson plans, use of the school garden as a learning laboratory, and use of the 'nutri school-home connection' approach where projects assigned to students require application at home. Nutrition education for the community or parents includes nutrition education sessions during parent-teacher association meetings, participatory activities such as cooking demonstrations or recipe development during the nutrition awareness month, and use of information, education, and communication materials (Figure 4.5). Different forms of information, education, and communication materials were developed to promote key nutrition and gardening messages. Teachers were provided with simplified reference materials

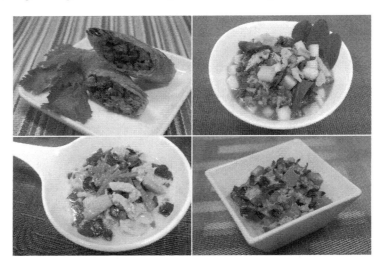

FIGURE 4.4 Photo of recipes with indigenous vegetables.
Source: FNRI-DOST.

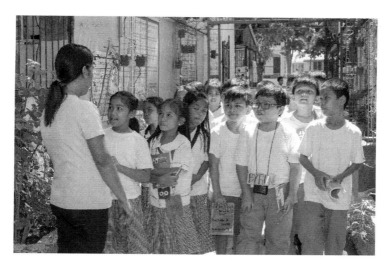

FIGURE 4.5 Photo of a nutrition education activity in a school.
Source: IIRR.

(nutrition modules) and teaching aids to help them better incorporate nutrition topics into their daily lesson plans and to facilitate short sessions with parents during their regular parent-teacher meetings.

Research results and outcomes

The following are the results as presented in the final research report from the project. The first part describes the different ways to enhance the link between the three components of school nutrition programme – school garden, school feeding, and nutrition education. The second part presents the results of interventions.

Mechanisms to enhance integration of components

School garden – school feeding link

The research identified the following conditions and mechanisms that contributed to improving the link between school gardens and school feeding:

- Familiarization of the feeding cycle menu by garden coordinators allowed them to plan accordingly
- Year-round garden diversity
- Incorporation of the recommended recipes with indigenous vegetables into the 20-day cycle menu of schools
- Effective coordination by the garden coordinator and the school feeding coordinator
- Sustained technical support from the division school health personnel

70   Emilita Monville-Oro et al.

Utilization of garden produce in the feeding programme was recorded in 56 schools. In the 21 lighthouse schools with complete data, 42% of the total garden produce was used in the feeding programme, 24% was distributed for free to parent volunteers, students, and teachers who helped out in garden activities, 17% was given to the school canteen, and 17% was sold.

In the three sentinel schools with intensive coaching and mentoring and detailed documentation, higher utilization of garden produce was observed as compared to the rest of the 55 lighthouse schools. School 1 (Julugan Elementary School) used at least 82% of the harvest in feeding programmes, with leafy vegetables (71%) contributing the most. School 2 (Sunny Brooke Elementary School) used 66% of the garden produce in the feeding programme, which are also mostly leafy vegetables (41%). School 3 (Tinabunan Elementary School) was able to use 54% in the feeding programme wherein 26% were leafy vegetables and 22% were fruit-bearing vegetables.

When schools grow vegetables in their gardens and when menus feature diverse vegetables, schools can reduce the cost of feeding. Savings accumulate over a typical feeding cycle. Tables 4.1 and 4.2 show the savings that were generated by schools with the use of garden produce within 120 days (Php 56.92/USD 1.14) and 200 days (PhP 126.48/ USD 2.53) respectively.

TABLE 4.1 Savings on expenses in a 120-day feeding cycle in sentinel schools

School	Total no. of beneficiaries	Total cost (PhP) (no. of beneficiaries × 16.00 × 120 days)	Peso value of garden produce used to SBFP (PhP)	Savings per student in 120 feeding days (PhP)
JES	278	533,760.00	18,398.63	66.18
SBES	769	1,476,480.00	20,578.02	26.76
TES	131	251,520.00	10,194.88	77.82
Average	393			56.92

Source: IIRR, FNRI-DOST, and DepEd, 2018.

TABLE 4.2 Savings on expenses in a 200-day feeding cycle in sentinel schools

School	Total no. of beneficiaries	SBFP total food cost for 120-day feeding (PhP) (a × PhP16 × 200 days)	Peso value of garden produce used in SBFP (PhP)	Savings per student in 200-days feeding (PhP) (c/a)
JES	278	889,600.00	35,127.63	126.36
SBES	769	2,460,800.00	36,389.64	47.32
TES	131	419,200.00	26,953.57	205.75
Average	393			126.48

Source: IIRR, FNRI-DOST, and DepEd, 2018.

TABLE 4.3 Total number of children that can benefit from the garden produce shared to SBFP in the three sentinel schools

School	Total vegetables needed in recipe per child in 120-day feeding (kg)	Total Garden Produce within 120-day feeding period (kg)	Total garden produce used in SBFP recipe (kg)	Percentage of garden produce used in SBFP (c/b)	Estimated number of beneficiaries (c/a)
JES	7.72	388.47	294.18	75.7	38
SBES	8.94	580.59	349.25	60.1	39
TES	8.82	412.69	168.87	40.9	19
Average	8.50		270.76	58.8	32

Source: IIRR, FNRI-DOST, and DepEd, 2018.

Table 4.3 shows the number of children that can benefit from a 200-square meter garden. On average, 32 students are estimated to be served with a vegetable meal in 120 days considering that about 270 kilograms of various vegetables are produced in the school garden.

On the use of iron-fortified rice, consultation meetings with retailers and at least 10 school administrators revealed that scaling up of iron-fortified rice within the school setting requires strong partnership (and engagement) with local businesses and local government units. Each school has their own supplier; thus, iron-fortified rice should be made available to these suppliers via local rice distributors. Rice varieties that are acceptable among children in terms of aroma and texture must also be considered to avoid plate waste among school feeding beneficiaries (as observed in schools).

School garden – education link

Use of gardens for school learning is strengthened if the following conditions are met:

- Gardens are functional all year round. Year-round availability of vegetables in the garden can be achieved with cultivation of diverse crops combining both annuals and perennials and drought and pest/disease tolerant crops.
- There is availability of information, education, and communication materials about BIG practices and indigenous vegetables within the garden.
- Garden visits as a class activity or methodology are incorporated into the lesson plans of teachers.
- There is continuous monitoring and technical support from school administrators and division level supervisors.

Fifty-two schools were able to utilize school gardens in other learning areas aside from agriculture. In the 36 schools with complete data, the garden was mostly used in the following areas – Science (Grades 4–6), EsP – *Edukasyon sa Pagpapakatao* or

Values Education (Grades 1–6), Mathematics (Grades 1–6), and Meeting time 2 (Kindergarten) where children are gathered by the teacher as a whole group. Few schools reported to have used the garden in Social Science, English, Filipino, Mother Tongue (language used within the locality), and other minor subjects. On a wider scale, institutionalization and sustainability can be achieved if use of the school garden is incorporated in the DepEd curriculum guide.

Nutrition education – school feeding link

Feeding centres can be used as venue to conduct creative nutrition education activities. Food served can be a medium to discuss food value and functions, which reinforces the actual feeding that happens. The following are the facilitating factors identified:

- Inclusion of nutrition education in the SBFP guidelines
- Provision of nutrition education modules to grade level coordinators and SBFP coordinators
- Capacity building of SBFP coordinators
- Availability of ready-to-use materials such as flash cards, posters, and flipcharts
- Inclusion of nutrition sessions during parent-teacher meetings and conferences
- Technical assistance and follow up

Of the 58 lighthouse schools, 44 were able to continuously deliver nutrition education during feeding activities via lectures, teacher demonstrations, games, audio-visual presentations, cooking demonstrations, nutrition quiz, peer teaching, puzzles, cooking festivals, and garden tours. Different nutrition education modalities improved the knowledge of children and parents, which resulted in no plate waste among schoolchildren, thereby increasing vegetable consumption. The nutrition education activities have also built a sense of cooperation among parents to help in the feeding activities and in maintaining the vegetable gardens as observed in schools.

Outcomes

Improvement in soil quality in school gardens

BIG techniques help regenerate the soil and replenish its capacity to grow healthy crops. Two years after the introduction of BIG, soils were tested in the three sentinel research schools. Two types of soil samples were collected and analyzed: (1) soil collected from sites without intervention; and (2) soil collected from sites where BIG practices were used. Table 4.4 provides evidence of the improvement in soil fertility status (availability of essential soil nutrients) in soils. The implications of these changes are important. For example, a decrease in soil pH from 7.6 to 7.2 can be expected to result in improved availability of most essential elements (N, P, K, Ca, and Mg) needed for growing vegetables. However, especially significant were the high amounts of nitrogen, phosphorus, and organic matter in gardens that

TABLE 4.4 Results of soil analysis in the three sentinel schools

	Non-bio-intensive garden area			Bio-intensive garden area		
	JES	TES	SBES	JES	TES	SBES
Soil pH	7.6	7.6	7.8	7.2	7.2	7.5
Nitrogen (N)	Low	Low	Low	High	High	High
Phosphorus (P)	Medium	Medium	Low	High	High	High
Potassium (K)	Sufficient	Sufficient	Sufficient	Sufficient	Sufficient	Sufficient
Organic matter (OM), %	1.56	1.37	0.92	2.23	5.68	1.46
Calcium (Ca) cmo$_{lc}$/kg soil	21.19	15.75	17.25	15.41	16.31	18.02
Magnesium (Mg) cmo$_{lc}$/kg soil	15.41	4.5	5.17	5.62	6.14	2.2

Source: IIRR, FNRI-DOST, and DepEd, 2018.

employed BIG practices. The use of climate- and nutrient-smart practices, that is, application of organic matter and fertilization (compost and liquid fertilizer), cover cropping, crop rotation, green manuring, mulching, and crop diversification, has contributed to overall improvement of soil nutritional status and health.

Diversification of school gardens and conservation of indigenous vegetables

Garden diversity was identified as one of the factors that influenced garden functionality and sustainability. Continuous and intensive promotion of indigenous vegetables and substantial distribution efforts contributed to achieving garden diversity. Different types of vegetables such as leafy, fruit-bearing, legumes, root crops, fruit trees, and herbs were grown in schools. After the intervention, an average of 26 crops was recorded in the 58 schools. Crop diversification led to availability of different types of vegetables with varied nutrients and provided teachers the flexibility in the choice of ingredients. A small number of schools reported having difficulty achieving crop diversity (10%) all year round due to seed saving and seedling propagation challenges. One of the mechanisms introduced and being practiced in the model is the yearly seed exchange among schools within a district or province to address such challenges.

Improvement in the nutrition status of undernourished children

DepEd's regular feeding programme runs for 120 days from July to December of every school year. A 20-day menu was developed combining recipes developed by the project and *Moringa*-based recipes from DepEd. Iron-fortified rice was used in the three sentinel schools and was procured directly from Nutridense, a private company that partnered with FNRI-DOST to produce and distribute iron-fortified rice. The following are the results of the 120-day feeding and the additional 80-day feeding as presented in the final research report:

Benefits gained from the 120 feeding days:

- There was a significant increase in the mean weight (p-value=0.000) and height (p-value=0.000) of children both male and females.
- The increment in the mean height of the male students aged 5 to 10-year olds (y.o.) from baseline to midline (after 5 months with only 60 feeding days) was 1.99 cm while for females 2.05 cm. These increments are lower than the normal increase of 2.21 cm for males and 2.48 cm for females of the same age group. However, the increment from midline to endpoint (after another 3 months with 60 feeding days) was 1.51 cm (males) and 1.70 cm (females), which are higher compared to the normal increase of 1.32 cm and 1.51 cm, respectively. The same result was observed in the female students aged 10.1 to 19 years, the increment (1.83) was higher compared to the normal increase of 1.46 cm. However, the increment in the mean height of the male students from midline to end point is similar (1.68 cm) compared to the normal increase of 1.69 cm.
- There was a significant decrease in the proportion of undernourished students aged 5.1–10 and 10.1–19 y.o. from baseline (100%) to end point (65%).

Improved use of gardens for learning and sharing nutrition and environment information

Gardens have the potential to serve as focal points for learning and education in relation to science, environment, health, nutrition, and food education. The integration of garden visits into different learning or subject areas, especially in *Edukasyong Pantahanan at Pangkabuhayan* (EPP) or Home Economics and Livelihood and Science for demonstration (50%), was taken on for the reason that gardens are functional year-round (33%) and because school heads had encouraged the use of gardens as venues for learning (7%) (Table 4.5).

Table 4.6 shows the different learning areas where garden visitation was integrated in the 36 lighthouse schools with complete records for school year 2016-2017. EPP (100%), Science (100%) and *Edukasyon sa Pagpapakatao* or Values education (94%) are the regular subjects that use gardens as demonstration and learning venues. This additional role of gardens is considered a significant finding.

TABLE 4.5 Garden use as platform for learning and sharing nutrition and environment information in 58 lighthouse schools

	No. of schools	% N = 58
Schools using garden as learning laboratory	52	89.66
Schools NOT using garden as learning laboratory	6	10.34
TOTAL	**58**	**100.00**

Source: IIRR, FNRI-DOST, and DepEd, 2018.

TABLE 4.6 Integration of garden visitation in different learning areas of 36 lighthouse schools for SY 2016–2017

Learning area	Grade level	Schools with garden visits integrated	
		No. of schools	%
Edukasyon	4 – 6	31	100.00
Science	3 – 6	31	100.00
EsP or Values Education	1 – 6	29	93.55
Mathematics	1 – 6	12	38.71
Meeting time 2	Kinder	12	38.71
Araling Panlipunan or Social Studies/HEKASI/ Agham/MAPEH/English/Filipino/Mother Tongue or Local Language/Work period 2	1 – 6	Less than 8	< 25.81

Source: IIRR, FNRI-DOST, and DepEd, 2018.

TABLE 4.7 Use of gardens as learning venues in different learning areas of the sentinel schools for school year 2016–2017 and 2017–2018

School 1	School 2	School 3
• *Edukasyong Pantahanan at Pangkabuhayan* (EPP) or Home Economics and Livelihood • Science • Filipino • Music, Arts, Physical Education and Health (MAPEH) • *Araling Panlipunan* (Social Studies) • English • Mother Tongue Base (Local Language) • Mathematics • *Edukasyon Sa Pagpapakatao* (Values Education)	• EPP or Home Economics and Livelihood • Science • Filipino • MAPEH • *Araling Panlipunan* (Social Studies) • English • Mother Tongue Base (Local Language)	• EPP or Home Economics and Livelihood • Science • Filipino • MAPEH

Source: IIRR, FNRI-DOST, and DepEd, 2018.

Table 4.7 shows data on the integration of garden visitation into different learning areas in three sentinel schools for school years 2016–2017 and 2017–2018. The garden is used for learning and sharing consistently in EPP, Science, and Filipino subjects across Grades 1–6.

Conclusion

Schools are effective platforms to generate multiple nutrition and environmental outcomes from a mix of nutrition-sensitive agriculture and nutrition-specific interventions. School gardens can be enhanced and sustained using low-external input agricultural approaches. Bio-intensive school gardens can contribute to diversifying nutrient sources provided that the feeding programme relies on recipes featuring indigenous vegetables. School-based supplementary feeding for 120-days using vegetable produce from school gardens and iron-fortified rice effectively improved nutritional status of feeding programme beneficiaries. Utilization of garden produce in the feeding programme can also help lower the cost of foods to be served while supporting nutrition and environmental education. Integrating agriculture and nutrition programmes at the local level requires policy support, multi-level capacity building, coordination among programme focal persons, development of technical guides, and a wide range of information, education, and communication materials and monitoring.

Acknowledgements

The action research project was made possible through the funding support from the International Development and Research Centre. The scaling up of the integrated school nutrition model was achieved through the collaborative efforts of school administrators and teachers from the Department of Education Region IVA and Department of Education – Support Services and research staff of IIRR and FNRI-DOST.

References

Bundy, D., Burbano, C., Grosh, M., Jelli, A., Jukes, M. and Drake, L. (2009) 'Rethinking school feeding: Social safety nets, child development, and the education sector', Washington, DC, World Bank.

Department of Education (2007) 'DepEd Memorandum No. 293, s. 2007, *Gulayan sa Paaralan*'.

Department of Education (2014) 'DepEd Memorandum No. 5, s. 2014, – Implementing Guidelines on the Integration of *Gulayan sa Paaralan*, Solid Waste Management, and Tree Planting under the National Greening Program'.

Department of Education (2016) 'DepEd Memorandum No. 51, s. 2016, "Implementation of School-based Feeding Program for School Year 2016–2917"'.

Department of Education (2017) 'School Health and Nutrition Programs', Power Point Presentation.

IIRR, FNRI-DOST and DepEd (2018) 'Improving food and nutrition security in the Philippines through school interventions: School nutrition brief', accessible from https://schoolnutritionphils.files.wordpress.com/2018/10/school-nutrition-brief-final_soft-copy.pdf.

IDRC (2018) 'Final technical report: Improving food and nutrition security through school interventions', accessible from https://idl-bnc-idrc.dspacedirect.org/bitstream/handle/10625/57234/57288.pdf.

IIRR (2011) 'Sustainable agriculture technical vocational education expansion to schools and communities project report', International Institute of Rural Reconstruction.

IIRR (2017) 'Bio-intensive Gardens (BIG): A climate and nutrition-smart agriculture approach', International Institute of Rural Reconstruction, accessible from https://schoolnutritionphils.files.wordpress.com/2017/04/big-primer.pdf.

Philippine Senate (2011) 'Angara launches *Oh my gulay*! To fight 'hidden hunger'', Press Release, February 11, 2011, accessible from www.senate.gov.ph/press_release/2011/0211_angara1.asp.

5
SCHOOL GARDENS IN NEPAL
Design, piloting, and scaling

Dhruba Raj Bhattarai and Pepijn Schreinemachers

Introduction

The nutritional status of the Nepalese population, particularly in rural areas, remains poor. A nationwide survey showed that 36% of children under five years of age are stunted (i.e. have a low height for their age), 10% are wasted (i.e. have a low weight for their height) and 27% are underweight (Ministry of Health et al., 2016). The prevalence of anaemia among children is 35% while 41% of women age 15–49 are anaemic (ibid.). The government of Nepal has formulated various policies, plans and strategies to address the problem, including the National Nutrition Policy and Strategy (Government of Nepal, 2014) and the National School Health and Nutrition Strategy (Government of Nepal, 2006). Recognizing that malnutrition is a multidimensional issue that requires the involvement of various sectors including health, education, and agriculture in synergistic ways, the government of Nepal developed the Multisector Nutrition Plan (Government of Nepal, 2012).

School garden programmes fit well into this thinking because it is an intervention that involves education, health, and agriculture. In Nepal, the concept of school vegetable gardens has been implemented as a learning tool to generate knowledge, behaviour change and possibly increase the consumption of nutritious vegetables. The assumption is that an increase in the awareness and knowledge of healthy food such as vegetables, will incline children towards healthier eating habits. Furthermore, school gardens are also seen as a strategy to promote production and consumption of a diverse range of nutrient-dense vegetables in families and in communities. Along with good health practices, it can contribute to the improved nutritional status of schoolchildren and their families.

In the programme, nutritional education is considered as important as hands-on work in the school garden, though both are usually combined in the school garden activities. By engaging in school gardens, students learn about the variety of vegetables that can grow in their local environment. They can also learn the value of nutritious vegetables in their daily diet, the consequences of good and bad food habits on human health and the effect on the environment. A school vegetable garden is a 'living lab' that can provide a place for the children to connect with the natural world as a true source of food and nutrition. School gardening can also teach children about other important subjects that can be integrated: science, health, and social studies. Ultimately, school vegetable gardens can make learning more enjoyable for children and more effective by offering opportunities for creative and critical thinking.

The Nepal school garden programme started with the project *Vegetables Go to School* (VGtS), which was funded by the Swiss Agency for Development and Cooperation (SDC) through a grant to the World Vegetable Center. The intervention was jointly designed by the Nepal Agricultural Research Council (NARC), the Ministry of Education, and the Ministry of Health and Population with technical support of the World Vegetable Center. Strengthening the collaboration between three ministries with the aim of improving child nutrition was an important aspect of the project. The actual implementation was led by NARC in close collaboration with the Ministry of Education.

The project piloted school gardens at ten schools per year over a three-year period in two districts in the mid-hills of Nepal. The pilot was combined with a research component to generate high-quality evidence for the impact of school gardens on nutritional outcomes. Key government people were engaged to promote the concept of school gardens and to share the research results. The school garden activities were promoted through national television and other national media. The project interacted with national policy makers, which helped to move the pilot to a programme that can be scaled nationwide.

The objective of this chapter is to provide details of how the Nepal school garden programme was designed, piloted in two districts, and subsequently scaled at a national level. The chapter is organized based on three major themes.

School garden design

School selection

Nepal is a mountainous country with much variation in agroecological conditions. In mountainous areas, suitable land for setting up a school garden is often limited as the terrain can be steep and rocky. Water availability is generally a constrained because it is often not technically possible to drill to the groundwater level while rainwater storage requires costly infrastructure. Furthermore, there are seasonal weather constraints as the winter may be too cold to grow vegetables in the open field, especially at higher altitudes. Another constraint is the damage by domestic animals and especially wild animals such as deer and monkeys, which can be a problem if the school is near a forested area. Although it is possible to grow vegetables in small areas, in containers, or make vertical gardens, these methods can be more costly and are generally more challenging to maintain than a field-based garden. School gardens may therefore not be a suitable intervention for all schools. In our project we therefore selected schools based on a minimum available area of 300 m^2 for gardening and access to a source of water for irrigation. Another important consideration is the support and motivation of school principals and teachers, which is essential for successful implementation of the intervention.

School garden components

The intervention had three complementary components as described in the following. More details are provided in Bhattarai et al. (2016a) and (2016b).

First, a 23-week curriculum was designed which included the following topics: school garden establishment, garden design, soil testing, compost making, crop selection, nursery techniques, planting method, integrated nutrient management, integrated pest management, identification of natural enemies and pests of vegetables, seed saving, harvesting, vegetable cooking techniques, vegetable consumption, importance of vegetables in human nutrition, and personal hygiene for promoting vegetable intake among children of grades 6 and 7. The curriculum is publicly available (Bhattarai et al., 2016b).

Second, a school garden was established on the school grounds. The standard design had 10 raised planting beds of 3 m × 1.5 m with 1 m space in between (Figure 5.1). The space between the beds and fence was 1 m on three sides and 2 m in front where a water tank and compost pit were placed. Sufficient space between the planting beds is important to accommodate a group of children working in the garden. Some schools used bricks, wooden planks, or bamboo to create the raised beds and prevent the soil from washing off. Raised beds also provide better drainage and allow children to easier reach and observe the plants without stepping on them.

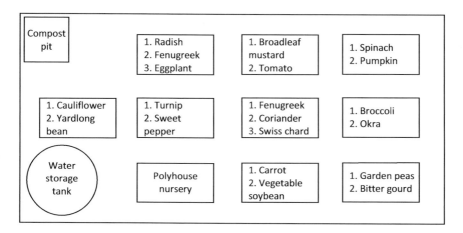

FIGURE 5.1 Example of the standard garden design with crop calendar.

The school gardens were fenced using steel wire or plants to protect the school garden from domestic animals (goats, cows, chickens) and wild animals (deer, monkeys). The land was well-levelled and proper drainage was installed to prevent water stagnating in the garden. The location of the garden was important as it should have direct sunlight and not be shaded. However, the planting of fruit trees like lemon, papaya and banana was encouraged as long as this did not shade the vegetable plots. A compost pit was created in a corner of the garden so that children would learn how to recycle green waste to create organic fertilizer. Low soil fertility was a serious constraint to garden production at most schools.

A standard cropping calendar was designed, separating between the winter and summer seasons. Each school was provided a small polyhouse nursery to raise seedlings, which helped to start vegetable production earlier in the year and increase the survival of young plants. Vegetables were selected by the project team based on local preferences, nutritional value and short growing periods so that they could be harvested more frequently. Table 5.1 shows the vegetables selected for the garden for each season. In addition, spice crops such as ginger, coriander, turmeric, chilies and garlic were planted around the garden. The project provided vegetable seed of good quality, along with the gardening tools and other basic equipment as required.

Teachers were instructed to inspect the garden regularly for insect pests and diseases and other agronomic problems. Teachers were told not to use pesticides in the school garden, but apply botanical pesticides such as extracted from neem leaves, garlic roots or chili pods. Proper crop rotations were an important part of the teaching curriculum: a legume crop would be followed by a leafy vegetable, followed by a fruit vegetable, and followed by a root vegetable.

TABLE 5.1 Standard cropping calendar used for the Nepal school gardens

Plot	Aug	Sep	Oct	Nov	Dec	Jan	Feb	Mar	Apr
1	–	Radish (*40 days*)		Fenugreek (local variety)		Brinjal (*Pusa Purple Long*)			
2	–	Broad Leaf Mustard *(Kumal Red)*				Tomato (*Sirjana*)			
3	–	Spinach (local variety)				Pumpkin/squash (local variety)			
4	–	Cauliflower (*Kumal Jyapu*)				Yard long bean (*Kumal Thane*)			
5	–	Turnip (*Kathmandu Red*)				Capsicum (*California Wonder*)			
6	–	Fenugreek (local variety)		Coriander (local variety)		Swiss chard (*Susag*)			
7	–	Broccoli (*Green Sprout*)				Okra (*Parbhani Kranti*)			
8	–	Carrot (*Nantes*)				Vegetable soybean (local variety)			
9	–	Garden Peas *(Arkle)*				Bitter gourd (*Green Karela*)			
10	Polyhouse nursery								

Third, community involvement and promotional activities were developed to strengthen the involvement of parents and emphasize the lessons learned. There was a contest for the best managed school garden. Schoolchildren established a small vegetable garden at their home and were given small packets of seed for this purpose. They were also stimulated to share the lessons learned with their family members. Teachers visited the children's homes to observe their home gardens. During the harvesting period parents and other community members were invited to the school and a harvesting event was organized. Harvested vegetables were distributed to the students for own consumption.

Training and follow-up

The project implementation started by first informing the local administrators of the Department of Education about the project and seeking their support. Subsequently, each selected school was visited to explain the project to the school principal and to identify a school garden focal teacher. The responsibility of this focal teacher was to implement garden activities as suggested by the project team, to provide security to the garden, allocate working time to different classes, support the data collection, organize promotional activities, facilitate parent visits and other related project activities. The visit was done jointly by a staff of the Department of Education and of the Nepal Agricultural Research Council (NARC). A memorandum of understanding was signed between the project and the schools.

A one-time training was provided for two teachers per school. It was important to train two persons to reduce the risk of staff turnovers, which are common in rural areas. The training was conducted in one location in the study area and lasted two days. The project team would visit each school after the training to assist with the setup of the school garden. A technical staff of NARC made regular follow-up visits to provide assistance.

Piloting

Pilots in Dolakha and Ramechhap districts

The above design was implemented in 10 schools per year for three subsequent years from 2014 to 2016. All schools were selected from Dolakha and Ramechhap Districts – two neighbouring districts in the mid-hills of Nepal. These districts were selected because they have high levels of malnutrition, yet are relatively easy to reach from Kathmandu, which facilitated the implementation of the project. The intervention targeted children 10–15 years old in grades 6 and 7 (Figures 5.2 and 5.3). The total budget per school was US$ 950, excluding the cost of teacher training and project management, which translates to about US$16 per child (Schreinemachers et al., 2017).

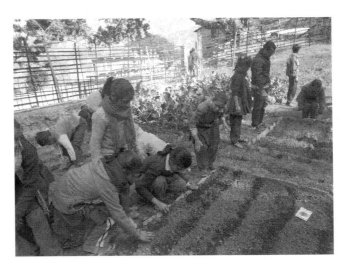

FIGURE 5.2 School gardening activities in Ramechhap district of Nepal.
Source: Bhattarai et al. (2016b).

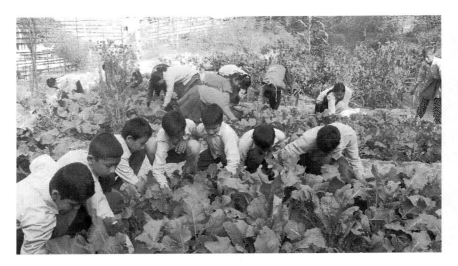

FIGURE 5.3 School gardening activities in Ramechhap district of Nepal.
Source: Bhattarai et al. (2016b).

The feedback from students and teachers was generally positive. Students engaged in hands-on gardening lessons, showed an increase in positive attitude towards content material and learning. Teachers believed that implementing these new learning styles were highly effective.

The project also generated quantitative data to test the hypothesis that school gardens linked to complementary teaching in gardening and nutrition and related promotional activities contributes to improvements in nutritional awareness, knowledge, perceptions, and eating behaviour of 10–15-year-old schoolchildren in Nepal. To do this, it used a cluster randomized controlled trial design (with schools as clusters). Data were collected at the start and at the end of the 2014 and 2015 school years from the project schools and a set of control schools. Further details are provided in Chapter 12 of this book, which compares the Nepal pilot to similar pilots conducted in Bhutan and Burkina Faso.

The study found a significant increase in children's awareness about fruit and vegetables, their knowledge about agriculture, nutrition, and WASH, and their stated preferences for eating fruit and vegetables. However, the study did not find a significant effect on vegetable consumption. Results are described in Chapter 8 of this book.

Pilot in Sindhupalchok district

The lack of impact of school gardens on children's vegetable consumption was confirmed by parallel studies for Bhutan and Burkina Faso. Two dominant explanations that emerged from discussions with stakeholders were that: (a) healthier food items such as fruit and vegetables were perhaps insufficiently available within children's households, which prevented them from eating these, even if they wanted to; and (b) children were perhaps unable to make food choices independently as their mothers and fathers largely decided what they ate and the food behaviour of parents was perhaps insufficiently affected by the intervention. An ongoing pilot project implemented in 15 treatment schools in Sindhupalchok District is currently testing these hypotheses using an experimental design in which the school gardens are linked to a complementary home garden programme aimed at promoting household-level vegetable production and consumption. Results are expected in 2020.

Challenges encountered

In the project districts public schools are located at great distances because of the hilly terrain. Moreover, many of the schools have very poor or no road and communication connectivity, which complicated the project implementation. Another challenge was that school teachers were generally familiar with developmental projects, but lacked understanding of the added research component and the need to generate evidence, which was tackled by familiarizing school staff with the research approach. Since school gardening is a new concept in Nepal, suitable land for gardening was not always readily available. In most cases some barren land was available, but it required extensive improvements such as levelling, fencing, removal of stones or construction materials, and soil fertility improvement. Limited availability of water for garden irrigation was an important constraint in some cases.

Lessons learnt

Based on the experience of the project team, the following key lessons were learned regarding the implementation of school gardens in Nepal:

- Focal teachers are key to the success of the project. In addition, to successfully implement schools garden, early discussions with school management committees and school teachers is essential to get buy-in and ownership.
- Only students of grades 6 and 7 were involved in the school garden activities, which created some envy among other students; sometimes these other students damaged the vegetables and garden structures. It would be more ideal to give all students at a school the opportunity to participate, if possible.
- The produce from the school garden was not nearly enough to make a significant contribution to the daily consumption needs of children. A much larger area would be required to produce more, but this is unrealistic. Therefore, the main purpose of the school garden is educational.
- A more integrated, holistic approach is required to complement the school garden programme and which aims to make changes to food production and food behaviour at the household and the community level.

Scaling up

The project was implemented through a close collaboration between the Nepal Agricultural Research Council (NARC), the Ministry of Education, and the Ministry of Health and Population. Representative of these departments participated in a two-week training-of-trainers workshop at World Vegetable Center headquarters in Taiwan in August 2013, which helped to strengthen the country team. The team members were continuously involved in project implementation which ensured strong collaboration.

The fact that government departments were leading the project in addition to the multi-sectoral nature of school gardens was conceptually appealing and fitted with the government's strategy to address malnutrition, ensured high visibility of the project, particularly within the Ministry of Agriculture and the Ministry of Education.

Project activities were promoted though national television and other media and a policy brief was published (Bhattarai et al., 2017). At the end of the project, in May 2017, a policy workshop was organized to share experiences and research results with stakeholders including senior officers of the involved government departments, members of parliament, and the national planning commission.

The Nepal project team was subsequently invited to contribute to the preparation of guidelines for the Green School Program which was released by the Ministry of Education, Science, and Technology in 2018. The results and documented materials of this project have also been used effectively by the Centre for Education and Human Resource Development under the Ministry of Education, Science and Technology for developing new reading materials and other activities of the Green School Program in Nepal which has recently been initiated.

Conclusion

The Nepal school garden programme aims to address malnutrition through an innovative multi-sectoral approach involving the ministries of agriculture, health, and education. As such it serves as a model intervention that uses a holistic approach to create nutritional outcomes through agriculture and education. Careful design and piloting of the intervention was conducted and this provided an important foundation to scale up the programme.

Acknowledgements

Funding for this research was provided by the Swiss Agency for Development and Cooperation (SDC) under grant number 81017189 and the Drivers of Food Choice (DFC) Competitive Grants Program, which is funded by the UK Government's Department for International Development (DFID) and the Bill & Melinda Gates Foundation, and managed by the University of South Carolina, Arnold School of Public Health, United States.

References

Bhattarai, D.R., Subedi, G.D., Acharya, T.P., Schreinemachers, P., Yang, R.-y., Luther, G., Dhungana, U., Poudyal, K.P. and Kashichwa, N.K. (2016a) 'Effect of school vegetable gardening on knowledge, preference and consumption of vegetables in Nepal', *International Journal of Horticulture* 5, 1–7.

Bhattarai, D.R., Subedi, G.D., Kashichwa, N.K., Dhungana, U., Yang, R.Y., Schreinemachers, P., Mecozzi, M., Luther, G., Luoh, J.W., Palaniswamy, U., Holmer, R., Cissé, G. and Drescher, A. (2017) 'Vegetables go to school NEPAL: School vegetable gardens: Linking nutrition, health and communities project documentation', World Vegetable Center, Shanhua, Taiwan.

Bhattarai, D.R., Subedi, G.D. and Schreinemachers, P. (2016b) 'School Vegetable Gardening: Concept, Curriculum & Action', Government of Nepal, Nepal Agricultural Research Council (NARC), Khumaltar, Lalitpur, Nepal.

Government of Nepal (2006) 'National school health and nutrition strategy, Nepal', Government of Nepal, Ministry of Health and Population, Kathmandu.

Government of Nepal (2012) 'Multisector Nutrition Plan for Accelerating the Reduction of Maternal and Child Under-nutrition in Nepal 2013–2017 (2023)', Government of Nepal, National Planning Commission, Kathmandu, Nepal.

Government of Nepal (2014) 'National Nutrition Policy and Strategy', Government of Nepal, Kathmandu, Nepal.

Ministry of Health, New ERA and ICF (2016) 'Nepal Demographic and Health Survey 2016', Ministry of Health, Kathmandu, Nepal.

Schreinemachers, P., Bhattarai, D.R., Subedi, G.D., Acharya, T.P., Chen, H.-p., Yang, R.-y., Kashichhawa, N.K., Dhungana, U., Luther, G.C. and Mecozzi, M. (2017) 'Impact of school gardens in Nepal: A cluster randomised controlled trial', *Journal of Development Effectiveness* 9, 329–343.

6

TREES NURTURE NUTRITION

An insight on how to integrate locally available food tree and crop species in school gardens

Stepha McMullin, Barbara Stadlmayr, Erick Ngethe, Brendah Wekesa, Ken Njogu, Agnes Gachuiri, Ben Mbaya, Agnes Katiwa, and Ramni Jamnadass

Introduction

Indigenous and underutilized fruit/food trees have an important role in providing vital minerals and micronutrients to growing children, as well as the wider community. The diversity of indigenous and underutilized fruit/food trees also means that they have an important role to play in addressing seasonality and hunger periods facing many rural communities by ensuring the availability of nutritious foods for a healthier diet year-round. This chapter will highlight the role of a diversity of indigenous and underutilized fruit/food trees, and their food composition and contribution to micronutrient and wider dietary needs. It will also highlight the 'portfolio approach' – for addressing seasonal food and nutrient-specific gaps in local diets. And an example of the inclusion of these portfolios in school gardens initiatives is presented to highlight the relevance of such a platform for anchoring learning, providing practical demonstration space and for wide community engagement for including a greater diversity of available food trees and crops in local food systems.

Food and agriculture systems for better nutrition and health

Malnutrition in all its forms, including under-nutrition, micronutrient deficiency and over-nutrition, affects one in three people worldwide, and is the major risk factor of non-communicable disease (Development Initiatives, 2018; Forouhi and Unwin, 2019). While the causes of malnutrition are complex, a common denominator of all types of malnutrition is often a nutritionally inappropriate diet, characterized by low diversity of nutritious foods, derived from food and agriculture systems that have been shaped for delivering sufficient calories rather than a broad range of nutrients over previous decades (Hawkes, 2007; Burchi et al., 2011; Global Panel on Agriculture and Food Systems for Nutrition, 2016; HLPE, 2017a). The associations between food, health, and environment, and their role in addressing chronic vitamin and mineral deficiencies, has been discussed for some time (Johns and Eyzaguirre, 2006; Burchi et al., 2011). The need for a profound change of the global food and agriculture system away from simply supplying food, towards providing healthy diets is increasingly recognized in recent global policy frameworks and commitments (FAO and WHO, 2014; United Nations, 2015; Global Panel on Agriculture and Food Systems for Nutrition, 2016). With the Sustainable Development Goals, specifically SDG 2 – Zero Hunger, the world has committed to ending all forms of malnutrition by 2030 by simultaneously ensuring sustainable food production and maintaining the genetic diversity of seeds, plants, and animal species. To achieve a better nourished world, actions throughout the entire food system, from production, to processing, transport, and consumption and across sectors including agriculture, health, social protection, and education are required (Ruel and Alderman, 2013; FAO and WHO, 2014; Development Initiatives, 2017). Nutrition-sensitive agriculture is one part of nutrition-sensitive programming that addresses the underlying causes of malnutrition, including poverty, food insecurity, health, water, and sanitation. It is a food-based approach, recognizing the importance of nutritionally rich foods and dietary diversity for overcoming malnutrition and micronutrient deficiencies (FAO, 2014). One example is agroforestry, the integration of a diversity of trees into landscapes for greater productivity and resilience and which plays an increasingly important role in diversifying agricultural production systems (Hillbrand et al., 2017). It has received global appreciation over the past decade for its potential impact on rural livelihoods, climate-smart agriculture, biodiversity conservation, and land restoration, as stated in the recent report of the State of the World's Biodiversity for Food and Agriculture (FAO, 2019).

The role of agroforestry for diversified production, diets and improved health

Tree-based agroforestry systems and forests provide a wide variety of foods and contribute substantially to food and nutrition security in multiple ways (Jamnadass et al., 2015; Bioversity International, 2017; HLPE, 2017b). Trees provide fruits, leafy vegetables, nuts, seeds, and oils into local farming systems (Stadlmayr et al., 2013; ICRAF, 2019). Tree foods can increase the nutritional quality of local diets, mostly due to their micronutrients (mineral and vitamins), but also macronutrients (protein, carbohydrates) and phytochemicals (e.g. antioxidants) (Stadlmayr et al., 2013). Trees also provide timber, fodder, fuel, and medicinals – for home use or income generation and can contribute to the resilience of resource-constrained households (Jamnadass et al., 2015). Additionally, they enhance productivity and ecological resilience by supporting ecosystem services such as watershed management, soil health, carbon sequestration, and biodiversity while restoring degraded landscapes (Jamnadass et al., 2015; Prabhu et al., 2015). Due to their high tolerance to drought, owing to the deep and extensive roots, trees are important also at times when other food sources are not available (Jamnadass et al., 2011). Tree foods thus have the potential to complement and diversify staple-based diets throughout the year, thereby improving diet quality and health.

Nutritional contributions of tree foods

In a World Agroforestry (ICRAF) recent research project 'Food Trees for diversified diets, improved nutrition, and better livelihoods for smallholders in East Africa',[1] 90 food tree and shrub species were identified across eight sites as important food sources from local food systems. Among the aim of the project was to target harvest and nutrient gaps through location specific food tree and crop portfolios (see section 3: How to fill harvest and nutrient 'gaps' through site-specific Food Tree and Crop species: An insight to the development of Food Tree and Crop Portfolios). To fill 'nutrient gaps' in a site, food tree and shrub species identified in local harvest calendars were mapped with food composition data from scientific articles and food composition databases. Food composition data play a key role in linking agriculture to nutrition. Knowing what people eat and which nutrients the consumed foods contain is key for assessing and improving diet quality and health, and it is equally important for agriculture, including domestication and breeding programmes, to select not only high-yielding but highly-nutritious species (Welch and Graham, 1999; Toledo and Burlingame, 2006; Burlingame et al., 2009).

Table 6.1 provides an overview of selected food tree and shrub species and their nutrient composition. The nutrients iron, folate, vitamin A, and vitamin C were selected because of their public health concerns (iron, folate, vitamin A), their supportive functions (vitamin C supports the uptake of non-haem iron from plant foods) and their natural high quantity in tree foods. Extended nutrient profiles, including data for macronutrients, vitamins, and minerals, are available at ICRAF's priority food tree and crop food composition database (ICRAF, 2019; Stadlmayr et al., 2019).

As shown in Table 6.1, trees and shrubs provide a variety of nutritious foods, which can be categorized in different food groups even by individual species, as they provide different edible parts. *Anacardium occidentale* and *Vitellaria paradoxa,* for example, are sources of nuts and fruits, and *Vigna unguiculata* is a supplier of green leafy vegetables and pulses.

While fruits and vegetables are characterized by their high micronutrient density by low energy content, pulses and nuts are known as sources of protein, energy, and minerals. Vitamin C is the main nutritive component in most fruit species, as shown in Table 6.1. The component is a good antioxidant protecting the body from radicals and it improves the absorption of non-haem iron in plant foods such as green leafy vegetables or nuts (Latham, 1997; FAO and WHO,

TABLE 6.1 Nutrient composition of selected tree and shrub foods (expressed per 100 g edible portion (EP) of fresh weight)

Food name in English	Scientific name	Water (g)	Iron (mg)	Vitamin A RE* (mcg)	Folate (mcg)	Vit C (mg)
Fruits						
Baobab, pulp, raw	Adansonia digitata	11.0	5.0	0	50	273
Cashew apple, raw	Anacardium occidentale	86.5	0.8	13	n.a	123
Azanza, pulp, raw	Azanza garckeana	47.2	4.4	n.a	n.a	n.a
Desert date, raw	Balanites aegyptiaca	70.4	1.6	n.a	18	51
Bird cherry, raw	Berchemia discolor	78.8	2.2	n.a	n.a	50
Papaya, pulp, raw	Carica papaya	89.8	0.7	161	25	58
Orange, pulp, raw	Citrus sinensis	86.8	0.1	22	30	53
Mango, pulp raw	Mangifera indica	82.7	0.7	227	25	36
Marula, pulp and skin, raw	Sclerocarya birrea	86.1	3.4	n.a	n.a	168
Sorindeia, raw	Sorindeia madagascariensis	80.5	1.9	n.a	n.a	107
Shea, fruit pulp, raw	Vitellaria paradoxa	73.3	1.9	n.a	n.a	1-196
Green leafy vegetables						
Spiderwisp, leaves, boiled	Cleome gynandra	85.7	7.3	794	76	37
Cassava, leaves, boiled	Manihot esculenta	71.7	4.4	542	62	16
Moringa, leaves, boiled	Moringa oleifera	75.7	3.8	2080	26	44
Spinach, boiled	Spinacia oleracea	90.5	2.5	775	93	15
Cowpea, leaves, boiled	Vigna unguiculata	85.9	4.0	283	68	24
Pulses						
Hyacinth bean, mature, whole, boiled	Lablab purpureus	78.6	1.4	<1	3	0
Mung bean, mature, whole, boiled	Vigna radiata	78.7	1.0	3	80	<1
Cowpea, mature, whole, boiled	Vigna unguiculata	79.7	1.1	1	80	<1
Nuts						
Cashew nut, raw	Anacardium occidentale	5.3	6.4	<1	46	<1
Macadamia, nut, raw	Macadamia integrifolia	1.4	3.7	0	11	1.2
Shea nut seed kernel, raw	Vitellaria paradoxa	6.3	3.4	0	n.a	n.a

*Vitamin A-RE expressed in retinol equivalent: retinol + 1/6 beta-carotene + 1/12 alpha-carotene + 1/12 beta-cryptoxanthin).

2004). Tree and shrub leaves, like those of *Cleome gynandra*, *Manihot esculenta*, or *Vigna unguiculate*, are not only sources of iron (required for growth, cognitive development and as an oxygen carrier) but also of folate (required for growth and foetal development) and vitamin A (indispensable for the visual circle and functioning of cells) – all key micronutrients often lacking in staple-based diets (Latham, 1997; FAO and WHO, 2004).

Nutritional differences exist not only between food groups but between species and within species, at variety or cultivar level and for underutilized and wild foods (Charrondière et al., 2013). Factors impacting the nutrient content of foods are manifold and include climate (Fischer et al., 2019), geography and soil, maturity stage, the preparation and processing stage (raw, cooked, dried, boiled), post-harvest handling of foods (Greenfield and Southgate, 2003), methods used for analyzing (Greenfield and Southgate, 2003; FAO/INFOODS, 2013), and the expression of components and genetics (Toledo and Burlingame, 2006; Charrondière et al., 2013).

A focus in World Agroforestry's (ICRAF) programmes is the promotion and cultivation of indigenous and underutilized species.[2] These are foods with underexploited potential for food and nutrition security and have received little attention by researchers and private industry in the past (Hawtin, 2007; Armstead et al., 2009; FAO and Bioversity International, 2017; Dawson et al., 2018). Many of these species have the potential to provide needed micronutrients and are often also superior in minerals and vitamins compared to mainstream or exotic species. A good example is the comparison of the vitamin C values of the indigenous species *Adansonia digitata* (baobab fruit), *Sclerocarya birrea* (marula fruit), and *Sorindeia madagascariensis* to that of the exotic species *Citrus sinensis* (orange), which is regarded as a reference source high in vitamin C. With on average 273 mg, 160 mg, and 107 mg/100 g EP, respectively, the indigenous species contain up to 5 times higher vitamin C values than oranges (53 mg/100 g EP). This does not mean that oranges should not be consumed anymore but rather that the diversity of locally available foods, particularly indigenous and underutilized species, has great potential to contribute to nutrient adequacy, and that these species should be further invested in and researched and promoted as locally appropriate and sustainable solutions. Important for the promotion of these foods is the knowledge of their nutrient content, but unfortunately this information, particularly on vitamins, is often missing in the literature (Stadlmayr et al., 2013). As shown in Table 6.1, data on vitamin A and folate are missing for many, particularly indigenous species. Hence, it is important that analysis of high-quality food composition data, particularly for under-researched indigenous species are conducted, so that these species can better be promoted and integrated in domestication programmes and for dietary assessments to improve diet quality from local food systems. Without this information, it could mean that certain crops rich in micronutrients are overlooked in agriculture – nutrition development planning, projects and policies. The importance of underutilized and wild species is increasingly recognized in international frameworks and guidelines (FAO and WHO, 2014; FAO, 2019).

As is the promotion of underutilized species in crop diversification explicitly stated as a recommendation[3] in the Framework of Action, of the International Nutrition Conference (ICN2). Additionally, the incorporation of underutilized species into locally adapted food based dietary guidelines is recommended by the 'Voluntary Guidelines for Mainstreaming Biodiversity into Policies, Programs and National and Regional Plans of Action on Nutrition', endorsed by the Commission on Genetic Resources for Food and Agriculture (FAO, 2016).

How to fill harvest and nutrient 'gaps' through locally available species: an insight to the development of Food Tree and Crop Portfolios

Among the main reasons for food insecurity in rural areas is the lack of seasonal availability of foods, particularly for smallholders relying mostly on foods from own production (Ng'endo et al., 2016; McMullin et al., 2019a). To overcome seasonal hunger gaps and diversify predominant staple-based diets in rural areas, World Agroforestry has developed a methodology to identify location specific seasonal food calendars with food tree species available in local food systems (McMullin et al., 2019b). These 'Food Tree and Crop Portfolios', based on the original Fruit Tree Portfolio concept (Jamnadass et al., 2015; Kehlenbeck and McMullin, 2015; McMullin et al., 2019b) (Figure 6.1), have been developed with the intended use of selecting socio-ecologically suitable and nutritionally important food tree species and complementary vegetable, pulse and staple crops for

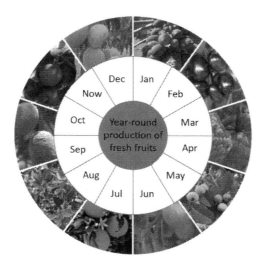

FIGURE 6.1 Based on the original methodology developed by World Agroforestry, a Fruit Tree Portfolio – providing for year-round harvest of at least one fruit rich in vitamins A or C, illustrated by a calendar wheel.

Source: World Agroforestry/Fruiting Africa Project.

production. These portfolios are combinations of indigenous/underutilized, and exotic species that can potentially provide year-round nutritious foods to address food harvest gaps and nutrient gaps in local diets (Dawson et al., 2018; McMullin et al., 2019b). Indigenous and underutilized food species are an important feature of the portfolios because they are more adapted to landscapes – to local soils and climatic stress (McKay et al., 2005) and their mainstreaming into wider use is relevant to ensure the total value of these foods are harnessed for meeting current and future dietary needs (Bioversity International, 2017).

The portfolio approach uses location-specific data on food tree and crop species phenology, months of household's food security, individual level food consumption data and nutrient composition data to target harvest and specific micronutrient gaps in local food systems.

The harvest months of prioritized food tree and crop species (Figure 6.2, part a) are mapped against periods of food insecurity (Figure 6.2, part b). In addition to filling harvest 'gaps', the portfolio addresses certain nutrient 'gaps' by matching the identified foods with nutrient content data (Figure 6.2, part c).

In Kenya, eight site-specific food tree and crop portfolios have been developed for different agroecological zones[4] (Figure 6.3). To adequately address food production and nutrient gaps, a greater diversity of foods could be cultivated on farms and in public spaces such as schools and religious grounds. However, for sustainable production, only the most ecologically suitable and preferred species should be recommended to farmers. An important component of the portfolio approach is that communities participated in the identification and prioritization of foods which can be used to meet food harvest and nutrient gaps in their local food systems. The discussion with community members around the local foods used and their seasonal availability filled information gaps on indigenous and underutilized food species. This was particularly important for tree foods, for which less is known and particularly the months of availability based on ecological suitability and tree phenology, as harvest times can show great inter-annual variability and large spatial differences (WMO, 2009).

The portfolio approach also makes use of several tools including the vegetationmap4africa (http://vegetationmap4africa.org/) to support food tree species selection. These maps are based on natural vegetation and potential distribution maps of useful tree species for many functional uses. Understanding the distribution of natural vegetation provides a good approximation of where wider planting of indigenous and underutilized tree species will contribute to ecosystem services, and food and nutrition security.

The recommended portfolios must also be made available to communities where they are promoted, this requires that farmers have access to quality planting material. Several entry points such as Agroforestry Innovation Hubs and schools (see section 4) are used to facilitate the distribution of quality planting material with training on agroforestry and tree management. *Seeds of Nutrition* packs are one example from the Food Tree Project of seed and seedling distribution. These packs are a selection of the portfolio seeds and seedlings distributed

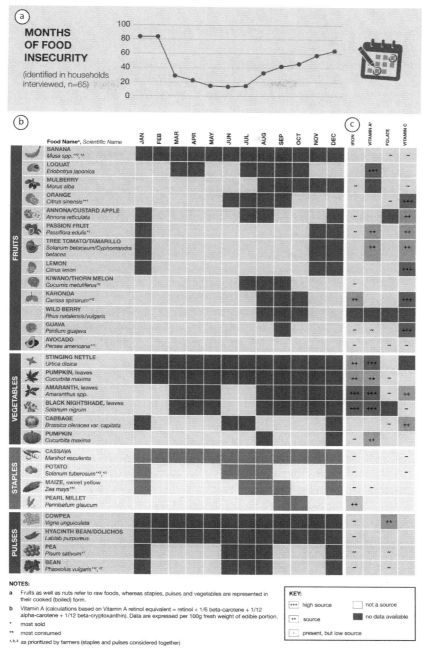

FIGURE 6.2 An example of a Food Tree and Crop Portfolio for Ngobit, Laikipia County, Kenya. This portfolio provides a recommendation for a diversity of socio-ecological suitable indigenous/underutilized and exotic food trees and crops (vegetables, pulses, and staples) that can be cultivated for addressing year-round food harvest and providing key micronutrients (iron, folate, vitamins A and C) in local diets.

Source: World Agroforestry/Food Trees Project.

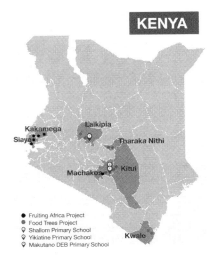

FIGURE 6.3 Project sites and counties where food tree and crop portfolios have been developed, and school garden locations used as demonstration sites in Kenya (Shalom Primary School, Ngobit, Laikipia County; Yikiatine Primary School and Makutano DEB Primary School, Machakos County. World Agroforestry/Food Trees Project.).

with accompanying agriculture-nutrition information. The portfolios not only support direct food production – consumption pathways, but also support diversified income generating pathways through engagement in nursery enterprises and the supply of tree seed and seedlings, and the potential to sell surplus produce. Increased income is important as the role of markets for meeting dietary needs should not be ignored, even in rural areas – as many households depend on a combination of own production and purchasing of foods, particularly foods that may not be seasonally available on-farm (Sibhatu and Qaim, 2017).

Training, education and practical 'hands-on' agricultural activities in school gardens as an important entry point for leveraging production diversity to consumption diversity

Diversity of agricultural production can be a relevant predictor of dietary diversity (and therefore diet quality) (Kumar et al., 2015). Nevertheless, increasing dietary diversity as a strategy for addressing micronutrient deficiencies requires the need for behaviour change and for outreach and education about how foods, and a diversity of foods meet multiple nutrient and dietary needs for optimum health. Integrating agriculture and nutrition messaging through training, education and practical 'hands-on' gardening activities in schools can deliver necessary outreach and learning on the cultivation and use of nutritious foods at the household level (FAO, 2010). Moreover, including school garden activities is going beyond just theoretical nutrition education. The social interaction of harvesting, sharing, preparing and eating, positively influences young people's food awareness and eating habits, with greater interest in eating fruits and vegetables shown by pupils who participated in school garden activities (Morris and Zidenberg-Cherr, 2002; Libman, 2007; McAleese and Rankin, 2007; Robinson-O'Brien et al., 2009). Socio-cultural practices and preferences and the desirability and convenience of certain foods (Hawkes et al., 2017) impact food choices (Oniang'o et al., 2003; Ruel et al., 2005; Keats and Wiggins, 2014; Keding et al., 2017). There has been a declining interest in 'traditional' foods associated with an intergenerational loss of knowledge about these foods and their importance in local diets (Turner and Turner, 2007; Reyes-García et al., 2013), and as a result, they are often stigmatized as being for those less well off, and for those 'left behind' in rural landscapes (Abukutsa, 2010). Through the promotion of healthy diet and eating practices and the social interaction during adolescence, there is the potential to mitigate nutritional deficits generated during the first decade of life, break intergenerational cycles of malnutrition, and limit the epidemic of obesity and non-communicable diseases in adulthood.

Planting seeds for nutrition: the application of the Food Tree and Crop Portfolios in school gardens – a case study from Machakos and Laikipia Counties, Kenya

To tackle the behavioural challenges associated with inadequate consumption of healthier foods and inadequate production and seasonal availability – in World Agroforestry's Food Trees Project, schools were selected as an essential entry point to reach target communities and harness the food and environmental benefits of integrating a diversity of food trees into landscapes, through the portfolio approach described previously.

Schools provide an excellent platform for influencing positive behaviour change and provide a ready framework for peer to peer learning amongst the pupils, parents and local communities (Box 6.1). This platform provides an opportunity to support integrated agriculture and nutrition training – through curriculum-based learning, transfer and exchange of technologies and information, reinforced by practical activities and interactive demonstration sites.

With partners, World Agroforestry implemented a school garden programme in several of its project sites in Kenya – two in Machakos county and one in Laikipia county (Figure 6.3). The programme was designed and implemented with multiple stakeholders including local government agencies – Ministries of Education, Agriculture, and Health, local school management, parent committees, the wider farming communities, and an international NGO – Feed the Children[5]– based in Kenya. The main purpose of the programme was to promote the cultivation of a greater diversity of ecologically suitable, nutrient-dense, and seasonally available foods, and, through targeted nutrition education and awareness campaigns, to promote the relevance of indigenous and underutilized foods for increased consumption to deliver healthier diets. This was achieved by

> **BOX 6.1: SCHOOLS OFFER A PLATFORM FOR PRACTICAL ACTION, A CASE STUDY FROM MACHAKOS COUNTY KENYA**
>
> **Kenyan students blaze a trail for 'planetary health' diet**
>
> Children have been working hard to grow nutritious food in their school garden, boosting community health. Fruit, vegetables, pulses, and nuts provide essential micronutrients for good health. But in East Africa, as in many other parts of the world, diets are dominated by starchy foods, with low consumption of nutrient-rich fruits and vegetables.
>
> In rural Machakos, about 100 km southeast of Nairobi, school student clubs have been focussed on establishing school gardens which provide a diversity of healthy foods. With the help of agroforestry researchers, a green-fingered teacher committee and a local NGO, the barren plot behind their school was carefully divided up to plant climate-adapted, nutritious fruits, vegetables, and pulses. The purpose is not only to educate youth on the important link between agriculture and healthy diets but also to link to surrounding farmers who visit the schools as demonstration sites to see how the approach has worked.
>
> Vitamin A and C-rich mango and potassium-rich indigenous chocolate berry and desert date trees grow alongside vegetables high in iron and vitamin A, like spinach and black nightshade.
>
> Including indigenous fruit trees like chocolate berry is important as these fruits are harvested several times a year and children enjoy the juicy 'chocolate' pulp. Once established these trees do not need much care, but one of the challenges is the initial seed germination, which can be difficult.
>
> The big idea is to show communities that normally suffer nutrient gaps in their diets how growing the right combination of food can provide year-round essential nutrition, as well as opportunities to generate income.
>
> Full story: https://news.trust.org/item/20190129123413-jgqh9

(i) strengthening the capacities of the target groups, mainly pupils and parents, on the production and utilization of indigenous and underutilized tree foods, and other foods available in the site-specific portfolios; (ii) reinforcing the organizational capacity of the programme's school management committees and the 4K club – *Kuungana, Kufanya, Kusaidia Kenya*, Swahili for 'Coming together, to Act, in order to Help Kenya' – members through agriculture and nutrition education training; and (iii) establishing school gardens based on the site-specific food tree and crop portfolios to act as demonstration and interactive learning spaces for the pupils, parents, and their wider communities (Figure 6.4).

To increase outreach at the community level, groups of lead farmers were selected based on interest and availability of space and water on their farms, to

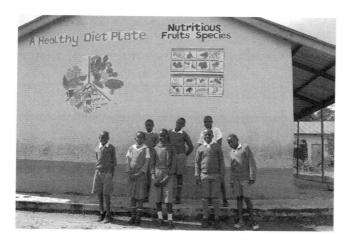

FIGURE 6.4 4K Club pupils standing in front of their 'Talking Wall' at school painted with the diversity of healthy foods they have sown in their communal garden.
Source: World Agroforestry/Alina Paul-Bossuet.

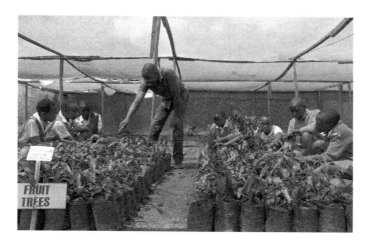

FIGURE 6.5 School children participating in a training module on tree planting and management.
Source: World Agroforestry/Alina Paul-Bossuet.

establish portfolios and use them as demonstration sites and to promote the programme to their community and encourage co-learning. Additionally, the established school demonstration gardens were used during community open days to provide training. Theoretical and practical training demonstrations on optimum agronomic practices and food and nutrition training were provided. The agronomic training module included topics such as tree and crop planting and management, soil fertility, pest and disease management, and water use (Figure 6.5).

The food and nutrition training module included topics such as food for nutrition and healthier diets, safe and nutrient-sensitive food preparation, and cooking demonstrations with nutritious recipes. Several customized training tools were developed by the programme partners for optimizing the delivery of information to the pupils and local communities (Figure 6.6).

BOX 6.2: ESTABLISHING LOCATION-SPECIFIC FOOD TREE AND CROP PORTFOLIOS IN SCHOOL GARDENS FOR TARGETING FOOD HARVEST AND NUTRIENT GAPS

How to develop a portfolio using location-specific data on food tree species phenology, months of household's food security, individual level food consumption, and tree food nutrient composition data to target harvest and specific micronutrient gaps in local food systems (McMullin et al., 2019b).

School garden establishment

Step 1. Site and school selection – Select school based on criteria such as availability of farming space, access to water resources, secured land and interest/motivation of school committee.

Step 2. School garden committee – Establish a school garden management committee which comprises of students, parents, teachers, school board of management members and local technical personnel from relevant ministries including agriculture, health, and education.

Step 3. Sensititization – Hold a sensitization meeting with school garden management committee and wider community stakeholders. During this meeting, the purpose of the school garden is explained, the requirements to establish and manage a school garden are detailed, and the expectations of stakeholders are discussed as well as the roles and responsibilities to ensure ownership and commitment to and sustainability of the garden project.

Step 4. Training – Undertake a comprehensive school health and nutrition training with all stakeholders (listed previously) to create awareness of these concpets and the purpose of the school garden and the location-specific portfolio.

Step 5. Land preparation – Prepare school garden by clearing the land, install required infrastructure including fencing, water support (water tank etc.), and prepare land for planting of food trees and complementary crops based on the location-speific portfolio and with advice and technical backstopping porvided by agricultural techncial staff.

Step 6. Planting – Procure quality planting material in prepartion for onset of the rains and plant seeds and seedlings, based on good agronomic practices such as hole depth, width and position for seedlings, and with adequate soil coverage, watering etc.

Step 7. Garden management – Monitor the porgress of the planted seed and seedlings, maintain adequate watering and weeding, and inspect the crops for any early signs of pest and disease.

Challenges for establishing location-specific portfolios in school gardens

- Access to quality inputs, seed and seedlings.
- Access to water for establishment of the garden and survival of the crops, partciuarly tree seedlings.
- Occurrence of pests and diseases, and subseqeunt management of these to esnure the health of crops and the garden.
- Appropriate technical know how for ensuring good agronomic practices for optimally establishing and managing the garden.

School gardens are established with educational goals to engage students and their families, school staff and the wider community to make the connection between growing a diversity of foods and healthy diets, develop life skills and increase environmental awareness. The success of school gardens is due to a good understanding of the purpose and multiple benefits of the garden and consistent engagement of the school and community in managing the garden.

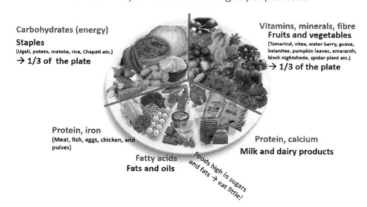

FIGURE 6.6 Customized food and nutrition education training tools developed by programme partners for use in schools and with communities.
Source: World Agroforestry/Fruiting Africa Project.[6]

With a combined population of over 1,000 pupils, the three project pilot schools have established school gardens. These are managed by pupils – specifically members of the schools' 4K clubs with support from the schools' management committees including parents. The school gardens not only provide a direct learning site for the pupils – but also facilitate wider community engagement and learning for greater adoption of the portfolios into farms. The school's gardens consist of site-specific portfolios which recommend ecologically suitable food trees, vegetables, pulses and staple crops including both indigenous/underutilized and exotic food tree species. Some of the indigenous and underutilized food tree species included in the portfolios; *Vitex payos* (chocolate berries), *Azanza garckeana* (azanza), *Balanites aegyptiaca* (desert dates), *Berchemia discolor* (bird cherry), *Vangueria madagascariensis* (common wild medlar), *Tamarindus indica* (tamarind), *Rhus natalensis* (wild berry), and *Euclea divinorum* (magic gwarra), to list a few. As mentioned in section 2 (The role of agroforestry for diversified production, diets and improved health), trees provide a variety of nutritious foods and particularly indigenous and underutilized fruits and vegetables are rich in vitamins and minerals and have a great potential to combat micronutrient deficiencies by diversifying staple based diets.

Conclusion

The development of food tree and crop portfolios using a diversity of locally adapted species, seasonal availability and their nutrient content information is an example of a sustainable food-based approach to address micronutrient deficiencies by promoting these nutritious foods in local diets and particularly the diets of children through school garden initiatives. Indigenous and underutilized tree foods and other crops have the potential to provide much needed micronutrients and are often also superior in minerals and vitamins compared to exotic species. The inclusion of site-specific portfolios in school programmes provides an excellent platform to engage pupils and their communities in interactive learning and practical demonstrations for positive behaviour change related to enhanced food production, and increased consumption of healthy foods. The social interaction of planting, harvesting, sharing, preparing, and eating can positively influence young people's food awareness and eating habits.

To date, sixteen portfolios have been established for site-specific locations in Kenya, Uganda, and Ethiopia. This approach can be further expanded geographically and scaled using school programmes for greater community outreach and long-term, intergenerational behaviour changes towards more sustainable food systems and healthier diets.

Notes

1 Food Tree Project in short, Project web page: www.worldagroforestry.org/project/food-trees-diversified-diets-improved-nutrition-and-better-livelihoods-smallholders-east, funded by EC/IFAD.
2 Indigenous, underutilized, orphan, or wild crops – many definitions exist for these crops (Hawtin, 2007; Armstead et al., 2009; FAO and International, 2017; Dawson

et al., 2018). What they have in common is that these are foods with underexploited potential for food and nutrition security, and they have received little attention from researchers and businesses. For this chapter, we use the terminology 'indigenous and underutilized species', referring to the adapted definition above, noting that we also include orphan and wild species.
3 Recommendation 10: Promote the diversification of crops including underutilized traditional crops, more production of fruits and vegetables, and appropriate production of animal-source products as needed, applying sustainable food production and natural resource management practices (FAO and WHO, 2018).
4 The original fruit tree portfolio concept was developed for three sites: Machakos, Kakamega, and Siaya counties, Kenya within the Fruiting Africa Project funded by EC/IFAD.
5 www.feedthechildren.org/our-work/around-the-world/kenya/.
6 Modified from www.kids-cooking-activities.com/healthy-portion-size.html.

References

Abukutsa, M.O.O. (2010) 'African indigenous vegetables in Kenya: Strategic repositioning in the horticultural sector', Jomo Kenyatta University of Agriculture and Technology, Nairobi.

Armstead, I., Huang, L., Ravagnani, A., Robson, P. and Ougham, H. (2009) 'Bioinformatics in the orphan crops', *Briefings in Bioinformatics*, vol 10, no 6, pp 645–653.

Bioversity International (2017) 'Food biodiversity for healthy, diverse diets', in 'Mainstreaming Agrobiodiversity in Sustainable Food Systems: Scientific Foundations for an Agrobiodiversity Index', Bioversity International, Rome, Italy, accesible from www.bioversityinternational.org/mainstreaming-agrobiodiversity/.

Burchi, F., Fanzo, J. and Frison, E. (2011) 'The role of food and nutrition system approaches in tackling hidden hunger', *International Journal of Environmental Research and Public Health*, vol 8, no 2, pp 358–373.

Burlingame, B., Charrondiere, R. and Mouille, B. (2009) 'Food composition is fundamental to the cross-cutting initiative on biodiversity for food and nutrition', *Journal of Food Composition and Analysis*, vol 22, no 5, pp 361–365.

Charrondière, U., Stadlmayr, B., Rittenschober, R., Mouille, B., Nilsson, E., Medhammer, E., Olango, T., Eisenwagen, E., Persijn, D., Ebanks, K., Nowak, V., Du, J. and Burlingame, B. (2013) 'FAO/INFOODS food composition database for biodiversity', *Food Chemistry*, vol 140, no 3, pp 408–412.

Dawson, I. K., McMullin, S., Kindt, R., Muchugi, A., Hendre, P., Lilleso, J-P.B. and Jamnadass, R. (2018) 'Delivering perennial new and orphan crops for resilient and nutritous farming systems', in T. S. Rosenstock and A.G.E. Nowak (eds), *The Climate-Smart Agriculture Papers*, Springer, Cham.

Development Initiatives (2017) 'Global Nutrition Report: Nourishing the SDGs', Development Initiatives, Bristol.

Development Initiatives (2018) 'Global Nutrition Report: Shining a light to spur action on nutrition', Development Initiatives, Bristol.

FAO (2010) 'Promoting lifelong healthy learning habits. A new deal for school gardens', accessible from www.fao.org/3/i1689e/i1689e00.pdf.

FAO (2014) 'ICN2 Second International Conference on Nutrition: Improving diets through nutrition-sensitive agriculture', www.fao.org/about/meetings/icn2/news-archive/news- detail/en/c/261494/, accessed January 2019.

FAO (2016) 'Voluntary guidelines for mainstreaming biodiversity into policies, programmes and national and regional plans of action on nutrition', FAO, Rome.

FAO (2019) 'The state of the world's biodiversity for food and agriculture', J. Bélanger and D. Pilling (eds), FAO Commission on Genetic Resources for Food and Agriculture Assessments, Rome.

FAO and Bioversity International (2017) 'Guidelines on assessing biodiverse foods in dietary intake surveys', FAO, Rome.

FAO and WHO (2004) ' Vitamins and mineral requirements in human nutrition: Report of a joint FAO/WHO expert consultation', 2nd edition, FAO, WHO, Geneva.

FAO and WHO (2014) 'Framework for action. Second International Conference on Nutrition (ICN2)', Conference Outcome Document, FAO, Rome.

FAO/INFOODS (2013) 'FAO/INFOODS e-Learning Course on Food Composition Data', FAO, Rome.

Fischer, S., Hilger, T., Piepho, H.P., Jordan, I. and Cadisch, G. (2019) 'Do we need more drought for better nutrition? The effect of precipitation on nutrient concentration in East African food crops', *Science of the Total Environment*, vol 658, pp 405–415.

Forouhi, N.G. and Unwin, N. (2019) 'Global diet and health: Old questions, fresh evidence, and new horizons', *The Lancet*. doi:10.1016/S0140-6736(19)30500-8.

Global Panel on Agriculture and Food Systems for Nutrition (2016) 'Food systems and diets: Facing the challenges of the 21st century', London.

Greenfield, H. and Southgate, D.A.T. (2003) 'Food composition data: Production, management and use', 2nd edn, FAO, Rome.

Hawkes, C. (2007) 'Promoting healthy diets and tackling obesity and diet-related chronic diseases: What are the agricultural policy levers?', *Food and Nutrition Bulletin*, vol 28, no 2, pp S312–S322.

Hawkes, C., Harris, J. and Gillespie, S. (2017) 'Changing diets: Urbanization and the nutrition transition', in 'Global Food Policy Report', International Food Policy Research Institute, Washington, DC.

Hawtin, G. (2007) 'Underutilized plant species research and development activities - review of issues and options, GFU/ICUC', International Plant Genetic Resources Institute, Rome.

Hillbrand, A. Borelli, S. Conigliaro, M. and Olivier, A. (2017) 'Agroforestry for landscape restoration. Exploring the potential of agroforestry to enhance the sustainability and resileince of degardded landscapes', Food and Agriculture Organization of the United Nations, Rome.

HLPE (2017a) 'Nutrition and food systems. A report by the High Level Panel of Experts on Food Security and Nutrition of the Committee on World Food Security', Rome.

HLPE (2017b) 'Sustainable forestry for food security and nutrition: A report by the High Level Panel of Experts on Food Security and Nutrition', FAO, Rome.

ICRAF (2019) 'ICRAF priority food tree and crop food composition database', ICRAF, Nairobi.

Jamnadass, R., McMullin, S., Iiyama, M. and Dawson, I., et al. (2015) 'Understanding the roles of forests and tree-based systems in food provision', in B. Vira, C. Wildburger, and S. Mansourian (eds), *Forests, Trees and Landscapes for Food Security and Nutrition*, A Global Assessment Report (p. 172), Vienna: IUFRO World Series, Volume 33.

Jamnadass, R.H., Dawson, I.K., Franzel, S., Leakey, R.R.B., Mithöfer, D., Akinnifesi, F.K. and Tchoundjeu, Z. (2011) 'Improving livelihoods and nutrition in sub-Saharan Africa through the promotion of indigenous and exotic fruit production in smallholders' agroforestry systems: A review', *International Forestry Review*, vol 13, no 3, pp 338–354.

Johns, T. and Eyzaguirre, P.B. (2006) 'Linking biodiversity, diet and health in policy and practice', *Proceedings of the Nutrition Society*, vol 65, no 02, pp 182–189.

Keats, S. and Wiggins, S. (2014) 'Future diets: Implications for agriculture and food prices', ODI, London.

Keding, G.B., Kehlenbeck, K., Kennedy, G. and McMullin, S. (2017) 'Fruit production and consumption: Practices, preferences and attitudes of women in rural western Kenya', *Food Security*, vol 9, no 3, pp 453–469.

Kehlenbeck, K. and McMullin, S. (2015) 'Fruit tree portfolios for improved diets and nutrition in Machakos County, Kenya', ICRAF, Nairobi.

Kumar, N., Harris, J. and Rawat, R. (2015) 'If they grow It, will they eat and grow? Evidence from Zambia on agricultural diversity and child undernutrition', *The Journal of Development Studies*, vol 51, no 8, pp 1060–1077.

Latham, M. (1997) 'Human nutrition in the developing world', FAO, Rome.

Libman, K. (2007) 'Growing youth growing food: How vegetable gardening influences young people's food consciousness and eating habits', *Applied Environmental Education & Communication*, vol 6, no 1, pp 87–95.

McAleese, J.D. and Rankin, L.L. (2007) 'Garden-based nutrition education affects fruit and vegetable consumption in sixth-grade adolescents', *Journal of the American Dietetic Association*, vol 107, no 4, pp 662–665.

McKay, J.K., Christian, C.E., Harrison, S. and Rice, K.J. (2005) 'How local is local?- A review of practical and conceptual issues in the genetics of restoration', *Restoration Ecology*, vol 13, no 3, pp 432–440.

McMullin, S., Stadlmayr, B., Roothaert, R. and Jamnadass, R. (2019a) 'Fresh fruit and vegetables: Contributions to food and nutrition security', in P. Ferranti, E.M. Berry and J.R. Anderson (eds), *Encyclopedia of Food Security and Sustainability*, Elsevier.

McMullin, S., Njogu., Wekesa, B., Gachuiri, A., Ngethe, E., Stadlmayr, B., Jamnadass, R., Kehlenbeck, K. (2019b) 'Developing fruit tree portfolios that link agriculture more effectively with nutrition and health: A new approach for providing year-round micronutrients to smallholder farmers' *Food Security: The Science, Sociology and Economics of Food Production and Access to Food* 10.1007/s12571-019-00970-7.

Morris, J.L. and Zidenberg-Cherr, S. (2002) 'Garden-enhanced nutrition curriculum improves fourth-grade school children's knowledge of nutrition and preferences for some vegetables', *Journal of the American Dietetic Association*, vol 102, no 1, pp 91–93.

Ng'endo, M., Bhagwat, S. and Keding, G.B. (2016) 'Influence of seasonal on-farm diversity on dietary diversity: A case study of smallholder farming households in Western Kenya', *Ecology of Food and Nutrition*, vol 55, no 5, pp 403–427.

Oniang'o, R.K., Mutuku, J.M. and Malaba, S.J. (2003) 'Contemporary African food habits and their nutritional and health implications', *Asia Pacific Journal of Clinical Nutrition*, vol 12, no 3, pp 331–336.

Prabhu, R., Barrios, E., Bayala, J., Diby, L., Donovan, J., Gyau, A., Graudal, L., Jamnadass, R., Kahia, J., Kehlenbeck, K., Kindt, R., Kouame, C., McMullin, S., van Noordwijk, M., Shepherd, K., Sinclair, F., Vaast, P., Vågen, T.G. and Xu, J. (2015) 'Agroforestry: Realizing the promise of an agroecological approach', Biodiversity and ecosystem services in agricultural production systems, Agroecology for food security and nutrition Proceedings of the FAO International Symposium, 18–19 September 2014, Rome, Italy.

Reyes-García, V., Guèze, M., Luz, A.C., Paneque-Gálvez, J., Macía, M.J., Orta-Martínze, M., Pino, J. and Rubio-Campillo, X. (2013) 'Evidence of traditional knowledge loss among a contemporary indigenous society', *Evolution and Human Behavior*, vol 34, no 4, pp 249–257.

Robinson-O'Brien, R., Story, M. and Heim, S. (2009) 'Impact of garden-based youth nutrition intervention programs: A review', *Journal of the American Dietetic Association*, vol 109, no 2, pp 273–280.

Ruel, M. Minot, N. and Smith, L. (2005) 'Patterns and determinants of fruit and vegetable consumption in sub-Saharan Africa: A multi-country comparison', Background paper – FAO/WHO Workshop on fruit and vegetables for health, Kobe, Japan, WHO, Geneva.

Ruel, M. T. and Alderman, H. (2013) 'Nutrition-sensitive interventions and programmes: How can they help to accelerate progress in improving maternal and child nutrition?', *The Lancet*, vol 382, no 9891, pp 536–551.

Sibhatu, K. T. and Qaim, M. (2017) 'Rural food security, subsistence agriculture, and seasonality', *PLoS One*, vol 12, no 10, pp e0186406.

Stadlmayr, B., Charrondière, U.R., Eisenwagen, S., Jamnadass, R. and Kehlenbeck, K. (2013) 'Nutrient composition of selected indigenous fruits from sub-Saharan Africa', *Journal of the Science of Food and Agriculture*, vol 93, no 11, pp 2627–2636.

Stadlmayr, B. McMullin, S. and Jamnadass, R. (2019) 'User Guide of ICRAF's priority food tree and crop food composition database', ICRAF, Nairobi.

Toledo, Á. and Burlingame, B. (2006) 'Biodiversity and nutrition: A common path toward global food security and sustainable development', *Journal of Food Composition and Analysis*, vol 19, no 6–7, pp 477–483.

Turner, N.J. and Turner, K.L. (2007) 'Traditional food systems, erosion and renewal in Northwestern North America', *Indian Journal of Traditional Knowledge (IJTK)*, vol 6, no 1, pp 57–68.

United Nations (2015) 'Transforming Our World: The 2030 Agenda for Global Action', United Nations, New York.

Welch, R.M. and Graham, R.D. (1999) 'A new paradigm for world agriculture: meeting human needs: Productive, sustainable, nutritious', *Field Crops Research*, vol 60, no 1–2, pp 1–10.

WMO (2009) 'Guidelines for plant phenological observations', O. Baddour and H. Kontongomde (eds), *World Climate Data and Monitoring Programme*, World Meteorological Organization (WMO), Geneva.

7
THE ROLE OF SCHOOL GARDENS AS CONSERVATION NETWORKS FOR TREE GENETIC RESOURCES

Francesca Grazioli, Muhabbat Turdieva, and Chris J. Kettle

Introduction

Trees play an important role in children's development and learning. We all remember climbing trees as children as well as the excitement that this brought and the trees' important role in our outside play. Trees are critical to human health and well-being in multiple ways, supporting biodiversity; providing important food and medicine; and helping to ensure climate amelioration, both locally and globally. Trees can be living climbing frames but also living laboratories for learning. It is estimated that we have about 3 trillion trees on the planet, which amounts to about 400 trees per person of the global population; this is about 50% of the trees present prior to human population expansion and industrialization (Crowther et al., 2015). Indeed, increasing human pressure on planetary ecosystems is leading to a massive depletion of forest cover and biodiversity as well as declining human health. Large-scale agriculture focussing on only a few crops is leading to environmental degradation and habitat fragmentation as the most significant driver of biodiversity loss (IPBES, 2019). This is having a devastating impact on global tree species, with 10,000 species[1] threatened with extinction. We currently have around 60,000 species of tree on our planet, but less than half of these have any documented conservation status[2] (see Botanic Gardens Conservation International).

School gardens or environs can play a key role in counterbalancing some of these challenges, acting as repositories for biological diversity. They provide a place where native tree species can be safeguarded and cultivated, and traditional knowledge about the different uses of trees can be shared (Cousins and Witkowski, 2015). For example, the recent Lancet report on food in the Anthropocene and the role of healthy diets from sustainable food systems shows that increasing our consumption of fruit and nuts (the majority of which are produced from trees) will be critical to ensuring more sustainable global diets for both humans and the planet (Willet et al., 2019). Trees planted and preserved in school gardens or environs can have additional functions, providing shade and improving local climate but also providing green spaces vital to mental well-being.

The aim of this chapter is to explore the potential of school gardens as a multidisciplinary tool used to address continued threats to tree biodiversity. We discuss how school gardens can increase students' familiarity with tree conservation issues, identification, and sustainable use when used in curricula. In addition to supporting and providing evidence of the benefits of the conservation and restoration of traditional and threatened tree species, school gardens can be a way to support the recommendations of international agencies, which are increasingly including the role of underutilized species in food policies to fight hunger and malnutrition, and in environmental policies to enhance biodiversity.

Linking appreciation of trees to better diets, livelihoods, and learning

Collecting fruit and nuts from edible trees is commonplace to some children, but in more urban environments, the planting of edible fruit or nut species is not common. Enhancing the planting of native fruit and nut trees within school gardens, as well as encouraging children to bring seeds and fruits of native trees to school as part of class activities, can raise awareness of their value. This also offers learning opportunities for botany, ecology, and biology. Children can discuss what might disperse the seeds in nature, germinate seeds at school, and record the seeds' growth and development.

School gardens that include indigenous fruit trees can be a source of extra income for schools as well as a place to conserve, register, and study genetic diversity. Linking indigenous vegetables and fruit to markets can be an incentive towards their inclusion in school gardens. A recent study shows a shift in production trends towards traditional products in Tanzania (70% increase) and Kenya between 2002 and 2006, once producers were linked to informal and formal markets (Ojiewo et al., 2013). Additionally, in the Chivi district of Zimbabwe, a participatory planting test was conducted on indigenous trees, such as *Afzelia quanzensis*, not only for timber but also for carving sculptures and utensils (Gerhardt and Nemarundwe, 2006). Depending on regrowth rate and the timing of trees, manual activities like these can be listed as one of the advantages of having indigenous trees besides for food or shade. Indigenous fruit trees are also considered providers of regular and low-risk returns (Schreckenberg et al., 2006), another reason to include them in school gardens.

Another example of regional tree domestication with an important socioeconomic role is the *marula* (*Sclerocarya birrea* subsp. *caffra*) in Southern Africa, which is used by local communities for many purposes: kernels are eaten or used to extract oil, fruits are eaten fresh or fermented for alcoholic beverages, leaves are to feed livestock, and so on (Shackleton, 2002). More specifically to school gardens, in the Ugandan Slow Food school garden in Kiboobi Village, Lwengo district, black jack (*Bidens pilosa*) is used to treat cuts and help stop blood flow, while stinging nettle (*Urtica massaica*) is used for urinary problems. Cultivation of local cultural trees increases the diversity and complexity of the territory (Lin et al., 2015), with multiple health benefits. In sub-Saharan Africa, growing domesticated and wild local fruit tree species is one smallholder strategy used to increase economic revenue and health and ecosystem services, as in the case of tree species such as guava (*Psidium guajava*), baobab (*Adansonia digitata*), and moringa (*Moringa oleifera*). By increasing the number of indigenous fruits and vegetables in school gardens that are made accessible to the community, students can reduce exploitation pressure on the natural habitat, helping to support in situ conservation of native trees. Researchers found that students exposed to school gardens can educate their parents and siblings about what they have learned, thereby influencing the eating habits of their whole household (Heim et al., 2009) and changing eating preconceptions, as in a case study in Kenya (Kehlenbeck et al., 2013) which showed that adults see fruits as food mainly for children and consume only those with a perceived higher energetic value, such as tamarind or baobab fruits.

BOX 7.1: MORINGA TREES TO IMPROVE DIETS AND ENVIRONMENTAL AWARENESS IN BRAZIL

Despite the country's rapid economic growth, people in Brazil continue to suffer from hunger and malnutrition, and rural areas are consistently worse off than urban areas. In 2010, field staff of Trees for the Future (TREES) noted that schoolchildren were eating their main meals at school because there was not enough food at home. Furthermore, local markets lacked the necessary options to provide children with a diverse diet. TREES identified moringa (*Moringa oleifera*) as a species with the potential to overcome some of these challenges and began integrating it into school curriculum and meals. Moringa is often referred to as the magical tree because of its rapid growth and resistance to drought and poor soils, and its nutritional leaves, rich in antioxidants, vitamin A, and vitamin C.

TREES introduced moringa trees into two schools in Marília, Brazil, through a three-step programme. First, teachers created a curriculum that included topics such as recycling, sustainability, and food security to help students understand their relationships with the environment, and help them develop 'an environmental conscience'. Second, students brought empty food packages to recycle into plant pots. TREES staff provided moringa seeds and supervised the students as they planted the seeds. The school designated a nursery area for the seedlings, which were pruned of leaves about once a month. As a third step, at the end of the school year, children took their moringa saplings home to plant in their home gardens and thereby also

(*Continued*)

leave the nursery empty and ready for the following year's students. During this last step, parents were invited to participate in TREES workshops at the schools, during which they were taught how to grow a variety of plants in a small space and how to use moringa in their cooking. After the saplings had been planted in the home gardens, TREES staff visited the families to measure the trees and give additional advice. Parents were encouraged to report back on how they put moringa to use in their kitchens and how the trees were benefitting their families.

The project showed positive results: environmental awareness increased both for children and for their parents in terms of more considerations of good environmental practices, such as recycling. An increased nutritional awareness was also detected, with 90% of the families experimenting with moringa recipes at home and 55% eating homemade moringa powder three times per week. The project even showed some positive impact on education, with overall better attendance and higher grades. Students who had problems in class often became responsible for nursing the moringa trees, which gave them a valued role in class and increased their self-esteem.

Read more about the project: www.b4fn.org/case-studies/case-studies/moringa-leaves/

Role for enhancing connectivity with home gardens and other reserves of forest genetic resources

Schools can offer an important space in urban or peri-urban landscapes to enhance tree cover. This can increase tree population sizes and connectivity, and consequently help conserve local genetic diversity. There is a growing network of arboreta (Arbnet.org) across the globe. Arboreta have long been part of university campuses, botanic gardens, and city parks, but only recently are schools recognizing the value of establishing arboreta and initiatives to integrate restoration activities into their curricula (Hall and Bauer-Armstrong, 2010). Moreover, trees around schools have even been linked to higher student cognitive function (Tallis et al., 2018; Bratman et al., 2019). Typically arboreta have been established by wealthy landowners, but Yongneng et al. (2006) found a positive correlation between household income and species richness in southernmost Yunnan Province, China; the lower the income level, the higher the number of species in the garden had to be to counterbalance risks and increase the level of food security or income generating products. In peri-urban environments of the Yucatan Peninsula Mexico, school gardens have been valuable in raising awareness of conservation and food security related to native trees (Poot-Pool et al., 2018). The presence of different trees can also depend on their products and their use for construction, foods, medicines, fuels, or fodder.

School gardens are highly heterogeneous in terms of size, scope, and structure. They exist under different environmental, geographic, and socio-economic conditions as well as different history and ethno-cultural traditions, all of which influence their socio-ecological role. School garden networks' abilities to cover wide geographic and environmental variation means that they can be useful locations for planting a broad diversity of trees. This can both help to conserve genetic diversity and also enable research on provenances across regions to better understand the importance of genetic differences. Therefore, school gardens offer not only a very valuable platform for demonstrating the great diversity of native trees but also a way to institutionalize the transfer of traditional knowledge on the uses of different species and varieties in order to conserve important knowledge.

School gardens can be a place not only to ensure urban greening and for education or food production but also for the restoration and ex situ conservation of rare and underutilized trees (Poot-Pool et al., 2018). These gardens can play an important role in mobilizing action for the conservation of plant genetic resources; especially for native tree species that have highly fragmented and degraded habitats, they can help in increasing population sizes, increasing connectivity, reducing extinction risk, and reducing pressure on other tree populations by demonstrating sustainable use.

Kuzevanov and Sizykh (2006) have demonstrated that botanic gardens enhance the establishment of gene banks for indigenous plants and seed banks as well as the development of scientific studies and the involvement of local communities in plant protection and decision-making processes with regards to environment conservation. As mentioned by Moreno-Black (1996), 'the home garden plot is also important as an informal experimental station where indigenous species can be transferred, encouraged and tended as the women try to adapt them for use'. School gardens can become experimental stations and ex situ conservation places for such research purposes.

Active contributions to conservation using school gardens could include students being encouraged to propagate and plant native trees in their school gardens: this can be viewed as a strategy to increase biodiversity and explore different aspects of conservation biology, such as the minimum size of conservation unit needed to sustain a viable population (Galluzzi et al., 2010); it can also help with, as in Kehlenbeck et al. (2013), considering local preferences, the nutrition values of planted species, seasonality, resilience to climate change, and the available market or value chain process. In the context of school gardens, it is more likely that trees are planted for their renewable products, such as food and medicine, shade, and soil fertility, than for a one-off function, such as timber (Boshier et al., 2017), so this helps to maintain population sizes.

Geldenhuys (2007) shows that many edible and medicinal plants usually harvested from the wild can be grown as small-scale agricultural crops. Both seeds and vegetative propagation techniques have been tested, and especially trees, in the framework of the 'Commercial Products from the Wild Innovation Fund

Project' in South Africa, could be included in school gardens, considering their low risk and relatively large harvesting window.

In research conducted by Shackleton et al. (2007), the authors investigate incentives to promote the diversity of trees in rural areas of South Africa; these findings can shed light on what drives decisions on how to optimize the level of tree diversity in school gardens. The study examines correlations between household characteristics and the density of both indigenous and exotic trees, and number of tree species. Important variables affecting the density and number of varieties of trees included access to space, gender of the household head, and level of wealth. Female-headed households had significantly less trees than their male equivalents. This highlights how school gardens can be a great equalizer in terms of exposure to tree diversity if the activities are organized equally between boys and girls.

Together with diversity of species and varieties, there should be a level of diversity in terms of nutritional composition in fruit trees, vegetables, and medicinal trees planted in school gardens. To ensure this, schools can adopt garden diversity kits, which include seeds and samples of different species, depending on documented nutritional gap analysis, market demand, agroecology, and school capacity (Sthapit et al., 2008). Seeds, plants, and products can be exchanged to maintain diversity; an example of this is seen in the UK Garden Organisation and its Heritage Seed Library, where a network of volunteers contribute to the reproduction, conservation, and exchange of seeds. The same can be achieved by creating a network of schools participating in similar school garden programmes. The Plant for the Planet campaign, for example, now has 100,000 students from more than 26 countries leading a campaign to plant a trillion trees to tackle climate change (Plant-for-the-planet.org). Linking such school garden nurseries to local restoration projects could be a powerful tool for scaling the production of diverse and high-quality native trees. Different schools could exchange their germplasm or seed material, making conservation of neglected species more effective while also increasing the pool of people with the horticultural knowledge needed to grow them and scaling the production of native tree seeds, which is a major bottleneck in many restoration projects.

Finally, school gardens can be a good place to promote agrobiodiversity because they are a link within the community where tree breeders and farmers can access seeds and seedlings suitable for their environment and their needs. When biodiversity and ecosystems services are taken into consideration, school gardens can have a complex vegetation structure, hosting organisms that would not exist in the urban context.

In schools, tree identification can become an additional teaching tool to engage students with taxonomy and botany. Trees can be identified through registers, horticultural experts, interviews, and field observation, both by local and scientific names. Assessing the level of genetic diversity of trees within the garden, the identities of local cultivars, and the variation of the morphological characteristics of fruits and leaves can be the starting point (Galluzzi et al., 2010); a food web pathway can be used for a more comprehensive analysis, with indicators such as soil fertility, diversity and cover of plants at the plot level, and diversity of land use types (Remans and Smukler, 2013).

Finally, an interesting result from a study conducted in the Chivi district of Zimbabwe highlighted how the elderly interviewed about the planting and management of indigenous trees were more sceptical than middle aged people; this suggests that targeting young students with explanations of the properties and the benefits of conservation and diversity of indigenous trees can be more effective (Gerhardt and Nemarundwe, 2006).

BOX 7.2: SCHOOL GARDENS AND CONSERVATION OF IMPORTANT FRUIT TREE GENETIC RESOURCES IN CENTRAL ASIA

As part of a Bioversity International project entitled 'Improving seed systems for smallholder farmers' food security' in 2018, five orchards with 12 local varieties of apple, 9 of apricot, 9 of grape, and 7 of pomegranate were established in the field area of 3 rural schools and 2 colleges in Khorezm, Surhandarya, and Fergana Province, Uzbekistan. The objective of this project was to establish these school orchards in order to increase knowledge among school students about traditional varieties of fruit trees from Central Asia developed by their ancestors (Figure 7.1). These varieties, which are well adapted to local environmental stress factors, are superior in terms of taste and nutritional value, and have been passed from generation to generation of local farmers. Unfortunately, globalization in agriculture and food production has resulted in the erosion of the valuable diversity of important fruit tree species and the malnutrition of children due to reduced consumption of fruits.

In May 2018 the project team met with the staff and managers of rural schools and colleges located in the project sites where the establishment of Schools of Young Breeders and Seed Growers were discussed to spark young people's interest in working in agriculture and agricultural research. The staff and authorities of rural schools and colleges met these suggestions with enthusiasm. Subsequently, 'Young Breeders and Seed Growers' has been established in five rural schools and one college, including 92 school and 18 college students. Curators of 'Young Breeders and Seed Growers' schools were selected and appointed with the permission of school authorities. The project team collaborated with the appointed curators to develop a curriculum for the schools, which included topics on the basics of fruit tree breeding using local varieties and technologies to produce high-quality seeds and saplings.

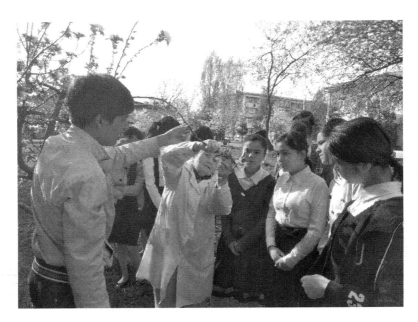

FIGURE 7.1 Dr Dorohova is explaining to schoolchildren technology of artificial cross-breeding of fruit trees used to create a new plant in a school orchard.
Source: Nodir Jalilov.

Conclusion and way forward

Unlike other underutilized species, trees require significant space, time, and resources to ensure their adequate conservation. Protected areas are often inadequate to capture the diversity of species as well as adequate numbers of individuals to conserve genetic diversity within those species. We have highlighted a number of ways in which school gardens could be employed not only to conserve knowledge and raise awareness but also to actually have an effective role in in situ and ex situ conservation of important tree genetic resources. The scale of the problem is great and requires large networks of stakeholders, who will need to consider a time frame that includes more than one generation of students. This is why schools with a long-term vision are so important.

School gardens can serve as tools to conserve not only genetic diversity but also traditional knowledge and skills in determining what trees are edible, how to cultivate them, and their socio-economic value in society. Using schools as a platform to broadly engage community members, including elders, through fairs or festivals can also enhance a sense of togetherness within the community, especially in a context of increasing urbanization.

These projects dismantle the traditional perception that farming and gardening are last choice activities, something seen as a punishment; school gardening can break barriers not only to a healthy diet but also to peer pressure and social stigmas. The stakeholders involved are not only students and teachers but farmers from the community; vegetable and fruit traders and processors; agricultural extension officers; and experts in agricultural economics, agronomy, ethnobotany, health, and nutrition.

School gardens have great potential to become places for the conservation and restoration of underutilized and threatened trees. Local edible species can be used to complement school feeding programmes. They can be easy to cultivate; can produce nutritious fruit, leaves, and vegetables; and are adaptable to different environmental conditions.

There is a growing movement towards using school gardens to inspire the next generation of tree breeders and conservation scientists (Hall and Bauer-Armstrong, 2010) but, more importantly, to demonstrate the vital role that trees play in agroecological systems and the necessity that they be maintained at adequate scales for resilient delivery of the broad ecosystem services that we all depend on.

Notes

1 http://globaltrees.org/threatened-trees/.
2 https://tools.bgci.org/global_tree_search.php.

References

Boshier, D., Loo, J. and Dawson, I.K. (2017) 'Forest and tree genetic resources', in D. Hunter, et al. (eds), 'Routledge handbook of agricultural biodiversity', London (UK), Routledge, p. 45–64, ISBN: 9780415746922.

Bratman, G.N., Anderson, C.B., Berman, M.G., Cochran, B., De Vries, S., Flanders, J., Folke, C., Frumkin, H., Gross, J.J., Hartig, T., Kahn, P.H. et al (2019) 'Nature and mental health: An ecosystem service perspective', *Science Advances*, 5(7), doi:10.1126/sciadv.aax0903.

Cousins, S.R. and Witkowski, E.T.F. (2015) 'Indigenous plants: Key role players in community horticulture initiatives', *Human Ecology Review*, 21(1), 59–86.

Crowther, T.W., Glick, H.B., Covey, K.R., Bettigole, C., Maynard, D.S., Thomas, S.M. and Tuanmu, M.N. (2015) 'Mapping tree density at a global scale', *Nature*, 525(7568), 201, doi:10.1038/nature14967.

Galluzzi, G., Eyzaguirre, P. and Negri, V. (2010) 'Home gardens: Neglected hotspots of agro-biodiversity and cultural diversity', *Biodiversity and Conservation*, 19(13), 3635–3654.

Geldenhuys, C.J. (2007) 'Weeds or useful medicinal plants in the rural home garden?', *Food and Nutrition Bulletin*, 28(2_suppl2), S392–S397.

Gerhardt, K. and Nemarundwe, N. (2006) 'Participatory planting and management of indigenous trees: Lessons from Chivi District, Zimbabwe', *Agriculture and Human Values*, 23(2), 231–243.

Hall, R. and Bauer-Armstrong, C. (2010) 'Earth partnership for schools: Ecological restoration in schools and communities', *Ecological Restoration*, 2010 Jun 1;28(2), 208–212.

Heim, S., Stang, J. and Ireland, M. (2009) 'A garden pilot project enhances fruit and vegetable consumption among children', *Journal of the American Dietetic Association*, 109(7), 1220–1226.

IPBES (2019) 'Summary for policymakers of the global assessment report on biodiversity and ecosystem services of the Intergovernmental Science-Policy Platform on Biodiversity and Ecosystem Services', S. Díaz, J. Settele, E.S. Brondizio E.S., H.T. Ngo, M. Guèze, J. Agard, A. Arneth, P. Balvanera, K.A. Brauman, S.H.M. Butchart, K.M.A. Chan, L.A. Garibaldi, K. Ichii, J. Liu, S.M. Subramanian, G.F. Midgley, P. Miloslavich,

Z. Molnár, D. Obura, A. Pfaff, S. Polasky, A. Purvis, J. Razzaque, B. Reyers, R. Roy Chowdhury, Y.J. Shin, I.J. Visseren-Hamakers, K.J. Willis and C.N. Zayas (eds), IPBES Secretariat, Bonn, Germany.

Kehlenbeck, K., Asaah, E. and Jamnadass, R. (2013) 'Diversity of indigenous fruit trees and their contribution to nutrition and livelihoods in sub-Saharan Africa: Examples from Kenya and Cameroon', in J. Fanzo, D. Hunter, T. Borelli and F. Mattei (eds) 'Diversifying food and diets: Using agricultural biodiversity to improve nutrition and health', Earthscan, 257–269.

Kuzevanov, V. and Sizykh, S. (2006) 'Botanic gardens resources: Tangible and intangible aspects of linking biodiversity and human well-being', *Hiroshima Peace Science*, 28(2006), 113–134.

Lin, B.B., Philpott, S.M. and Jha, S. (2015) 'The future of urban agriculture and biodiversity-ecosystem services: Challenges and next steps', *Basic and Applied Ecology*, 16(3), 189–201.

Moreno-Black, G., Somnasang, P. and Thamathawan, S. (1996) 'Cultivating continuity and creating change: Women's home garden practices in northeastern Thailand', *Agriculture and Human Values*, 13(3), 3–11.

Ojiewo, C., Tenkouano, A., Hughes, J. D.A. and Keatinge, J.D.H. (2013) 'Diversifying diets: Using indigenous vegetables to improve profitability, nutrition and health in Africa' in J. Fanzo, D. Hunter, T. Borelli and F. Mattei (eds), 'Diversifying food and diets: Using agricultural biodiversity to improve nutrition and health', Earthscan, 291–302.

Poot-Pool, W.S., Cetzal-Ix, W., Basu, S.K., Noguera-Savelli, E. and Noh-Contreras, D.G. (2018) 'Urban home gardens: A sustainable conservation model for local plants', *Urban Horticulture: Sustainability for the Future*, 18, 73.

Remans, R. and Smukler, S. (2013) 'Linking biodiversity and nutrition' in J. Fanzo, D. Hunter, T. Borelli and F. Mattei (eds), 'Diversifying food and diets: Using agricultural biodiversity to improve nutrition and health', Earthscan, 140–163.

Schreckenberg, K., Awono, A., Degrande, A., Mbosso, C., Ndoye, O. and Tchoundjeu, Z. (2006) 'Domesticating indigenous fruit trees as a contribution to poverty reduction', *Forests, Trees and Livelihoods*, 16(1), 35–51.

Shackleton, C.M. (2002) 'Growth and fruit production of *Sclerocarya birrea* in the South African lowveld', *Agroforestry systems*, 55(3), 175–180.

Shackleton, C.M., Paumgarten, F. and Cocks, M.L. (2007) 'Household attributes promote diversity of tree holdings in rural areas, South Africa', *Agroforestry Systems*, 72(3), 221–230.

Sthapit, B., Rana, R., Eyzaguirre, P. and Jarvis, D. (2008) 'The value of plant genetic diversity to resource-poor farmers in Nepal and Vietnam', *International journal of agricultural sustainability*, 6(2), 148–166.

Tallis, H., Bratman, G.N., Samhouri, J.F. and Fargione, J. (2018) 'Are California elementary school test scores more strongly associated with urban trees than poverty?', *Frontiers in Psychology* 2018;9, 2074, doi:10.3389/fpsyg.2018.02074.

Willett, W., Rockström, J., Loken, B., Springmann, M., Lang, T., Vermeulen, S. et al. (2019) 'Food in the Anthropocene: The EAT–Lancet Commission on healthy diets from sustainable food systems', *The Lancet*, 393(10170), 447–492.

Yongneng, F., Huijun, G., Aiguo, C. and Jinyun, C. (2006) 'Household differentiation and on-farm conservation of biodiversity by indigenous households in Xishuangbanna, China', *Human Exploitation and Biodiversity Conservation* (pp. 347–363), Springer, Dordrecht.

8
THE IMPACT OF SCHOOL GARDENS ON NUTRITION OUTCOMES IN LOW-INCOME COUNTRIES

Pepijn Schreinemachers, Ray-yu Yang, Dhruba Raj Bhattarai, Bal Bdr Rai, and Mamounata Sandaogo Ouedraogo

Introduction

Low quality diets have significant human health risks (Willett et al., 2019). Of the world's population of 7.2 billion, more than 2.1 billion people are overweight or obese and 2 billion people are micronutrient deficient. Hence there is a growing need to transform current food systems to ensure healthy diets. As part of this, there is a need for good policies and programmes that promote healthy eating habits.

This requires a sound understanding of drivers of eating habits. It is known that taste preferences and food attitudes are important drivers alongside lifestyles, convenience, affordability, nutrition awareness, and policies (Kearney, 2010; Traill et al., 2014). Taste preferences and food attitudes are established early in life and tend to persist through to adulthood (Kelder et al., 1994; Birch, 1999; Cooke, 2007). This understanding has stimulated interest in interventions that nudge children to adopt healthy eating habits. School garden programmes are one such type of intervention.

School garden programmes have become popular for improving food, nutrition, and health behaviour of schoolchildren in both high- and low-income countries (FAO, 2005; Ozer, 2007; Parmer et al., 2009; Christian et al., 2014a; Hutchinson et al., 2015; Triador et al., 2015; Nury et al., 2017). Such programmes usually bundle hands-on practical education in school gardening with nutrition education. School gardening training is expected to give children the knowledge and the ability to produce food, while nutrition education promotes children's demand for quality food. This combination of supply- and demand-side interventions is a key feature of school garden programmes.

The use of school gardens to promote healthy eating behaviour in low-income countries is conceptually appealing because of high rates of child malnutrition. As a result, there has been a substantial increase in such programmes in low-income countries. However, the evidence basis for their impact on food behaviour in low-income countries is very limited as there are no impact evaluations in the literature.

This chapter describes the results of three recent impact evaluations, each using a cluster randomised controlled trial design, of school garden programmes in Bhutan, Nepal, and Burkina Faso with the objective to assess the current evidence for the impact of school garden programmes in low-income countries. The three studies that this chapter is based on are the largest evaluation of school garden programmes to date.

The results show that school garden interventions significantly improved children's knowledge about food and agriculture in all three countries. For Bhutan and Nepal, the results showed improvements in children's awareness of fruit and vegetables and their stated preferences for eating them. In none of the countries did these changes translate into clear increases in fruit and vegetable consumption. The results therefore suggest that for school garden programmes to contribute to healthier food choices a more holistic intervention design may be needed that addresses the household-level supply of healthy foods and influences the food choices of parents, considering affordability and availability factors.

The chapter starts by reviewing the existing evidence for school garden programmes. It then presents the results of three recent studies from Bhutan, Burkina Faso, and Nepal. The chapter concludes with some recommendations on how to better design school garden programmes aimed at influencing food choices in low-income countries.

Current evidence for school garden programmes

School garden programmes need to be designed in response to the food environment and lifestyle of people in the target location. In high-income countries, school gardens often try to promote greater physical activity levels among children, encourage social interaction, promote healthier eating habits, and give children a better understanding of food production while trying to instil a love for nature. Such goals can also be found in lower income countries, but the emphasis is usually more on building children's resilience by giving them the ability to grow food in a sustainable way through the transfer of agricultural knowledge and skills, and increasing the consumption of healthy foods such as micronutrient-dense fruit and vegetables.

Virtually all the evidence for the impact of school gardens has come from higher-income countries (Ozer, 2007; Lineberger and Zajicek, 2009; Parmer et al., 2009; Morgan et al., 2010; Ratcliffe et al., 2011; Christian et al., 2014b), while there was no evidence for lower-income countries until this project was completed. In the following we will describe this evidence based on four review papers before turning our attention to lower-income countries.

Blair (2009) reviewed 12 quantitative impact studies of school garden programmes in the United States. All 12 quantitative studies collected pre- and post-intervention data, but none used an experimental design in which schools would be randomly assigned to a treatment or control group. These 12 studies used samples of 1 to 5 schools and no more than 500 schoolchildren. The review showed that 9 out of the 12 studies showed positive outcomes in the area of science achievement, but only one study showed a significant increase in fruit and vegetable consumption that could be attributed to the school garden programme.

Robinson-O'Brien et al. (2009) reviewed 11 studies for the United States that examined the impact of garden-based nutrition education programmes on preferences, willingness to taste, and intake of fruit and vegetables. Of these 11 studies, four reported effects on fruit and vegetable intake and three of these reported a significant increase. Six studies reported results on fruit and vegetable preferences, and two of these reported a significant increase. Three studies reported results on willingness to taste fruit or vegetables, and two of these reported a significant increase. The authors therefore concluded that, based on the limited evidence available, garden-based nutrition-education programmes may have the potential to lead to improvements in fruit and vegetable intake, willingness to taste, and preferences among students.

Langellotto and Gupta (2012) specifically reviewed the evidence of garden-based nutrition education programmes on student's nutrition knowledge, preferences for fruit and vegetables, and consumption of fruit and vegetables. They reviewed 20 studies from the United States and found that nutrition education programmes that included a gardening component were more effective at increasing vegetable consumption in children than nutrition education programmes without such gardening component.

Ohly et al. (2016) conducted a systematic review of quantitative and qualitative evidence of school gardening programmes. The review identified 21 quantitative studies, 16 qualitative studies, and 3 mixed methods studies. The 40 studies all came from high-income countries (United States, United Kingdom, Australia, and Portugal). Thirteen studies reported the effect on healthier food preferences and eight found a significant effect. Ten studies reported effects on food knowledge and attitudes, and seven of these reported a significant increase. Thirteen studies reported the effect on fruit and vegetable consumption, and only two found a significant increase. Hence, this review shows that school garden programmes are more capable of influencing children's food preferences, knowledge, and attitudes but less able to influence actual food behaviour in terms of a significant increase in children's fruit and vegetable consumption.

These reviews for high-income countries point out that there is no strong evidence that school garden programmes improve children's consumption of fruit and vegetables. School garden programmes are more likely to improve science scores, food knowledge, and food preferences than they are able to influence actual behaviour towards healthier food choices.

Results of three recent experimental studies for low-income countries

To fill the evidence gap for the impact of school garden programmes in low-income counties, the Swiss Agency for Development and Cooperation (SDC) funded the project 'Vegetables Go to School: Improving Nutrition by

Agricultural Diversification' (2013–2017). Through this project, the World Vegetable Center worked with national partners in Burkina Faso, Tanzania, Indonesia, Bhutan, Nepal, and the Philippines to design and implement school garden programmes. Quantitative evidence for impact was generated for three of these countries – Bhutan, Nepal, and Burkina Faso. Results have been published previously (Schreinemachers et al., 2017a; Schreinemachers et al., 2017b; Schreinemachers et al., 2019) and the purpose of this chapter is to synthesise and highlight the evidence from these studies.

Research design and data collection

Each study used a cluster randomised controlled trial design. Treatment and control schools were selected randomly from a larger list of primary schools in a particular region of the country. For each school, baseline data were collected at the start of the school year, next the intervention was implemented, and end line data were collected at the end of the school year for the same students (Table 8.1). In Nepal and Burkina Faso the study was repeated to increase the robustness of the results. For these two countries, control schools in year-1 became treatment schools in year-2. In Bhutan the data collection started only in the second year of the project.

TABLE 8.1 Data collected for the study

	Bhutan			Nepal			Burkina Faso		
	C	T	A	C	T	A	C	T	A
Year-1:									
# schools	–	–	–	20	10	30	10	10	20
# students, baseline	–	–	–	904	466	1,370	500	500	1,000
# students, endline	–	–	–	882	454	1,336	499	501	1,000
# students, total[1]	–	–	–	846	429	1,275	491	488	979
Year-2:									
# schools	9	9	18	10	10	20	10	10	20
# students, baseline	265	260	525	433	394	827	400	400	800
# students, endline	258	259	517	385	428	813	400	400	800
# students, total[1]	235	233	468	416	369	785	389	392	781

Source: (Schreinemachers et al., 2017a; Schreinemachers et al., 2017b; Schreinemachers et al., 2019).
Notes: C = Control; T = Treatment; A = Sum of Control and Treatment.
1 Students outside an age range were dropped from the sample with the age range being 9–15 years old for Bhutan, 10–15 years old for Nepal, and 8–14 years old for Burkina Faso.

Outcome indicators were selected from a review of previous impact studies of school garden programmes. The selected outcome indicators represented stepwise changes in the intervention's impact pathway from increased awareness about fruit and vegetables to improved knowledge of food, nutrition, and WASH (water, sanitation, and hygiene) as well as knowledge of sustainable agriculture and increased preferences for healthy foods and food behaviour in terms of increased fruit and vegetable consumption. Details about variable definitions and measurement can be found in the published papers. Data were collected using relatively simple questionnaires with photos and multiple-choice questions to aid children's comprehension. The text was brief, and the phrasing was simple. The questionnaire was designed in English and translated into the local language.

Intervention designs

The school garden programmes in each country were designed in collaboration between the Ministry of Agriculture and the Ministry of Education. For details see (Bhattarai et al., 2016; Bhattarai et al., 2017; Ouedraogo et al., 2017; Rai et al., 2017). This collaboration across ministries was an important aspect of the project. A nutrition expert from the Ministry of Health in Burkina Faso and Nepal and from a local university in Bhutan also contributed to the project. Each programme design included three intervention components that were concurrently implemented in all treatment schools and targeted children in elementary education:

School garden component: School gardens were established in each treatment school for the cultivation of about eight different vegetables. Emphasis was given to vegetables that were culturally accepted, nutrient-dense, and easy to grow. The school garden designs generally included raised planting beds, fences to prevent livestock from entering the garden. Irrigation water tanks were installed where water availability was a constraint. Other improvements were made depending on the local situation.

Education component: Complementary education was provided about agriculture, nutrition, and hygiene. A curriculum was developed for 23 weeks and teachers received training on how to use it. Topics covered were food groups, the health benefits of vegetables, food and body hygiene, and school and environmental sanitation. The school garden and its products were used by teachers to illustrate mathematics, biology, moral education, and language. The agricultural education emphasised learning by doing and was regularly conducted in the school garden.

Involvement of parents, local farmers and other community members: Parents helped preparing the school garden and fencing it with locally available materials. Depending on the local situation, vegetables were supplied to the school canteen or given to the children to bring home. In many instances, local farmers helped with making nurseries and preparing seed beds and local extension officers visited the schools to provide technical advice as needed.

The three intervention components are jointly expected to raise children's awareness about vegetables and increase their knowledge. This increased knowledge is then expected to stimulate their preferences for healthier food choices including vegetables, which should then lead to better food choices and improved nutrition status.

Results

Table 8.2 shows the average treatment effects, which is the difference in mean outcomes between students assigned to the treatment and students assigned to the control. For means and standard errors we refer to the original papers.

TABLE 8.2 Impact of the school garden intervention on nutrition outcomes in Bhutan, Nepal, and Burkina Faso, average treatment effects showing marginal effects at means

Outcome variable	Bhutan	Nepal		Burkina Faso	
	Year-2	Year-1	Year-2	Year-1	Year-2
Awareness:					
% of fruit and vegetables correctly named	17.9 ***	29.4 ***	12.8 ***	3.3	2.5
Knowledge:					
% of correct answers on sustainable agriculture	15.2 **	21.7 ***	16.7 ***	4.5	5.7
% of correct answers on food, nutrition, and WASH	−5.2	13.8 ***	14.6 ***	6.1 **	7.7 **
Preferences:					
% of fruit and vegetables liked	9.5 **	15.8 ***	19.1 ***	−1.4	12.3
Behaviour:					
% of children that ate vegetables	11.7 **	2.35	0.91	20.2 *	2.7
% of children that ate fruit	−3.6	−0.75	7.11	−6.5	−3.9
# of different vegetables eaten	0.19	0.09	−0.04	0.3	0.2
# of different fruits eaten	−0.09	0.07	0.08	NA	0.1
Students (n)	468	1,275	785	979	781

Source: (Schreinemachers et al., 2017a; Schreinemachers et al., 2017b; Schreinemachers et al., Under review).

Notes: ***$p < 0.01$, **$p < 0.05$, *$p < 0.10$. NA = Not available (the average treatment effect could not be estimated as the number of different fruits eaten in the sample of students in Burkina Faso in year-1 was near zero).

The results show that the school garden programme, which was similarly designed and implemented in each country, had more significant effects on nutrition outcomes in Bhutan and Nepal than in Burkina Faso. For the latter country, only one of the eight outcome variables showed a significant increase.

For Bhutan and Nepal, the school garden programme increased students' awareness of fruit and vegetables. For Nepal and Burkina Faso, the school garden programme increased students' knowledge of food, nutrition, and WASH. For Bhutan and Nepal, but not for Burkina Faso, the school garden programme also enhanced students' knowledge of sustainable agriculture. It is, however, noted that for Burkina Faso, when pooling the two years together, the effect on agricultural knowledge was also significant ($p < 0.05$).

For Bhutan and Nepal, but not for Burkina Faso, the school garden programme promoted children's preferences for eating fruit and vegetables. Only in Bhutan, did the school garden programme increase the percentage of children eating vegetables. The effect of the school garden programme on fruit consumption or the number of different fruits or vegetables consumed was insignificant for all years and all countries.

These studies therefore broadly show that school garden programmes in low-income countries can be effective in increasing students' awareness of fruit and vegetables, their knowledge of food and agriculture, and their preferences for eating fruit and vegetables, but school garden programmes appear less effective in changing students' actual food behaviour towards the increased consumption of fruit and vegetables, at least in the short-term.

Discussion

The finding that school garden programmes in low-income countries are more effective in increasing students' awareness, knowledge, and preferences and less effective in increasing students' actual consumption of fruit and vegetables confirms the findings of two major reviews on the effect of school garden programmes on nutrition outcomes in high-income countries (Blair, 2009; Ohly et al., 2016).

In explaining the reasons for this lack of impact, it is important to bear in mind that school gardens themselves cannot supply students with a daily serving of vegetables. The size of a school garden is just too small for this and trying to do this would seriously distract students and teachers from the school curriculum. Hence, the purpose of a school garden is usually purely educational while vegetable harvests are small and irregular. Therefore, school gardens can only make an indirect impact on nutrition outcomes through stimulating students' awareness of fruit and vegetables and enhancing their knowledge about the importance of eating a diverse range of fruit and vegetables for good health. The combination of these effects is assumed to nudge students to adjust their food behaviour and eat more fruit and vegetables.

The problem in this assumed impact pathway is that the school garden intervention does not adequately address the supply of fruit and vegetables to students. This is likely the main reason why none of the three impact studies showed convincing evidence for increased fruit and vegetable consumption. This constraint was also identified by the country implementation teams when reviewing the results of the programme.

The availability of vegetables in students' homes may be very limited in many countries, while schools may not serve a school meal that includes vegetables. If school meals are served at all, then this is usually a combination of staple food grain and pulses with very small quantities of fresh vegetables. However, if vegetables are unavailable in the home or in the school then students do not have a real choice of eating fruit and vegetables, even if they wanted to.

To accomplish this and give children a healthy food choice, school garden programmes may need to be coupled to a school meals programme that serves fruit and vegetables as part of a mid-day meal, or to an intervention that promotes the availability of fruit and vegetables within the household or within the community. It is also important that primary caregivers understand the importance of serving vegetables to their children, which may not always be the case, especially in low-income countries.

Home gardens are an intervention that address both the household-level demand and supply of vegetables (World Vegetable Center, 2016). Home garden interventions typically couple training in garden management with nutrition education of mothers. There is evidence that home garden interventions have a significant effect on increasing household production and consumption of vegetables (Olney et al., 2009; Galhena et al., 2013; Schreinemachers et al., 2016). However, there is no evidence to date that such interventions influence the food attitudes, knowledge, or food behaviour of children 8-15 years old. It therefore appears ideal to couple a school garden programme – which has a proven effect on raising children's interest in vegetables, to a home garden programme – which has a proven effect on increasing household production and consumption of vegetables.

The impact of such coupled intervention is currently unknown. Several of this paper's authors are involved in an ongoing project in Nepal (2018–2020), titled 'Nudging children toward healthier food choices: An experiment combining school and home gardens', that pilots such coupled intervention in 15 schools. This project is part of the Drivers of Food Choice Competitive Grants Program funded by the UK Government's Department for International Development and the Bill & Melinda Gates Foundation.

The 'Vegetables Go to School' project was successful in raising the interest of the governments of Bhutan and Nepal in school-based programmes combining agriculture, nutrition, and health. As a result of this project, Bhutan has adopted an integrated approach of tackling child malnutrition through a holistic approach combining school feeding, WASH, and school gardening. Also, as a result of this project, the government of Nepal launched the 'Green School Program' to roll out school gardens to public schools across the country and the Department of Education has meanwhile designed a school garden curriculum that integrates nutrition, agriculture, and health. There is a need to closely study these initiatives to gain a better understanding for how these programmes can optimally influence the healthy eating behaviour of children and parents and to draw lessons that can be applied to other countries considering similar programmes.

Conclusion

The evidence for high-income countries suggests that school garden programmes are more effective in improving knowledge and attitudes about healthy eating than at changing short-term actual food behaviour. The findings of three impact studies of school garden programmes in Bhutan, Burkina Faso, and Nepal, as presented in this chapter, confirm that school garden programmes are more effective in changing knowledge and attitudes than in changing actual food behaviour. Improvements in knowledge and attitudes can, of course, have long-term positive effects on food behaviour, which are difficult to measure. Yet, to achieve also short-term effects in terms of increased vegetable consumption, it may be necessary to couple school garden programmes to other interventions that raise the nutrition awareness among parents and increase the availability of vegetables in students' homes and the community. Coupling school gardens with home gardens appears as one suitable combination to accomplish this.

Acknowledgements

Funding for this research was provided by the Swiss Agency for Development and Cooperation (SDC) under grant number 81017189 and the Drivers of Food Choice Competitive Grants Programs, which is funded by the UK Government's Department for International Development (DFID) and the Bill & Melinda Gates Foundation, and managed by the University of South Carolina, Arnold School of Public Health, United States. Funding was also provided by core donors to the World Vegetable Center: Republic of China (Taiwan), DFID, United States Agency for International Development (USAID), Australian Centre for International Agricultural Research (ACIAR), Germany, Thailand, Philippines, Korea, and Japan.

References

Bhattarai, D. R., Subedi, G. D., Kashichwa, N. K., Dhungana, U., Yang, R. Y., Schreinemachers, P., Mecozzi, M., Luther, G., Luoh, J. W., Palaniswamy, U., Holmer, R., Cissé, G. and Drescher, A. (2017) 'Vegetables go to school NEPAL: School vegetable gardens: Linking nutrition, health and communities project documentation', Shanhua, Taiwan: World Vegetable Center.
Bhattarai, D. R., Subedi, G. D. and Schreinemachers, P. (2016) 'School Vegetable Gardening: Concept, Curriculum & Action', Khumaltar, Lalitpur, Nepal: Government of Nepal, Nepal Agricultural Research Council (NARC).
Birch, L.L. (1999) 'Development of food preferences', *Annual Review of Nutrition* 19, 41–62.
Blair, D. (2009) 'The child in the garden: An evaluative review of the benefits of school gardening', *The Journal of Environmental Education* 40, 15–38, doi:10.3200/joee.40.2.15-38.

Christian, M., Evans, C., Nykjaer, C., Hancock, N. and Cade, J. (2014a) 'Evaluation of the impact of a school gardening intervention on children's fruit and vegetable intake: A randomised controlled trial', *International Journal of Behavioral Nutrition and Physical Activity* 11, doi:10.1186/s12966-014-0099-7.

Christian, M. S., Evans, C. E. L. and Cade, J. E. (2014b) 'Does the Royal Horticultural Society Campaign for School Gardening increase intake of fruit and vegetables in children? Results from two randomised controlled trials', *Public Health Res* 2, doi:10.3310/phr02040.

Cooke, L. (2007) 'The importance of exposure for healthy eating in childhood: A review', *The Journal of Human Nutrition and Dietetics*, 20, 294–301.

FAO (2005) 'Setting up and running a school garden: A manual for teachers, parents and communities', Rome: Food and Agriculture Organization of the United Nations.

Galhena, D., Freed, R. and Maredia, K. (2013) 'Home gardens: A promising approach to enhance household food security and wellbeing', *Agriculture & Food Security* 2, 8.

Hutchinson, J., Christian, M. S., Evans, C. E. L., Nykjaer, C., Hancock, N. and Cade, J. E. (2015) 'Evaluation of the impact of school gardening interventions on children's knowledge of and attitudes towards fruit and vegetables. A cluster randomised controlled trial', *Appetite* 91, 405–414, doi:10.1016/j.appet.2015.04.076.

Kearney, J. (2010) 'Food consumption trends and drivers', *Philosophical Transactions of the Royal Society B: Biological Sciences* 365, 2793–2807, doi:10.1098/rstb.2010.0149.

Kelder, S.H., Perry, C.L., Klepp, K-I., Lytle, L.L. (1994) 'Longitudinal tracking of adolescent smoking, physical activity, and food choice behaviors', *American Journal of Public Health* 84(7), 1121–1126.

Langellotto, G. A. and Gupta, A. (2012) 'Gardening increases vegetable consumption in school-aged children: A meta-analytical synthesis', *HortTechnology* 22, 430–445.

Lineberger, S. E. and Zajicek, J. M. (2009) 'School gardens: Can a hands-on teaching tool affect students' attitudes and behaviors regarding fruit and vegetables?', *HortTechnology* 10, 593–597.

Morgan, P. J., Warren, J. M., Lubans, D. R., Saunders, K. L., Quick, G. I. and Collins, C. E. (2010) 'The impact of nutrition education with and without a school garden on knowledge, vegetable intake and preferences and quality of school life among primary-school students', *Public Health Nutrition* 13, 1931–1940, doi:10.1017/s1368980010000959.

Nury, E., Sarti, A., Dijkstra, C., Seidell, J. and Dedding, C. (2017) 'Sowing seeds for healthier diets: Children's perspectives on school gardening', *International Journal of Environmental Research and Public Health* 14, 688.

Ohly, H., Gentry, S., Wigglesworth, R., Bethel, A., Lovell, R. and Garside, R. (2016) 'A systematic review of the health and well-being impacts of school gardening: Synthesis of quantitative and qualitative evidence', *BMC Public Health* 16, 286, doi:10.1186/s12889-016-2941-0.

Olney, D. K., Talukder, A., Iannotti, L. L., Ruel, M. T. and Quinn, V. (2009) 'Assessing impact and impact pathways of a homestead food production program on household and child nutrition in Cambodia', *Food and Nutrition Bulletin* 30, 355–369.

Ouedraogo, M. S., Thiombiano, A., Kouamé, S. R., Yang, R. Y., Sobgui, C. M., Tignegre, J. B., Schreinemachers, P., Mecozzi, M., Luoh, J. W., Palaniswamy, U., Holmer, R., Cissé, G. and Drescher, A. (2017) 'Vegetables go to school BURKINA FASO: School vegetable gardens: Linking nutrition, health and communities', in *Vegetables go to school BURKINA FASO: School vegetable gardens: Linking nutrition, health and communities*: World Vegetable Center.

Ozer, E. J. (2007) 'The effects of school gardens on students and schools: Conceptualization and considerations for maximizing healthy development', *Health Education & Behavior* 34, 846–863, doi:10.1177/1090198106289002.

Parmer, S. M., Salisbury-Glennon, J., Shannon, D. and Struempler, B. (2009) 'School gardens: An experiential learning approach for a nutrition education program to increase fruit and vegetable knowledge, preference, and consumption among second-grade students', *Journal of Nutrition Education and Behavior* 41, 212–217.

Rai, B. B., Thinley, N., Dorji, D., Dukpa, T., Lham, P., Subba, A., Tshering, K., Wangchuk, N., Yang, R. Y., Schreinemachers, P., Mecozzi, M., Luther, G., Luoh, J. W., Palaniswamy, U., Holmer, R., Cissé, G. and Drescher, A. (2017) 'Vegetables go to school Bhutan: School vegetable gardens: Linking nutrition, health and communities', in 'Vegetables go to school Bhutan: School vegetable gardens: Linking nutrition, health and communities', Shanhua, Taiwan: World Vegetable Center.

Ratcliffe, M. M., Merrigan, K. A., Rogers, B. L. and Goldberg, J. P. (2011) 'The effects of school garden experiences on middle school-aged students' knowledge, attitudes, and behaviors associated with vegetable consumption', *Health Promotion Practice* 12, 36–43, doi:10.1177/1524839909349182.

Robinson-O'Brien, R., Story, M. and Heim, S. (2009) 'Impact of garden-based youth nutrition intervention programs: A review', *Journal of the American Dietetic Association* 109, doi:10.1016/j.jada.2008.10.051.

Schreinemachers, P., Bhattarai, D. R., Subedi, G. D., Acharya, T. P., Chen, H.-p., Yang, R.-y., Kashichhawa, N. K., Dhungana, U., Luther, G. C. and Mecozzi, M. (2017a) 'Impact of school gardens in Nepal: A cluster randomised controlled trial', *Journal of Development Effectiveness* 9, 329–343, doi:10.1080/19439342.2017.1311356.

Schreinemachers, P., Ouedraogo, M. S., Diagbouga, S., Thiombiano, A., Kouamé, S. R., Sobgui, C. M., Chen, H.-p. and Yang, R.-y. (2019) 'Impact of school gardens and complementary education in Burkina Faso', *Journal of Development Effectiveness* 11(2), 132–145, doi:10.1080/19439342.2019.1624595.

Schreinemachers, P., Patalagsa, M. A. and Uddin, N. (2016) 'Impact and cost-effectiveness of women's training in home gardening and nutrition in Bangladesh', *Journal of Development Effectiveness* 8, 473–488, doi:10.1080/19439342.2016.1231704.

Schreinemachers, P., Rai, B. B., Dorji, D., Chen, H.-p., Dukpa, T., Thinley, N., Sherpa, P. L. and Yang, R.-Y. (2017b) 'School gardening in Bhutan: Evaluating outcomes and impact', *Food Security* 9, 635–648, doi:10.1007/s12571-017-0673-3.

Traill, W. B., Mazzocchi, M., Shankar, B. and Hallam, D. (2014) 'Importance of government policies and other influences in transforming global diets', *Nutrition Reviews* 72, 591–604, doi:10.1111/nure.12134.

Triador, L., Farmer, A., Maximova, K., Willows, N. and Kootenay, J. (2015) 'A school gardening and healthy snack program increased aboriginal first nations children's preferences toward vegetables and fruit', *Journal of Nutrition Education and Behavior* 47, 176–180, doi:10.1016/j.jneb.2014.09.002.

Willett, W., Rockstrom, J., Loken, B., Springmann, M., Lang, T., Vermeulen, S., Garnett, T., Tilman, D., DeClerck, F., Wood, A., Jonell, M., Clark, M., Gordon, L. J., Fanzo, J., Hawkes, C., Zurayk, R., Rivera, J. A., De Vries, W., Majele Sibanda, L., Afshin, A., Chaudhary, A., Herrero, M., Agustina, R., Branca, F., Lartey, A., Fan, S., Crona, B., Fox, E., Bignet, V., Troell, M., Lindahl, T., Singh, S., Cornell, S. E., Srinath Reddy, K., Narain, S., Nishtar, S. and Murray, C. J. L. (2019) 'Food in the Anthropocene: The EAT-lancet commission on healthy diets from sustainable food systems', *Lancet* 393, 447–492, doi:10.1016/s0140-6736(18)31788-4.

World Vegetable Center (2016) 'The World Vegetable Center approach to household gardening for nutrition', Shanhua, Taiwan: World Vegetable Center.

9
PARENT ENGAGEMENT IN SUSTAINING THE NUTRITIONAL GAINS FROM SCHOOL-PLUS-HOME GARDENS PROJECT AND SCHOOL-BASED FEEDING PROGRAMMES IN THE PHILIPPINES

The case of the Province of Laguna

Blesilda Calub, Leila S. Africa, and Bessie Burgos

Introduction

School gardens have been promoted in the Philippines as early as the 1970s under various programme titles and priority focus for elementary, secondary, or vocational schools (Salita, 2002; Bauzon, 2009; Inocian and Nuneza, 2015). In 2010, the Department of Education (DepEd) and the Department of Agriculture (DA) promoted the 'Gulayan sa Paaralan Program' (GPP) (vegetable gardens in the schools programme) to address malnutrition by promoting vegetable production and consumption among schoolchildren (DepEd, 2007).

Likewise, the DepEd since 1997 has been implementing School-Based Feeding Programs (SBFP) initially to address short-term hunger among elementary schoolchildren. In 2013, the SBFP was refocussed to address also nutrition among public schoolchildren (DepEd, 2013). This was in response to survey results of the Food and Nutrition Research Institute (FNRI) of the Philippines, which revealed that, among 5- to 10-year-old children, 29% were 'underweight', while 30% were 'stunted' (FNRI, 2013). To further address both under-nutrition and short-term hunger, the DepEd School Health Division covered about 0.53M severely wasted[1] (SW) and 1.38M wasted (W) schoolchildren from Kindergarten to Grade 6 (DepEd, 2016). The main goals were to (1) improve the nutritional status of the beneficiaries by at least 70% at the end of the 120-day feeding period, (2) increase classroom attendance by 85%, and (3) improve children's health and nutritional values and behaviour. This DepEd Memorandum also mandated that '... all schools shall establish and maintain the "*Gulayan sa Paaralan* Program" as a source of ingredients for the SBFP and shall encourage the families of the beneficiaries to have their own home gardens'. However, effective implementation on the ground varied among schools.

The results of an impact study by the Philippine Institute for Development Studies (PIDS) for school year 2013–2014 showed that, among severely wasted children, about 62% attained normal nutritional status at the end of the feeding programme. This falls short of the 70% target due to factors beyond the control of the SBFP implementers, specifically characteristics and practices of beneficiary families, parents and the children themselves. Logistic regression analysis of the 1,081 families sampled indicated that severely wasted children living in rural villages with at least one parent or guardian having some college education, and whose family has access to safe water supply are more likely to improve normal nutritional status.

On the other hand, children who were less likely to gain normal nutritional status were those whose parents said that the SBFP food served was at times inadequate and those severely wasted children residing in rural villages who bring home some of their SBFP food to share with family members (PIDS, 2015; Tabunda et al., 2016). Thus, in the school years from 2012–2013 to 2013–2014, about 38% of the children who remained undernourished during the study became repeat beneficiaries for the next school year's SBFP. For three consecutive school years (2012–2013, 2013–2014, and 2014–2015), at least 14% of children under the SBFP were repeat beneficiaries. This means that among the undernourished children who gained normal status after the 120-day school feeding period, about half reverted back to being wasted or severely wasted (PIDS, 2015; Tabunda et al., 2016) due to inadequate and less nutritious food in their homes for the remaining days of the year.

Overview of the School Plus Home Gardens Project (S+HGP)

According to the World Health Organization, children with stunted growth could exhibit reduced cognitive, motor, and language development. Eventually, this translates to long-term consequences of poor school performance, reduced learning capacity, and unachieved overall potential (WHO, 2017).

The Philippines is one of 34 countries with the highest burden of stunting (Zulfiqar et al., 2013) due to malnutrition. Filipino children's malnutrition is a national concern due to its negative economic impact on the children's educational attainment (low grades attained and grade-level repetition), on future economic productivity (reduced productivity of stunted workforce and low wage prospects), the workforce population (45% of child mortality due to malnutrition results to complete loss of human resources), and health costs (susceptibility to diarrhoea, respiratory infections, and anaemia) (Lebanan et al., 2016). Another primary concern for the future of food security in the country is the youth's declining interest in agriculture (FAO-CTA-IFAD, 2014; AFA, 2015).

Thus, the Southeast Asian Regional Center for Graduate Study and Research in Agriculture (SEARCA), the University of the Philippines Los Baños (UPLB), and the DepEd in Laguna Province (DepEd Laguna) jointly implemented a participatory action research programme (Figure 9.1) to address these problems. This was piloted in six schools in Laguna with specific objectives: namely to increase the diversity and availability of food to meet the nutritional needs of

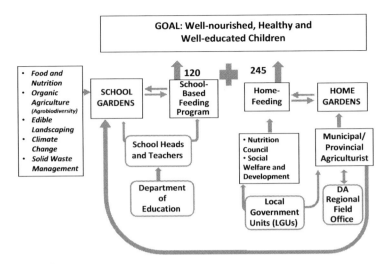

FIGURE 9.1 Operational model of the School-Plus-Home Gardens Project (S+HGP).
Source: Calub et al. (2017).

children; to increase the knowledge and improve the skills of students and teachers with regards to food production and nutrition through experiential learning activities; and to reduce food expenses, create savings, and provide an alternative source of income for families to alleviate poverty.

Initially known as the School Gardens Project (SGP), it was later renamed 'School-Plus-Home Gardens Project' (S+HGP) to draw attention to the 'plus' factors that significantly contributed to the key accomplishments and self-sustaining scaling up of the project. 'Plus' refers to the:

1. project's success in mobilizing parents to take on the challenge and develop a greater sense of responsibility to be involved in the nutrition of their children—by actively helping tend the school gardens and building their own home gardens;
2. project's success in complementing the 120-day SBFP by promoting year-round production of nutritious food coming from both the school and home gardens, particularly during the remaining period of the year that is not covered by the SBFP;
3. strong collaboration among stakeholders, particularly the local government units' (LGUs) committed support to the schools and homes—by allocating funds for garden inputs, providing capacity-building services, and directly assigning some personnel to assist teachers in maintaining the school gardens or helping parents establish food gardens in their homes;
4. multiple functions of the school and home gardens as a source of supplemental food, nutrition, and income (see Boxes 9.1 and 9.2 about learning gardens and inspirational pocket landscape); and project's contribution to stimulating children's interest in agriculture.

> **BOX 9.1: THE SCHOOL GARDEN AS A LEARNING GARDEN**
>
> The S+HGP promoted the use of the school garden for teaching Math, Science, English, and Home Economics/Technology Livelihood Education. The students enjoyed the walk to the gardens and easily learned the lessons on Math (i.e. counting seedlings, weighing the harvests – great lessons on fractions and decimal points!), Science (observing plant growth and development, comparing plant life cycles, decomposition/composting), and English (identification of local and English names of the plants, writing poems and short paragraphs about observations in the garden).

> **BOX 9.2: THE SCHOOL GARDEN AS AN INSPIRATIONAL POCKET LANDSCAPE**
>
> The S+HGP promoted 'Edible Landscaping', which gave an aesthetic dimension to the school garden. In schools with limited land area, they managed to convert small spaces into pocket gardens using diverse colours and shapes of vegetable plants. Both the big and pocket (small) gardens became attractive and interesting for students. Curious about how the gardens were evolving, the children visited the school gardens often, taking pictures of the growing flowers and fruits as well as their 'selfies'.

Mechanisms for sustaining and scaling up the initial success of the S+HGP were designed in a stepwise process where each of six pilot schools took the lead to pay forward and share their knowledge to at least three other sister schools. In turn, the sister schools also adopted other schools, particularly the small ones in remote areas. From the original six pilot schools in 2016, there is now a growing network of 40 adopted sister schools with corresponding partner parents and LGUs.

This chapter presents the project strategies that contributed to the success in engaging parents in the nutrition of their children and families. Parents' appreciation of the social, personal, family, economic, and environmental benefits they gained from engaging in school and home gardening, as well as some challenges and issues, is also discussed.

Profile of families of undernourished students

Most of the case study households ($n = 45$) of the undernourished schoolchildren from the six partner schools have 3–10 members, where 3 out of 4 children are 13 years old or younger (Calub et al., 2017). Parents' ages ranged from 32 to 58 years. Either one or both parents per household was able to work and earn wages as factory or building construction workers, delivery crew, cooks, bakers, sales staff, security personnel, teacher, house helpers, laundry staff, gardeners, tailor, beauty shop staff, or carpenters.

The household income ranged from about USD 60 to 700 per month with an average of USD 75. To augment this, particularly those in rural villages, some have vegetable gardens, raise pigs, go fishing, and sell clothes, food products, and charcoal. Some households occasionally received remittances from older children or their relatives working in the cities or abroad. Household income was mainly spent for food (74%), transportation (11%), house electricity and water (7%), children's education (4%), healthcare and medicines (3%), and other items. Most of these families lived in limited spaces (about 57–112 m^2) that were either owned or rented, or inherited or were allowed free use by relatives or friends. Almost half of the number of households have access to a nearby vacant lot for gardening. About 33% of the households have existing vegetable gardens; 16% used to have vegetable gardens, but now don't, while 51% never had a home garden. Of those who never had home gardens, 87% were actually interested to start their home gardens, while 13% were not interested for various reasons (Table 9.1).

About two years after the S+HGP ended, the number of households with established home gardens has doubled. They continued to maintain or expand their home gardens with or without malnourished children in their families.

TABLE 9.1 Home gardening experience of the respondent households

Experience with home gardens	Percentage of respondents	Respondents' reasons
Currently have home gardens	33	• Fondness for vegetable gardening was inherited from parents; It is a hobby; they know how to grow vegetables, so they started a garden; household received planting materials, so they decided to use them. • The family loves eating vegetables. • To encourage their children to eat vegetables. • To generate extra income.
Never had a home garden but interested to have one	44	• Can provide food for the family and generate savings. • Harvests can be sold to neighbours, thus augmenting household income. • To be able to ensure that their food source is clean. • To have a convenient, easily accessible, and almost unlimited source of vegetables. • Husband likes farming. • Household members like to eat vegetables.

Experience with home gardens	Percentage of respondents	Respondents' reasons
Used to have a home garden but now not anymore	16	• Husband who tends the garden went overseas to work. • The household member who tends the garden passed away. • The family moved to a new house which does not have space for a garden. • The family sold the lot that was once used for vegetable gardening. • They used to sell marketable produce from the garden but decided to shift to a more profitable income-generating activity.
Never had a home garden and not interested to have one	7	• Not interested. • More interested to raise pigs than vegetables. • No time because of household chores or paid work. • No available space for even a small garden.

Source: Calub et al. (2017).

Strategies to engage and sustain parents' participation

Strategies that contributed to the success in engaging parents in the nutrition of their children and families included a combination of participatory development approaches, capacity building of the key stakeholders (i.e. teachers and parents), and close collaboration with LGUs.

Participatory development approaches

Participatory development approaches facilitate the process where people can build their capacity towards self-management. Stakeholders are enabled to be actively involved in identifying and analyzing their problems, defining and refining strategies to address constraints and jointly make decisions to take action, and attaining agreed-upon goals and priorities (Chambers, 1994; Pretty et al., 1995)

The teachers underwent participatory planning and coordinating workshops together with their school heads, school garden coordinators, and teachers-in-charge of school feeding and school canteen. They then gained confidence in using the same participatory approaches to engage the parents in school gardening and feeding.

Stepwise capacity building of key stakeholders

Initially, a series of capacity building activities for teachers and school heads promoted better understanding about sustainability concepts and inter-relationships of food and nutrition, cultivation of traditional lesser-known crops, organic agriculture, edible landscaping, climate change, and solid waste management. Combined with practical experience, they were able to prepare a total of 120 lesson plans integrating those concepts. Towards the end of S+HGP implementation, the teachers gained enough confidence to be able to adopt sister schools and pass on to them their knowledge and experiences in promoting the S+HGP, including how to mobilize parents, LGUs, village heads, and village councillors.

Building on existing parent-teacher associations (PTA)

The teachers built upon the long-established PTA in the Philippines. The teachers mobilized the PTA in every grade level and every partner school to focus on helping set up and maintain the school gardens to supply harvests to the SBFP. During school card giving days, teachers used the opportunity for one-on-one talks with parents not just about children's school grades but informing them that academic performance is linked to their children's nutritional status. Teachers encouraged parents to establish their own home gardens to provide nutritious food for their children beyond the 120 days school feeding. Parents learned that better nutrition and food supply translated to better health and academic performance of their children. Thus, many parents with or without malnourished children voluntarily gave their time and labour for the school gardens as well as in establishing their home gardens. Some of the pilot schools allotted areas inside their campuses to enable landless parents to do group gardening. The parents organized themselves and agreed on a schedule for them to take turns in tending the gardens. In one school, the parents formed themselves into the 'Association of Parents with Gardens in the School'.

Extension services and supporting policies from government units

In order to support both the school gardens and parents' home gardens, the LGUs, and village heads were invited to join the participatory planning workshops with the teachers. As a result, the Municipal Agriculture Office provided the schools and parents with garden inputs, some infrastructure, and extension services usually allocated for farmers only. As the S+HGP gained momentum, the Department of Agriculture Regional Field Office – Organic Agriculture Program also included the schools in their list of beneficiaries of vermicomposting facilities, shredding machines, and greenhouses. Other LGU offices such as the Municipal Nutrition Action Office (MNAO), the Municipal Social Welfare and Development Office (MSWDO), and some Municipal/City Nutrition Councils also joined in. Existing school programmes of the Department of Health such as vitamin-mineral supplementation and deworming continued to complement the feeding programmes. The local school board of each of the municipalities where the pilot schools were located also provided financial support and inputs. Some village chiefs and village council members crafted village ordinances to strengthen the implementation of school policies. Some of these ordinances were even adopted at the Municipal Council level.

Contests, awards, and recognition

School-organized contests for best school gardens, best home gardens, parent-child cooking contests, and other similar activities promoted friendly competition, fun, and camaraderie among parents, children, and school teachers. During the end-of-school year closing programmes, outstanding parents who helped in the school programmes (particularly in the school gardens and feeding programmes) took pride in receiving recognition certificates. Both parents and teachers were further inspired to give their best when awards and recognition were given by the Municipal and Provincial government units. There was much more encouragement when the S+HGP received awards from a national civic group (Philippine Agriculture and Resources Research Foundation, Inc. [PARRFI] R&D Award: Development Category, 2018) and when one of the partner schools received international awards (SEAMEO-Japan Education for Sustainable Development Award, 2017 [3rd place] and the 2018 SEAMEO-RECFON Partnership in Nutrition Program Award [Best Partnership of Policy Commitment]).

Project accomplishments in improving children's access to food and nutrition

Nutritional gains among undernourished children

Comparison of the baseline and end line nutritional status assessments indicated significant increases in the height, weight, and body mass index (BMI) of students in the pilot elementary and secondary schools. Also, significant increase in knowledge was observed in the vegetables familiarity test, nutrient contents test (types of nutrients contained in vegetables and food group functions (Go, Grow, Glow foods). The schoolchildren likewise appreciated the benefits and importance of eating organic vegetables daily. There was a significant increase in the dietary diversity score of students, which implies that the higher the diversity of food intake, the better the quality of the diet.

Expanded coverage of the SBFP

Because of the improved supply of fresh vegetables from the school and home gardens, all the partner schools were able to complete the required 120-day SBFP. In some schools the SBFP was extended to 20 more days because of the continued availability of vegetables. With the extra harvests from the school gardens there was enough food for all children, and not necessarily only the undernourished children. Students who helped in harvesting vegetables and washing kitchen utensils were allowed to partake some of the food. In another school, 'non-reader' students were allowed to receive food as an incentive for them to attend remedial classes. School feeding coordinators also gave schoolchildren extra fresh or cooked vegetable meals to bring home to their families.

Extending school gardening to home gardening

The gardening-feeding linkage and active participation of teachers, parents, and other stakeholders contributed to food security in the undernourished children's homes particularly after the 120-day SBFP ended. By establishing home gardens, there was a greater chance of children being served some nutritious food in their homes for the remaining days of the year not covered by the SBFP. This also instilled among parents a greater sense of responsibility to be involved in ensuring good food and nutrition for their children.

Two of the six pilot schools directly assisted some parents in establishing and maintaining home gardens. Their workshop participated in by 40 households resulted in nine households immediately establishing their own gardens and applying the techniques they learned about organic vegetable production and edible landscaping. To support these households, the school regularly provided them with seeds saved from the school garden. Regular household visitations and consultations were conducted by the teachers. The school recorded more households inquiring about home gardens. Some households near the schools also requested to be invited to the school gardening training. In another school, through a joint initiative with their Municipal Agriculture Office (MAO), parents of undernourished children underwent training on organic agriculture.

School savings and income generation

About 45.5% of the school garden harvests were used for the 120-day SBFP for undernourished children. This translated to savings for the SBFP. About 19% were shared with students or parents who helped in gardening. Some 10% were used for classes in cooking and food preservation and processing. The remaining 17% was sold in the school canteens, thus providing it some income. About 8% of harvested food was damaged by pests, and this was given to livestock or composted.

Educational aspects of school gardens

Teachers, children, and parents now have better appreciation of the school garden and the feeding programme as they see the linkage between what they plant in the garden and food they can harvest and eat later. This observation indicates the importance of not only showing vegetables during the nutrition education classes or cooking classes but also undergoing the chain of activities involved between food production and consumption. Additionally, the school gardens were living laboratories for experiential learning about Science, Math, English, and Home Economics (Calub et al., 2018). Teachers prepared lessons plans that integrated the concepts of organic agriculture (including topics on agrobiodiversity and environmental sustainability), edible landscaping, solid waste management, and climate change. Both the school and home gardens gave children and parents some opportunities to learn business skills and entrepreneurship. Teachers, parents, children, and school guests also appreciated the edible landscaping of the school gardens.

They liked spending time in the garden taking 'selfies' for sharing in social media. Overall these contribute to increasing the youth's interest in agriculture.

Project outcomes enhanced by parent engagement in S+HGP

Assured supply of nutritious vegetables from the school and home gardens

As a key component under the S+HGP, teachers-in-charge of the feeding programmes and the school gardening programme were encouraged to coordinate closely with each other. Teacher coordinators of the feeding programme planned their menu and prepared meals based on the available vegetables harvested from their school gardens. The school garden teachers were encouraged to plant highly nutritious vegetables that were needed for the feeding programme. They were taught to prepare crop planting calendars where a large array of annual and perennial crops were planted and timed so that they can be harvested at different periods of the year (Table 9.2).

Many parents appreciated the crop planting calendar and applied it in their home gardens. This enabled them to produce vegetables year-round and ensure the availability of vegetables for their families.

Diet diversity through garden diversity

Where there used to be 1–2 crop species only, most of the school and home gardens now have 10–20 species of vegetables, like *'kulitis'* (*Amaranthus spinosus*); root crops, like *camote* (*Ipomoea batatas*) for tubers and young leaves; semi-perennial legumes, like pigeon pea, *Cajanus cajan*), and winged bean (*Psophocarpus tetragonolobus*); tree vegetables, like *malunggay* (*Moringa oleifera*); shrubs, like *lagikway* (*Abelmoschus manihot*), *saluyot* (*Corchorus olitorius*), and 'talinum' (*Talinum paniculatum*); and small-sized fruit trees, like guava, papaya, banana, and *calamansi* (*Citrus microcarpa*), an indigenous local citrus rich in vitamin C and A. The diversity in the crops planted and integration of perennial crops ensured diversity of the family's diet and year-round supply of nutritious food for the family. Some parents and teachers brought and exchanged seeds and planting materials as well as cooking techniques. This revived the interest and knowledge on lesser-known traditional but nutritious vegetables.

Reduced number of repeaters in the school feeding programme

Repeaters refer to students who participated in the SBFP, gained normal weight after the 120-day feeding period but became wasted again during the school break that in the next school year they were re-enrolled in the SBFP. The percentage of the SBFP repeaters in two of the 5 partner elementary schools (B and C) considerably decreased by the end of the S+HGP implementation and even one year after the S+HGP ended (Figure 9.2). These were the schools where parents have established

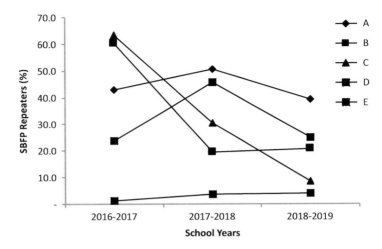

FIGURE 9.2 Trends in the percentage of SBFP repeaters among partner schools from school years 2016–2019.
Source: Original survey data of this paper.

their home gardens in 2016–2017 (S+HGP started) and continued until 2018–2019 (18 months after S+HGP ended). More parents got involved in home gardening in the succeeding years, thus the continued reduction in the number of repeaters.

In schools A and D, there was an increase in the number of repeaters in 2017–2018 (S+HGP ended). The teachers claimed that initially they focussed more on the school garden development. Later when they extended gardening to the homes the number of repeaters dropped considerably in the next school year. Meanwhile, School E is a big school in an urban area with the highest number of SBFP participants. Most parents were not able to establish home gardens due to no or very limited space to establish gardens. Other parents were preoccupied working for daily wages. For these urbanizing areas, container and vertical gardening are options, but it is also important to provide other supporting interventions so that parents can still be actively engaged in the nutrition of their children.

Improving children's consumption of vegetables

Among undernourished children, 85% continued to eat vegetables with an additional 8% who have learned to eat vegetables in their homes (Table 9.2). A previous SBFP beneficiary in 2016 claimed that he has now gained weight and is taller because he regularly eats vegetables cooked at home. As a child he did not like the taste of vegetables. Now he has learned to like them when he learned about the nutrients they contain. On the other hand, 6% of children used to eat vegetables, but at the time of survey, they did so rarely because their mothers were not always able to serve them in their meals. A remaining 1% still did not eat vegetables.

Benefits realized and challenges encountered

Parents realized that while they were actively involved in sustaining the nutritional gains of their children, they also gained social, personal, family, economic, and environmental benefits from their home gardens (Table 9.3).

TABLE 9.2 Changes in vegetable consumption among households of undernourished students from the start to the end of the project

Indicators	Changes from pre-assessment to post-assessment (after 14 months)	
	n	%
Children eating vegetable		
Yes to Yes	123	85
No to Yes	12	8
Yes to No	8	6
No to No	2	1

Source: Calub et al. (2017).

TABLE 9.3 Feedback from parents about benefits derived from and challenges faced in participating in school gardens and having their own home gardens

Benefits		Challenges
Social	• Sharing of harvested vegetables to family, neighbours, friends, and relatives (74.3%) • Met other parents, gained friends, and became closer to neighbours (8.6%) • Showed kindness to others by sharing seeds/planting materials (8.6%) • Able to set an example of doing good deeds for others (8.6%)	• Some stray animals from farms eat our crops • Some people pre-harvest our crops
Personal	• Realized that gardening as a form of exercise is good for their health, garden as a source of safe food, children gained normal weight and seldom got sick (38.3%) • Have positive feelings of happiness, accomplishment and sense of fulfilment, garden work is tiresome but worth the effort, receiving compliments from others and being recognized in the community, happy to teach others about gardening, enable production of own organic fertilizers and seeds, desire to expand home gardens (31.9%). • Gardening as stress reliever, provides mental relaxation, keeps us busy and is a productive pastime (29.8%).	• Requires diligence to work in the garden • We lack time to expand our garden because we have other work to do. • There were parents who were not much concerned with their children's food because they said anyway the school will feed them.

(*Continued*)

	Benefits	Challenges
Family	• Gardening strengthened family bonding, now a family hobby, family members work together and share the meal from their harvests. We feel assured to feed our family year-round with safe, clean, organic, and nutritious food (35.9%). • Children learned gardening, enjoying and being of help in the family. Gardens educate children better than being hooked to computer games (28.2%). • Whole family feels healthy with improved appetite for vegetables harvested from the garden and cooked at home (20.5%). • Children learned to eat vegetables more easily when they see other family members also eating vegetables; children now ask for vegetable dishes (15.4%).	• Some children take time to learn or have not really learned to eat vegetables • Some children like to eat vegetables but some parents do not cook them for family meals. Some parents do not eat vegetables.
Economic	• Provides savings on food purchases, we rarely buy vegetables (62.7%) • Provides additional income opportunity from the sale of extra harvests. Establishing gardens is not costly, requires minimal purchase of inputs because we can make our own organic fertilizers and produce own seeds, especially of traditional crops (33.3%) • Income from gardens was used for payment of some school needs (3.9%)	• Some pests and rats damage our plants, resulting in low yields • Where can we sell our harvests if we produce more? • We have low entrepreneurial skills • Limited space for garden expansion
Environmental	• Fresh air, no pollution, no pesticide spraying, thus better for our health (50.0%) • Conscious not to throw garbage anywhere, learned recycling and composting, kept surroundings clean (26.3%) • The landscaped gardens are attractive, encouraged children to go to the garden, children take 'selfies' in the garden. (23.7%) • The beautiful school gardens enticed parents to establish their home gardens to promote year-round supply of vegetables which they don't have to buy.	• Flooding • Heavy rains submerge our plots • We cannot plant during the dry season due to lack of water and strong sun.

Source: Original survey data of this paper.

Some challenges met were also expressed by the parents. Among the challenges mentioned by the parents, climate change manifestations (flooding, heavy rains, and drought tendency) and pest damage are the biggest threats to agricultural production and thus to food security. Marketing systems can open opportunities for households who can expand their home gardens for income generation. For families with limited or no access to land, technologies on container and vertical gardening can be considered. Strategies to overcome all these challenges will require at least start-up support for investments in protected agriculture structures.

Conclusions

The SEARCA-UPLB-DepEd Laguna S+HGP demonstrates a strategy where schools and parents were mobilized and engaged in school and home gardening towards food security and improved nutrition. It strengthened the coordinated implementation of two existing nation-wide programmes of DepEd, the school gardens programme and the SBFP for undernourished children. In addition to the school's efforts the need for greater parent engagement was emphasized. Activities were initiated for values and skills strengthening so that parents gained a greater sense of responsibility in ensuring nutritious food for their children through year-round production of vegetables from the school gardens and from their home gardens. Factors that contributed to successfully engaging parents included regular joint parent-teacher consultations; participatory planning; implementation and monitoring; hands-on training and seminars; parent-child tandem cooking contests using vegetables harvested from the school gardens; and close collaboration with the local government units in providing garden inputs, services, and supporting policies.

This approach is key to the currently continuing scaling up from the 6 original and 2 adopted partner schools to 46 adopted sister schools. While initially intended only for parents of undernourished children many other parents have joined in tending the school gardens and have also established their home gardens. Parents have come to realize that in actively sustaining the nutrition of their children they also gained additional social, personal, family, economic, and environmental benefits by having school and home gardens.

The S+HGP is flexible; thus, other schools would be able to adapt and tailor it into their localities. Interventions need not be totally new but can build upon existing school institutions: for example the PTA. It is also important to encourage the participation of LGUs and village institutions for their vital support and services in order to sustain the school and home gardens.

Through participatory engagement among teachers, parents, and LGUs, our children's and their families' food and nutrition, education, health, and economic well-being can be uplifted. This process is a first step in increasing and sustaining the availability of vegetables in children's homes and schools and in scaling up towards inclusive and sustainable community development that addresses food and nutrition security and poverty reduction in the Philippines and elsewhere.

Acknowledgements

Acknowledgement is expressed to the Asian Development Bank and the Japan Fund for Poverty Reduction through SEAMEO College for initial funding, SEARCA for continued fund support and overall coordination, UPLB for technical expertise and assistance, DepEd Division of Laguna, Education Program Supervisor (Mr Lamberto Perolina) for schools coordination, all the participating pilot school heads, teachers, parents, children, and LGUs, and SEARCA Staff (R. B. Lapitan, E. G. C. Sencida, X. G. B. Capiña, D. B. N. Malayang, L. A. M. Carandang, M. H. D Teve), UPLB staff (H. E. Carandang), University of California Santa Cruz graduate student S. Chiang, and UN University graduate student E. I. N. E. Galang for field survey assistance.

Note

1 A child is considered severely wasted when his or her body weight is below three standard deviations from the median weight-for-height or is considered wasted when the child's weight-for-height is lower than two standard deviations from the growth standard. The DepEd uses the World Health Organization (WHO) weight-for-age tables for pre-primary schoolchildren aged 5 years old and below, and the WHO body mass index-for-age tables from pre-primary, primary, and secondary students aged 6-19 years old in determining the nutrition status.

References

Asian Farmers' Association for Sustainable Rural Development (AFA) (2015) 'A Viable Future: Attracting the Youth to Agriculture', AFA Issue Paper Vol 7 (1), Quezon City, Philippines.

Bauzon, P.T. (2009) 'Foundations of Curriculum Development' 2nd ed, Rex Bookstore, Mandaluyong City, Philippines In Inocian and Nuneza, 2015.

Calub, B.M., Africa L.S., Burgos, BM., Custodio, H.M., Vallez A.G.C., Galang, E.I.N. (2017) 'SEARCA-UPLB-DepEd [Southeast Asian Regional Center for Graduate Study and Research in Agriculture, University of the Philippines Los Banos, and Department of Education Laguna] 2017 - A Participatory Action Research on School- and Community-based Food and Nutrition Program for Literacy, Poverty Reduction and Sustainable Development', Final Report, Laguna, Philippines.

Calub, B.B., Africa, L.S., Burgos, B.M., Custodio, H.M, Chiang, S.N., Galvez, A.G.Z. and Galang, E.I.N.E. (2018) 'Linking School Gardening and Feeding: Experience from the School-Plus-Home Gardens Project (S+HGP) in the Philippines', Proceedings of the 2018 Asia-Pacific Societies for Agricultural and Food Ethics (APSafe), Taipei City, Taiwan.

Chambers, R. (1994) 'Participatory Rural Appraisal (PRA): Challenges, Potentials and Paradigm', World Development, Vol. 22, No. 10, 1437–1454.

DepEd (2007) '*Gulayan sa Paaralan* (Vegetable Gardens in Schools), Memo # 293 s 2007', http://www.deped.gov.ph/wp-content/uploads/2018/10/DM_s2007_293.pdf, accessed May 2019.

DepEd (2013) 'DepEd Memorandum No. 191, Series of 2013. Implementation of the Health and Nutrition Center (HCN)-Funded *Gulayan sa Paaralan Program* (GPP) Assisted by the Department of Agriculture-Bureau of Plant Industry (DA-BPI)'.

DepEd (2016) 'DepEd Order No. 51, Series of 2016. Implementation of the School-Based Feeding Program for School Year 2016–2017. Issued by DepEd Secretary Br. Armin A. Luistro, FSC'.

Food and Agriculture Organization, United Nations (FAO), Technical Centre for Agricultural and Rural Cooperation (CTA) and International Fund for Agricultural Development (IFAD) (2014) 'Youth and agriculture: Key challenges and concrete solutions', FAO, Rome.

Food and Nutrition Research Institute, Department of Science and Technology (FNRI) (2013) '8th National Nutrition Survey: Philippines'.

Inocian, R.B. and Nuneza, L.M. (2015) 'The *Gulayan sa Paaralan* (School Vegetable Garden) in Response to Sustainable Development' *European Scientific Journal*, Vol. 11 No. 8, ISSN 1857-7881.

Lebanan, M.A., Antipolo, J.V., Lamac, M.R. and Borja, A. (2016) 'Cost of Hunger: Philippines', Save the Children Philippines.

Philippine Institute for Development Studies (PIDS) (2015) 'Policy Notes 15-01. Feeding severely wasted children in school: Examining processes in DepED's School Feeding Program' http://dirp4.pids.gov.ph/webportal/CDN/PUBLICATIONS/pidspn1501.pdf, accessed Mar 17, 2018.

Pretty, J.N., Guijt, I., Thompson, J. and Scoones, I. (1995) 'A trainer's guide for participatory learning and action', International Institute for Environment and Development (IIED), UK, accessible from https://pubs.iied.org/pdfs/6021IIED.pdf.

Salita, D.C. (2002) 'Environmental Geography', JMC Press, Inc. Quezon City, Philippines.

Tabunda, A.M.L., Albert, J.R.G. and Agdeppa, I.A. (2016) 'Results of an impact evaluation study of DepEd's school-based feeding program', PIDS Discussion Paper Series 2016-05, https://dirp3.pids.gov.ph/websitecms/CDN/PUBLICATIONS/pidsdps1605.pdf, accessed Mar 17, 2018.

World Health Organization (WHO) (2017) 'Stunted Growth and Development, Context, Causes and Consequences', World Health Organization.

Zulfiqar, A.B., Das, J.K., Rizvi A., Gaffey M.F., Walker N., Horton S., Webb, P., Lartey, A. and Black, R.E. (2013) 'Evidence-based interventions for improvement of maternal and child nutrition: what can be done and at what cost?' *The Lancet*, Vol 382, pp. 452–477.

10
SCALING UP THE INTEGRATED SCHOOL NUTRITION MODEL IN THE PHILIPPINES

Experiences and lessons learned

Emilita Monville-Oro, Imelda Angeles-Agdeppa, Irish P. Baguilat, Julian Gonsalves, and Mario V. Capanzana

Introduction

The Philippines' Department of Education (DepEd) instituted a school-based feeding programme (SBFP) as part of the national government's Accelerated Hunger-Mitigation Program (NNC, 2014) and a school gardening programme referred to as *Gulayan sa Paaralan* (Vegetable Gardens in School) Program or GPP (DepEd, 2007), to address hunger and promote better attendance and retention among schoolchildren. Unfortunately, implementation issues and weak links between the two programmes continue to affect the effectiveness and sustainability of the programme. Thus, there is a need to understand these issues and gaps, and try to address them via new models of implementation.

After three years of generating evidence through the integrated school nutrition model (ISNM) (Chapter 4), which features bio-intensive gardening (BIG), supplementary school feeding using iron-fortified rice and promotion of nutrient-rich indigenous vegetables from school gardens, and nutrition education, the model has been systematically expanded from one province (Cavite) in 2015 to 2017 to an entire region comprising 5 provinces (IV-A/Calabarzon) in the Philippines. Initially, 58 lighthouse schools (LSs), which now serve as focal points for research, learning and scaling, were established and are now influencing, at varying levels, 2,732 public elementary schools benefitting a total student population of 1,839,445.

Recognizing the value of the model, DepEd pursued a capacity-building programme to establish additional LSs, targeting at least one LS per school division, all over the Philippines. Through training of trainers, a total of 273 LSs are now installed in 17 regions of the Philippines. The ISNM is now being scaled up in schools across the nation via institutionalization and multi-stakeholder engagement and partnerships. Investments by the government and private sector have been important. Currently, national agencies like the Department of Agriculture, the Department of Social Welfare and Development and the National Nutrition Council of the Department of Health have adopted elements of the model in their own programmes (Oro, 2018).

Background

Schools provide strategic, targeted pathways for delivering nutrition interventions among children and, indirectly, to their families and communities. A 3-year action research project (Phase 1: 2012–2015) implemented by IIRR and the Food and Nutrition Research Institute of the Department of Science and Technology (FNRI-DOST), in partnership with DepEd, with support from the International Development Research Centre (IDRC), developed and tested an ISNM of school gardening, supplementary school feeding, and nutrition education among schoolchildren in Cavite province in the Philippines. Results showed that supplementary feeding of malnourished schoolchildren using iron-fortified rice and indigenous vegetables from school gardens significantly improved their nutritional status (chapter 4) (Oro and Angeles-Agdeppa, 2015a). Enhanced knowledge, attitude, and practices on gardening and nutrition were observed among parents (Oro and Angeles-Agdeppa, 2015b). The project tested and successfully sustained bio-intensive nutrition gardens and crop museums that aimed to retrieve and conserve traditional crop cultivars while improving year-round availability of a diverse range of climate resilient, locally adapted, and nutritionally important vegetables (Oro and Angeles-Agdeppa, 2015c).

Phase 2 (2017–2018) of this project focussed on more in-depth understanding and operationalization of the integrated model by expanding the number of research schools. The potential of schools as platforms for nutritional and environmental learning was investigated. Modalities by which local government and private sector, through public-private partnership, can support school nutrition were explored. A multi-scalar approach tested two pathways for scaling up. The first one was directed towards public elementary schools at a sub-national level. The second was directed at national agencies, policy makers, planners, and the media.

Research results were documented, packaged, and disseminated through publications, national and international forums, reports, policy briefs, and other communication materials (IIRR, 2018a). These knowledge products serve as the basis for advocating the ISNM for wider adoption and support by relevant government agencies such as DepEd, Department of Agriculture, Department of Social Welfare and Development, and the National Nutrition Council of the Department of Health. This chapter discusses the process of scaling and the lessons generated from the experience.

Understanding the concepts of scaling

Scaling up defined

Institutionalization and scaling up reflect wider adoption of a proven model, strategy, technology, or an intervention. Clark makes a distinction among three types of scaling up: project replication; building grassroots movements; and, influencing policy reform. The first two are linked to expansion. Fisher also defined scaling up as a process of influencing policy; she uses the term 'scaling out' to describe expansion (Uvin and Miller, 1999).

Scaling up is defined as 'more quality benefits to more people over a wider geographical area more quickly, more equitably and more lastingly' (IIRR, 2000). Going to scale, in general, connotes vertical movement across institutional levels and/or horizontal spread as shown in Figure 10.1.

Horizontal scaling up, sometimes referred to as *scaling out* means geographical expansion to include more communities, institutions, and people. Vertical scaling up refers to higher-level expansion and is institutional in nature. This reflects influence and advocacy to policy makers, donors, development institutions, and investors at national and international levels.

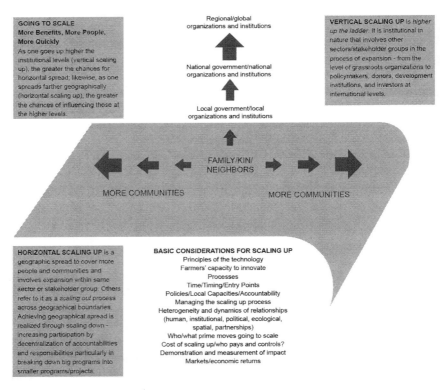

FIGURE 10.1 IIRR's scaling up framework.
Source: IIRR, 2000.

In a comparative review of scaling strategies for research in natural resources management, scaling up was linked to a people-centred vision and highlighted the 'value of time, equity and sustainability dimensions' (Gündel et al., 2001).

Implementing at scale

What to scale?

DepEd implemented two national programmes: the SBFP and the GPP to mitigate hunger and to increase attendance and retention of public elementary students in schools. However, the two programmes have been operating separately, limiting expected outcomes. Through the action research implemented by IIRR, in partnership with FNRI-DOST and DepEd, the ISNM, an innovative approach to school nutrition for better nutrition and educational outcomes, has been developed and is described in detail in chapter 4. The ISNM integrates three major components: (i) Bio-intensive gardens (Gonsalves et al., 2015), (ii) Supplementary feeding of underweight children using iron-fortified rice and indigenous vegetables from school gardens, and (iii) Nutrition education of students, parents/care providers/guardians, and teachers to promote the importance of nutrient dense food and good eating habits. The ISNM offers a way to achieve better nutritional outcomes, which are linked to good educational outcomes. It also ensures sustainability of the gains in school nutrition programmes while optimizing benefits from limited resources.

How to scale? The multi-scalar approach to scaling

The initial three-year (2012–2015) research generated evidence on the effectiveness of the ISNM in addressing under-nutrition among children. Based on lessons generated, the model was refined and implemented at a wider scale to achieve greater nutritional outcomes through institutionalization, wider adoption, better linkages, increased investments, and enabling policies to support integrated school nutrition programming.

Utilizing a multi-scalar approach, the ISNM was brought to scale through two pathways (Figure 10.2). The first pathway was via horizontal scaling where ISNM was institutionalized in public elementary schools in one province (Cavite) and expanded at sub-national level – that is from Cavite province to Region IV-A Calabarzon (comprising of five provinces – Cavite, Laguna, Batangas, Rizal, and Quezon). Schools were selected and designated as LSs, which are focal points for research, learning, sharing, and dissemination hubs of integrated school nutrition innovations (IIRR, 2018b). A critical mass of 58 LSs (40 in Cavite province and 18 in other provinces of Region IV-A) were established, from whom other public elementary schools in Cavite and Region IV-A learned. The LSs also served as crop museums (IIRR, 2017), which are relevant in reintroducing agrobiodiversity as nutritionally important to schools and surrounding communities.

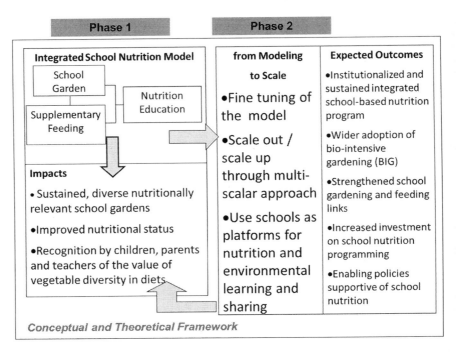

FIGURE 10.2 Research conceptual and theoretical framework.
Source: IIRR.

The second pathway (Figure 10.3) was via vertical scaling aimed at the national level, influencing relevant national agencies, policy makers, and decision makers through thematic presentations and related dialogue processes. Through partnership building and networking the wider nutrition community, which includes non-governmental organizations (NGOs), international donors, private (including corporate social responsibility pathways) and public sector, they were engaged towards building a community of practice for school-based nutrition. The platforms and associated knowledge products that came out of the action research influenced national government policy and planning processes to generate impact at the national level, including new policy guidelines in school-based feeding and additional resource allocation in the school nutrition programme.

Learning about scaling up

Experiences from the research project pointed to various issues and dimensions that need to be considered to ensure effective implementation and later up-scaling of an integrated nutrition programme in schools. A scalable, self-sustaining, and effective programme for integrated nutrition programming for Philippines schools must

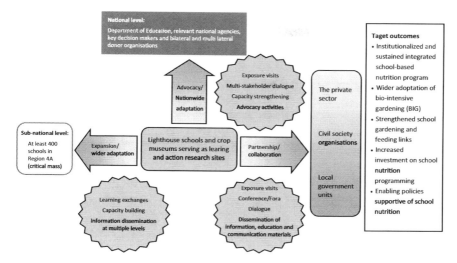

FIGURE 10.3 Multi-scalar scaling up strategy.
Source: IIRR.

have the following attributes: (1) the programme is supported by administrators, students, and parents at all relevant levels. For this to happen, schools must be able to gain capacity to adapt the programme based on their local context; (2) the programme is consistent with the governments' education and nutrition objectives and policies; (3) it is supported by appropriate educational resources including garden space, learning resources, linkages to curricula for different subjects; (4) it is supported financially, including contributions from school budgets, NGOs, local governments, and the private sector; and (5) it generates strong synergies among the different elements, including nutrition, agricultural, and environmental education.

Strategies, methods and lessons

It was the intent of the research project to establish a critical mass of schools implementing the ISNM and to generate evidence-based policy recommendations that would enhance existing school-based nutrition programmes to address school-aged malnutrition. Thus, at the outset, strategies for scaling out (to expand coverage of the adoption), as well as scaling up (influencing policies for national adoption), were developed and deployed. Below is a discussion of key strategies and methods, as well as lessons generated from them.

Enabling environment at the national and sub-national level is necessary for scaling up

The enabling policy environment is key to sustaining and implementing the school nutrition programme at a larger scale. This must be backed up by the commitment of school authorities headed by DepEd secretary, directors, supervisors, and principals, to ensure implementation. One of the important requirements for adoption and implementation of the model is the issuance of memorandum orders since DepEd still follows a centralized set-up. In 2016, memoranda were issued, which included the bio-intensive gardening approach in the national guidelines of the GPP (DepEd Memorandum No. 223, s. 2016) (DepEd, 2016a); use of iron-fortified rice and recipes with indigenous vegetables for feeding in the SBFP national guidelines (DepEd Order No. 39, s. 2017) (DepEd, 2017a); and establishment of crop museums in every school division (DepEd Memorandum No. 223, s. 2016). At the regional level, two government memoranda were sent to all the 19 divisions of Region IV-A in support of the implementation of the nutrition model and establishment of additional crop museums (Regional Memorandum No. 226, s. 2016 and Regional Memorandum No. 446, s. 2017) (DepEd, 2016b; 2017b). These served as legal documents that allowed school administrators to incorporate activities into their school improvement plan, and in turn allowed them to allocate resources to strengthen the programme. The results from the Phase 1 study as well as the information, education, and communication materials developed were instrumental in setting up a supportive enabling environment.

LSs: focal point for horizontal scaling

A LS is a designated focal point school used for establishing evidence (decentralized and location-specific action research site for the ISNM) to support the advocacy and out-scaling efforts of school nutrition by DepEd. Every LS is expected to demonstrate the ISNM, which features a regular feeding programme, a well-maintained and sustained bio-intensive garden, and related school-based nutrition education activities that are strongly linked with each other. For this to happen, a comprehensive capacity-building package, which includes training of trainers and learning exchanges, implementation guidelines, and starter diversity kits (seeds and planting materials) and innovative information, education, and communication materials, was provided to all LSs.

Fifty-eight LSs were established within Region IV-A (Figure 10.4). Learning and sharing events were conducted in LSs. Trained teachers were given the responsibility to train other teachers within their respective school districts or school divisions. A total of 1,598 schools and 626 parents were reached. Inter-division learning exchanges and benchmarking activities were conducted across the region. In addition, LSs shared seeds with other schools within their own division.

The role of crop museums

The 58 LSs were also designated as crop museums (Figure 10.5). Crop museums in schools serve as a focal point for collecting and saving varieties, especially nutritionally relevant crops. This is a garden where teachers, students, and community members can view a diverse range of nutritionally relevant and

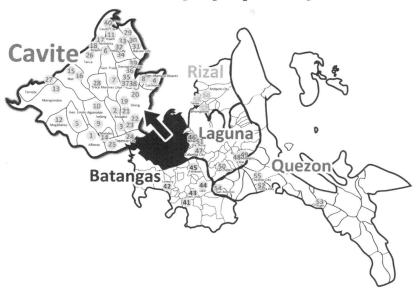

FIGURE 10.4 Distribution of LSs in Region IV-A.
Source: IIRR.

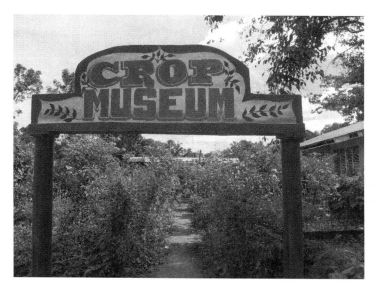

FIGURE 10.5 Crop museum.
Source: IIRR.

climate hardy vegetables. Crop museums also serve as nurseries (source of planting materials) for surrounding schools and communities.

School crop museums played a key role in the dispersal of planting materials across the 19 school divisions in Region IV-A. An additional 237 school crop museums were designated in Region IV-A. IIRR extended support including planting materials and information, education, and communication materials. The goal is to have one crop museum per school district (comprising around 10 schools).

Seed exchange was another event that was successfully institutionalized within Region IV-A to facilitate retrieval from farmers and households and popularization of indigenous/local vegetables and promote self-reliance among school divisions. Eighteen school divisions from Region IV-A were able to conduct seed exchange involving 1,359 schools during the duration of the Phase 2 of the project. Seed exchanges contributed to the conservation of agrobiodiversity and promoted garden diversification.

In 2018, DepEd invested in supporting the establishment of another 215 LSs and crop museums in each school division nationwide. Orientations and trainings, as well as provision of materials, that is, planting materials and information, education, and communication materials, were provided. This then expanded the network of the LSs and crop museums to 273 in 17 regions of the Philippines, already representing nationwide reach. In the next five years, it is anticipated that the ISNM will be implemented in every school in the Philippines.

Multi-level capacity-building programme for school programme implementers

The capacity-building programme was designed not only for school level implementers but also school officials and programme planners at various levels of DepEd. The programme includes training of trainers; consultative workshop with school principals; orientation of division-level school officials; learning and sharing events (Figure 10.6); and provision of information, education, and communication materials, basic garden tools, planting materials, and on-site coaching and mentoring of local actors. Prior to the training, the research team developed a training-of-trainers manual, which was provided to LSs. A series of orientation events for school officials were held at the national level to generate interest and support. For technical assistance of local actors, it is important to consider the staff movement within the DepEd system in planning and programming to avoid unplanned re-training/re-orientation.

Generating evidence for influencing policies

Evidence for the effectiveness of the integrated nutrition approach has to be established as a basis for adopting the approach on a wider scale. The project worked on the assumption that scaling up and institutionalization of innovations

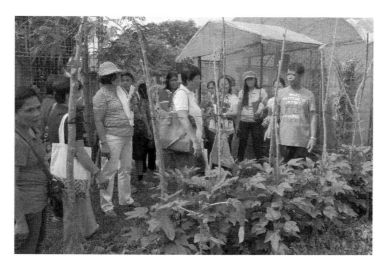

FIGURE 10.6 School visits/exchanges.
Source: IIRR.

rely on evidence of its effectiveness and scalability. Evidence generated in Phases 1 and 2 of the programme (IIRR, 2018c) played a major role in influencing national-level programme planners to adopt the model and allocate resources for nationwide dissemination. The establishment of 58 LSs led to wide-scale data collection. Baseline and end line data were collected and analyzed to serve as basis for recommendations and policy formulation. Teachers played a significant role in documenting activities and data within their respective schools. Results from the research were packaged into knowledge products that were shared with various stakeholders, sectors, and national agencies. Advocacy activities through roundtable discussions, exposure visits, multi-stakeholder dialogues, bilateral meetings, and active participation and sharing in national conferences have been effective platforms in raising interest and influencing other government agencies and programme plans.

Broad-based partnership for school nutrition

Scaling up efforts also paved the way for partnerships with the different national agencies. The Department of Agriculture – Bureau of Plant and Industry supported a national level training on the ISNM to regional representatives of DepEd and Department of Agriculture coming from the 17 regions of the Philippines. The Department of Social Welfare and Development (DSWD) saw the potential of the ISNM to day care centres (child development centres), which cater to younger children aged 3–5 years old. Within the last three years, DSWD Region IV-A has been investing in orienting select day care centre workers and local governments on the ISNM. Finally, the National Nutrition Council of the

Department of Health recognized the potential of the ISNM to contribute to efforts in scaling up nutrition interventions and to help the country achieve its commitments to the Sustainable Development Goals (SDGs), which included wider uptake of the model within the DepEd, as part of the country's PPAN – Philippine Plan of Action for Nutrition 2017–2022.

Fostering better information and resource sharing through dialogue platforms

Multi-stakeholder dialogue and advocacy events that increased awareness, improved coordination and enhanced convergence of the various stakeholders, targeting different segmented audiences are key elements of scaling up. Round table discussion and targeted discussion were organized with key decision makers and officials, and resulted in positive outputs. The project team met with different key officials of DepEd at the start of the project to secure needed support and to ensure adoption by schools. Study findings and recommendations were presented to different key officials at the national level.

Two key round table discussions with DepEd and the Department of Agriculture were facilitated. The discussions allowed both parties to share initiatives and identify similar objective and ways to collaborate. Partnership was forged and a technical working group was established composed of representatives from the Department of Agriculture – Bureau of Plant Industry (DA-BPI), DepEd's Bureau of Learner Support Services, and IIRR to strengthen the crop museums in Region IV-A and to promote a similar concept in another region as part of the scaling out strategy. A round table discussion was also organized with six private sector representatives. Information, education, and communication materials were shared to encourage the use of these outputs in their existing nutrition programmes. Round table discussions are also seen as an effective means to engage and solicit support from local government units.

Advocacy and dissemination via multiple platforms

The research team shared the project in several events. The project was showcased during the Food Security Forum at the Asian Development Bank in June 2016. Initial findings were also shared at the following events: Philippine Association of Nutrition Convention in July 2017 with more than 1,000 attendees; Philippine Society of Nutritionist-Dietitians, Inc. Convention in October 2017 with 250 participants; DepEd Region IV-A International Conference of Basic Education Researchers 2017 with 2,287 participants; and the DSWD MIMAROPA Review and Planning Workshop for Supplementary Feeding in 2017.

The research was also presented during DepEd national events such as the DepEd *Gulayan sa Paaralan* Program National Workshop in 2017 and the Consultative Workshop on Nutrition Services in January 2018.

Events organized by NGOs also served as a point of dissemination. The model was shared in a multi-stakeholder event organized by Green Peace in observance of the World Food Day with 373 participants and in a Campaign on Healthy Diet with 150 participants. Another event involved sharing among NGOs via the Philippine Coalition of Advocates for Nutrition Security. The project was also shared in the Southeast Asian Ministers of Education Organization-Southeast Asian Regional Center for Graduate Study and Research in Agriculture (SEAMEO-SEARCA) international conference on the multi-functionality of school gardens and training of trainers (2018) and at the national Nutrition Sensitive Food Systems workshop (2018).

In South East Asia, learning exchanges were conducted between government offices and civil society organizations in the Philippines and Myanmar. IIRR organized round table discussions on nutrition in Yangon, Myanmar attended by 50 participants from 46 agencies. This was followed by a learning and sharing activity among officials from IIRR, DepEd, and FNRI-DOST and officials from Myanmar's Ministry of Education and Health.

The complete package of information, education, and communication materials acted as a catalyst in the diffusion of the model and guidelines (Figure 10.7). Different forms of materials were developed as support to school implementers and as promotional materials to officials at various levels.[1] The use of educational and communication strategies to expand nutrition-oriented gardening programmes are very useful. The posters, flyers, primers, and modules used provided ready information to highlight the gardening and nutrition links, as well as the importance of good nutrition, especially to school-age children. The nutrition campaigns, especially during the nutrition month, provide a venue for wider dissemination of nutrition messages.

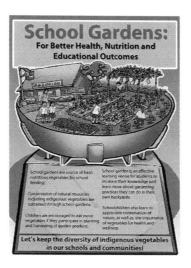

FIGURE 10.7 Package of information, education, and communication materials.
Source: IIRR.

The role of media

It is recognized that media have a major role in influencing the wider public. Reporters and writers were engaged in an attempt to draw the media's attention to important issues such as nutrition and food security, the role of agrobiodiversity, climate change, and food safety. A compilation of resource materials especially prepared for media personnel were distributed. Three media professionals were given additional and longer exposure visits and participated in events undertaken as part of this project. As a result, nine articles were written about the project.

Use of social media as platforms for information sharing

Social media is a significant and low-cost platform to disseminate new knowledge, lessons learned, accomplishments, activities, and innovations among a community of practice to sustain a movement. The project team created a Facebook group (GarNESupp – Gardening, nutrition education, and supplementary feeding) (GarNESupp, 2019) that has 1,047 members (at the time of writing) composed mostly of schoolteachers. The site is being utilized by schoolteachers to share activity photos, announcements, and training opportunities.

Results achieved at the sub-national and national level

Wide-scale adoption of innovations

Continuous capacity building through experiential training; provision of information, education, and communication material; and regular visits for technical input and monitoring led to adoption of various innovations introduced (Figure 10.8).

Data collected in 58 schools showed that there was a significant increase in the adoption of 12 BIG practices (IIRR, 2018d). To link gardens and supplementary feeding, 15 recipes with indigenous vegetables were developed and introduced in Phase 1 in addition to the moringa-based recipe recommended by DepEd. Schools were encouraged to adjust or explore other recipes or combinations of recipes to enable them to utilize the garden produce and to meet the needs of beneficiaries. The number of recipes adopted from those introduced by the project had increased to 9–10. Aside from the support given to schools, the issuance of memorandum that includes the endorsement of the 15 recipes led to increase in adoption.

Nutrition education strategies were divided into two main modalities – non-formal and formal. Non-formal nutrition education methods target parents, teachers, and the general community, whereas formal nutrition education modes are directed towards students. Records from schools showed that schools were able to deliver nutrition education activities using varied strategies. The most widely used mode is the participatory nutrition education activities for community and parents (83.64%), followed by nutrition education during feeding (74.55%), nutrition integration in lessons, and nutrition education during PTA/PTCs at 67.27%, and garden-based nutrition education (65.45%) (IIRR, 2018e).

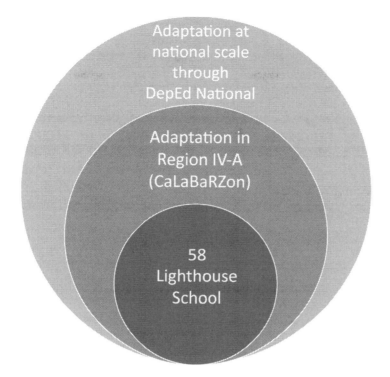

FIGURE 10.8 Adoption at national scale through DepEd National.

Collaboration and resource-sharing

Constructive dialogue with various government and non-government officials led to multiple trainings to disseminate the model. Two government agencies funded two training programmes – DA-BPI funded a 3-day training for 37 participants composed of 23 DA regional level staff from the 17 regions of the Philippines and 14 DepEd regional level representatives. It was followed by a training programme funded by DSWD Region IV-A for 88 participants in 2017 and a planned training for 177 child development workers from 4 provinces. Three other organizations engaged members of their project teams to train schools and child development workers in other provinces in the Philippines: Fostering Education & Environment for Development (FEED, Inc.), – *Angat Buhay* programme of the Office of the Vice President, and Adventist Development and Relief Agency.

Increased investment on school nutrition

At the sub-national level, the Education Support Services Division of DepEd Region IV-A, which oversees the school-based feeding programme, organized a three-day training in November 2016 for school health personnel composed of medical doctors and nurses and allocated funds for 17 sets of weighing scales and height boards for the schools and city divisions. This was in response to the findings presented to key personnel about the weak capacity of schools when it comes to nutrition assessment.

At the national level, DepEd made a commitment to promote the ISNM to all schools in the Philippines. So in 2017, DepEd allocated resources for teachers' training and reprinting of all information, education, and communication materials. A total of 220 schools, one from each school division across the Philippines, were designated and are being trained to be LSs.

Institutionalization of the model

Creating a DepEd Memorandum Order for schools to adapt and implement the ISNM is ongoing and once signed by the secretary, all 38,600 public elementary schools in the Philippines will be required to adopt the ISNM approach. This research project made the case for this to happen and will continue to provide the methodological and technical innovations to support DepEd via the knowledge products, working papers, primers, and information, education, and communication materials featuring research-derived recommendations. Most recently, RA 11037, an Act institutionalizing a national feeding programme for undernourished children in day care, kindergarten, and public elementary schools was enacted (Congress of the Philippines, 2018).

Improvement in nutritional status

In the recent Expanded National Nutrition Survey (ENNS) conducted by the FNRI-DOST, it was reported that stunting among school-aged children had reduced by 6.6% in the last three years. This had not been noted in the last 15 years, and it is believed that efforts in scaling the ISNM may have contributed to this improvement (Food and Nutrition Research Institute, 2018).

Conclusion

Schools can serve as centres for learning and sharing about nutrition, food security, agrobiodiversity conservation, and climate change. The ISNM that combines nutrition-specific and nutrition-sensitive interventions produced multiple nutrition outcomes. Effective scaling up requires demonstration of the ISNM's effectiveness and scalability and a combination of advocacy, education, and communication strategies directed at relevant agencies and sectors.

Acknowledgements

This chapter is based on the findings of the implementation of the Improving Food and Nutrition Security through interventions through Schools project, which was supported by IDRC, Canada.

Special acknowledgement is given to the other members of the research team: Maria Christy Jesusa G. Tacugue; Ma, Shiela S. Anunciado; Ronnie M. De Castro; Kirstein D. Itliong; Carmina Alicia N.Lainez; and Ian Curt R. Sarmiento.

Special acknowledgement is also given to the partners from the government: DepEd: Rizalino T. Rosales; Ella Cecilia G. Naliponguit; Maria Corazon C. Dumlao; Juan R. Araojo Jr.; Magdalene Portia T. Cariaga; Ferdinand M. Nunez; Mei-Ling V. Duhig; Diosdado M. San Antonio; Annaliza T. Araojo; Neil B. Evangelista; Romeo E. Endraca; Rolando B. Talon, Jr.; Virgilio O. Guevarra; Yolanda S. Oliver; and Galileo L. Go.

Department of Agriculture: Felix Joselito H. Noceda.

Sentinel Schools/LSs: Julugan Elementary School Personnel; Sunnybrooke Elementary School Personnel; Tinabunan Elementary School Personnel; and Region IV-A LS Personnel.

Note

1 Information, education, and communication materials are accessible at https://schoolnutritionphils.wordpress.com/.

References

Congress of the Philippines (2018) 'RA 11037: *Masustansyang Pagkain Para sa Batang Pilipino* Act', https://www.fnri.dost.gov.ph/images//sources/eNNS2018/Pre-school_and_School-Children.pdf, accessed Aug 2019.

DepEd (2007) 'Department of Education, Philippines DepEd Memo No. 293 s2007 *Gulayan sa Paaralan*', https://www.deped.gov.ph/wp-content/uploads/2018/10/DM_s2007_293.pdf, accessed July 2019.

DepEd (2016a) 'DepEd Memorandum No. 223, s. 2016', Republic of Philippines, Department of Education, https://www.deped.gov.ph/wp-content/uploads/2018/10/DM_s2016_223.pdf.

DepEd (2016b) 'Regional Memorandum No. 226, s. 2016', Republic of Philippines, Department of Education, http://depedcalabarzon.ph/wp-content/uploads/2016/07/Regional-Memorandum-No.-226-s.20161.pdf.

DepEd (2017a) 'DepEd Order No. 39, s. 2017', Republic of Philippines, Department of Education, https://www.deped.gov.ph/wp-content/uploads/2017/08/DO_s2017_039.pdf.

DepEd (2017b) 'Regional Memorandum No. 446, s. 2017' Republic of Philippines, Department of Education.

Food and Nutrition Research Institute (2018) 'Expanded National Nutrition Survey: Pre-school and School-Children', Department of Science and Technology, https://www.fnri.dost.gov.ph/images//sources/eNNS2018/Pre-school_and_School-Children.pdf, accessed Aug 2019.

GarNESupp (2019) 'GarNESupp: Integrated School nutrition', Facebook page, https://www.facebook.com/integratedschoolnutritionproject/, accessed Aug 2019.

Gonsalves, J., Baguilat, I., Oro, E., Tacugue, C. and Castro, R. (2015) 'Bio Intensive Gardens A climate & nutrition smart agriculture approach', https://schoolnutritionphils.files.wordpress.com/2015/11/big-primer.pdf, accessed Jan 2019.

Gündel, S., Hancock, J. and Anderson, S. (2001) 'Scaling up strategies for research in natural resource management: a comparative review', Greenwich: Natural Resources

Institute, University of Greenwich, https://www.ircwash.org/sites/default/files/Gundel-2001-Scalingup.pdf, accessed Jan 2019.

IIRR (2000) 'Going to Scale: Can we bring more benefits to more people more quickly?', International Institute of Rural Reconstruction, Y.C. James Yen Center, Silang, Cavite, Philippines.

IIRR (2017) 'Crop Museum in Schools: Conserving Agrobiodiversity of Nutritional Importance', https://schoolnutritionphils.files.wordpress.com/2017/04/crop-museum-primer.pdf, accessed Jan 2019.

IIRR (2018a). Integrated School Nutrition Project, https://schoolnutritionphils.wordpress.com/, accessed Aug 2019.

IIRR (2018b) 'Light houses Schools: Decentralized Platforms for Outscaling School Interventions', International Institute of Rural Reconstruction, https://schoolnutritionphils.files.wordpress.com/2018/05/ls-primer-final-draft.pdf, accessed Jan 2019.

IIRR (2018c) 'Integrated School Nutrition Project', https://schoolnutritionphils.wordpress.com/, accessed Jan 2019.

IIRR (2018d) 'Climate and Nutrition Smart School Gardens', https://schoolnutritionphils.files.wordpress.com/2018/10/climate-and-nutrition-smart-school-gardens-pdf.pdf, accessed Aug 2019.

IIRR (2018e) 'Enhancing Opportunities for Nutrition Education in Public Elementary Schools in the Philippines', https://schoolnutritionphils.files.wordpress.com/2018/10/enhancing-opportunities-for-nutrition-education-in-public-elementary-schools-in-the-philippines.pdf, accessed Aug 2019.

NNC (2014) 'Accelerated Hunger Mitigation Program (AHMP)', National Nutrition Council, http://www.nnc.gov.ph/index.php/plans-and-programs/accelerated-hunger-mitigation-program-ahmp.html, accessed July 2019.

Oro, E. (2018) 'Improving Food and Nutrition Security in the Philippines through School Interventions', IIRR, slideshow, *https://idl-bnc-idrc.dspacedirect.org › bitstream › handle*, accessed July 2019.

Oro, E. and Angeles-Agdeppa, I. (2015a) 'The Efficacy of Supplementary Feeding among 6 to 8 years old School Children in Selected Elementary Schools in Cavite', https://schoolnutritionphils.files.wordpress.com/2015/03/the-efficacy-of-supplementary-feeding-among-6-8-years-old-schoolchildren-in-selected-elementary-schools-in-cavite.pdf, accessed August 2019.

Oro, E. and Angeles-Agdeppa, I. (2015b) 'The Effects of Nutrition Education on Knowledge, Attitude and Practice among School Children and their Parents' https://schoolnutritionphils.files.wordpress.com/2015/03/the-effects-of-nutrition-education-on-knowledge-attitude-and-practice-among-schoolchildren-and-their-parents.pdf, accessed August 2019.

Oro, E. and Angeles-Agdeppa, I. (2015c) 'Enhancing the Nutrition and Agro-biodiversity Outcomes of School Gardens', Policy brief, https://schoolnutritionphils.files.wordpress.com/2015/03/enhancing-the-nutrition-and-agro-biodiversity-outcomes-of-school-gardens.pdf, accessed Aug 2019.

Uvin, P. and Miller, D. (1999) 'Scaling Up: Thinking through the Issues', http://www.brown.edu/Departments/World_Hunger_Program/hungerweb/WHP/SCALINGU.html, accessed Jan 2019.

CASE STUDY 1

THE STEPHANIE ALEXANDER KITCHEN GARDEN FOUNDATION PROGRAM

Stephanie Alexander Kitchen Garden Foundation

About the Stephanie Alexander Kitchen Garden Foundation

The Kitchen Garden Foundation was established by Stephanie Alexander AO, Australia's most recognized and iconic chef and food writer, in 2004. This was on the basis of the success of the Stephanie Alexander Kitchen Garden Program pilot that began in 2001. The pilot was a response to the growing childhood obesity crisis in Australia, and Stephanie's belief that involving children in the food production process in their school environment, and making sure their experience was pleasurable, fun and delicious, would change their attitude to fresh food and give them skills and understanding to last a lifetime.

Today the Kitchen Garden Foundation works with a growing number of over 2000 early childhood services and schools to run kitchen garden programmes and deliver pleasurable food education. The foundation provides professional development to educators, creates and shares educational resources that align kitchen and garden activities to the Australian curriculum, maintains a huge online community of kitchen garden teachers, and supports them with ongoing phone and email contact. We continually work on improving the accessibility and flexibility of the model, and on refining our support services for educators and communities.

The foundation is a small, dedicated team that works with all levels of government, philanthropic organizations, corporations, and community to further our work and the work of communities all over Australia to bring the joy of fresh, seasonal, delicious food to children and families.

Why did Stephanie start the Kitchen Garden Program?

> I believe that the way to change how kids feel about food is for them to have a hands-on experience and to learn about it from the very beginning

of popping a seed in the ground to coming into a kitchen and sitting around the table and eating with their friends.

– Stephanie Alexander AO

Stephanie had been aware of the growing obesity problem in Australia and internationally, and felt it was largely caused by people simply not knowing how to prepare fresh, nutritious food that is also delicious and fun to prepare. She believes the problem begins in childhood, and that the best way to address it is by means of early intervention. While many educational food programmes are well-intentioned, they neglect to involve children in an engaging, *pleasurable* model.

Inspired by her childhood memories of a kitchen garden, parents passionate about food and a family culture that focussed on the ritual of sharing a meal, Stephanie developed the Kitchen Garden Program to ensure children were enthusiastic about the food production process from start to finish, were encouraged to be proud of their achievements, and were given the skills and understanding that would inform them for life.

How the Kitchen Garden Program began[1]

In order to get children cooking and gardening in a way that taught them the pleasures and benefits of freshly grown food, Stephanie needed to find a primary school with the land to grow produce, as well as a principal with a shared concern for the food habits of young children. With her starting point, the belief that the idea could work and to 'just do it!', Stephanie started investigating sites for a kitchen garden programme.

Basil Natoli, the community gardens project manager from the Office of Housing, Department of Human Services, introduced Stephanie to the principal of Collingwood College, Frances Laurino. Frances came from a culture that valued eating and sharing food. She was also very aware of the disadvantage that some children faced and was absolutely convinced that teaching life skills would lead to improved circumstances and the possibility of better lives.

Collingwood College – situated in a Melbourne suburb of mixed fortunes, right next to a large public housing estate – exuded a sense of energy and ran a Steiner programme. It was both a primary and secondary school, and therefore had a home economics classroom.

The existence of the kitchen crystallized Stephanie's previously hazy notion of how the grown food would be used. She envisioned creating a 'seed to table' experience, which eventually developed into the mantra 'growing, harvesting, preparing, sharing'.

From these beginnings – a school, a willing principal, supportive school staff, and a link to the world of community gardening (in Basil) – a committee was formed. The committee worked hard on fleshing out and designing the Kitchen Garden Program; planning the garden; lobbying for and securing funding; and getting the community involved, including engaging Cultivating Community, a not-for-profit funded by the Office of Housing, to support community gardens on public housing estates.

On the ground, several working bees to build the garden followed in quick succession. A dedicated core of people turned up to every working bee, who shared a vision for a beautiful space for children and who remained indefatigable despite the hard work required.

In the office, the committee worked hard to follow up leads, enquiries and promises of help. A launch was planned to let the community know that the idea of a kitchen garden programme was becoming a reality.

On Friday, 27 July 2001, the kitchen garden was launched in pouring rain. Flyers calling out for volunteers and funds were handed out, children did the rounds as vegetables, and dignitaries were in attendance. Bronwyn Pike, then the Victorian minister for housing and aged care, launched the project. Despite the weather, the launch was a success and established the pilot programme at Collingwood College.

The Stephanie Alexander Kitchen Garden Foundation (SAKGF) was later established to increase the capacity to raise money and expand the Kitchen Garden Program to other schools.

The kitchen garden programme

In the Kitchen Garden Program, students are responsible for growing and maintaining productive vegetable gardens. They plan, help create beds, raise seedlings and harvest the produce – all while having fun. They take this harvest into the kitchen to prepare fresh, seasonal, *delicious* food (Figure C1.1).

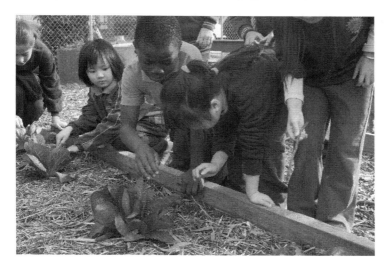

FIGURE C1.1 Students and raised beds in Sunshine North Primary School's kitchen garden.
Source: SAKGF.

The finished dishes are arranged with pride and care on tables set with flowers from the garden, and the *shared* meal is a time for students, helpers, teachers and specialists to enjoy each other's company and conversation. The programme is embedded in the school curriculum, becoming part of the school's timetable for at least two years of a child's life, and the practical learning is used to reinforce academic studies.

The kitchen garden at Collingwood College became a persuasive model for government support, and both state and national governments made commitments to helping schools start kitchen garden programmes. As the number of Kitchen Garden Program schools grew, different needs began to emerge – both from schools running the programme and those wanting to join.

Programme models

Before January 2013 schools could only run the 'Intensive' model of the programme, as described below.

- Only government schools could join the programme.
- Schools went through a rigorous application process in which they committed to building infrastructure and running weekly kitchen and garden classes.
- Schools were expected to hire external 'specialists' to run kitchen and garden classes.
- The foundation administered state and national government grants to facilitate schools building infrastructure or hiring specialists.
- Schools 'joined' the programme and signed a Memorandum of Understanding (MoU) with the foundation that committed them to running the programme, and the foundation to continue supporting them.

In 2012, in response to feedback from schools, the foundation made changes to make the programme more accessible, affordable, and flexible.

After January 2013, schools could run the 'flexible' model of the programme, as described below.

- All government and non-government schools became eligible to join the programme.
- Schools can use their existing teaching staff to run the programme, or use a mix of teacher- and specialist-led classes.
- Government grants are no longer intrinsic to the programme. Schools are encouraged to start small, using what they have.

Kitchen Garden Program schools decide which model works best for them. Before the flexible model was introduced, there were 267 schools running the Intensive model across Australia.

Kitchen Garden Classroom membership

Many schools and organizations were not eligible for government funding, but wished to benefit from the Kitchen Garden Program.

The membership model enables schools, organizations, and individuals to adapt the Kitchen Garden Program model and draw on the knowledge and expertise gained by the foundation and Kitchen Garden Program schools over many years of intensive practice.

Anyone can become a member. Early years centres, primary schools and secondary schools, and a growing community of food enthusiasts and educators from across Australia have joined the Kitchen Garden Classroom (Figure C1.2).[2]

The benefits of membership include:

- access to the 'Shared Table' online community and resource library with hundreds of planning guides, recipes and garden activities, examples and curriculum-aligned resources
- a vibrant online community of thousands of kitchen garden educators, who constantly post images and content on what their students are doing in their kitchen garden programme
- discounts on professional development and printed educational resources
- ongoing email and phone support from the foundation's friendly and professional team.

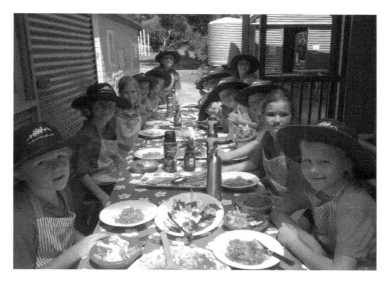

FIGURE C1.2 Students from Deans Marsh Primary School are sharing a meal with pasta and vegetables from the garden.

Source: SAKGF.

Pleasurable food education

Pleasurable food education is delivered through a kitchen garden programme. The model entails children gaining life skills, self-confidence, and a positive relationship with food through practical learning that is integrated with the curriculum. The model also provides meaningful opportunities to engage students and families, connect communities, and change local food cultures. Pleasurable food education brings an array of health, well-being, education, and community benefits, and is designed to achieve long-term change.

The pleasurable food education philosophy

Pleasurable food education emphasizes the flavours as well as the health benefits of fresh, seasonal, delicious food. Dishes cooked reflect the vegetables, herbs and fruits grown, season-by-season, by the children in their organic gardens, and also reflect the Australian dietary guidelines. Kitchen educators emphasize balance and moderation, and endorse the concept of preparing fruit-based desserts 'sometimes-only'. Pleasurable food education is designed to be fully integrated into the curriculum or learning framework as it offers infinite possibilities to reinforce literacy, numeracy, science, cultural studies and all aspects of environmental sustainability. In addition, pleasurable food education delivers observable social benefits to all children, including those with special needs. Pleasurable food education encourages critical thinking, teamwork, an understanding of cause and effect, and increased levels of observation (Figure C1.3).

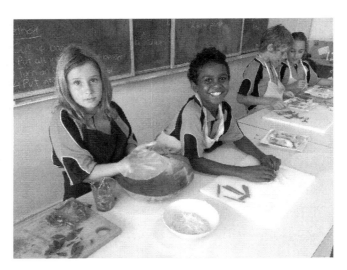

FIGURE C1.3 Primary students from Wyndham are learning about cutting vegetables and discovering that it is better to have good sharp knives.

Source: SAKGF.

BOX C1.1: IN CONVERSATION WITH DRIVER PRIMARY SCHOOL

Driver Primary School is located in the suburb of Driver in the city of Palmerston, Northern Territory. The school has a significant proportion of students from Defence Force families, Aboriginal students, and students who speak languages other than English. At Driver Primary School, the kitchen has become the indoor life skills classroom. The garden is called 'the Farm' and is used for the outdoor life skills programme. To maximize use of spaces, teachers are encouraged to use the kitchen and garden for cross-curricular activities.

Here we interview Sherrida Edgecombe, kitchen garden coordinator; Karen Johnson, garden specialist; and Trudy Dacey, kitchen specialist as part of the Schools' Stories series:

What does the Kitchen Garden National Program mean to Driver Primary School?

Sherrida: *The program is embedded in the school ethos. It brings joy and excitement to our students and to the school at large. We are headed by a very supportive principal in Rob Presswell. He believes it's the best thing he has seen in 30 years of teaching.*

Can you explain the learning process and how you integrate Australian Curriculum?

Sherrida: *We run 120-minute classes, rather than the 45-minute classes, because we find the extra time aids the learning process and no one is rushed. Taking the extra time means we can cover topics more thoroughly and kids can enjoy sharing the meal together. We are constantly learning from each other and sharing ideas. The Rosella plant was introduced to staff by some of our Aboriginal students who explained how it could be used to make cordial and jams. It's now planted at the Farm and considered a favourite. Non-academic kids, given the opportunity to learn by doing, thrive in the program. You see each kid play to their strengths.*

Curriculum is integrated. There are science lessons in the kitchen classes; literacy activities such as reading recipes and learning new vocabulary in ingredients lists; fractions when doubling recipes; mathematic problem solving covering topics like fundraising; and activities such as calculating the volume and area of garden beds.

Kids are working on their own cookbooks. These will include recipes and illustrations. And as part of their art classes they're designing their own scarecrow. They have won the prize Grand Champion at the Royal Darwin Show for the last 2 years.

(Continued)

Next year we plan to integrate the curriculum even further and discuss the best way to do this with our classroom teachers. Opportunities to learn arise from challenges too – for example, our kids have learnt about the behaviours and effects of rats, termites and cane toads on people and the environment.

Your school is represented by varied cultures – how do you celebrate and integrate them?

Sherrida: Our program acknowledges the importance of all students. It enriches the learning of our kids, our teachers and the whole school community. Leslie Gordon, our Aboriginal islander education worker, teaches students about the Larrakia people. Students learn about bush tucker and the Larrakia Country seasonal calendar which is based on the climate and when native plants fruit.

Karen: Parents of students from South East Asian countries regularly send their children in with cuttings from their own home veggie gardens. This has inspired us to plant things like lemongrass, bok choy, ginger, chilli, galangal and turmeric. Our tropical climate is perfect for these plants.

Trudy: Our students know how to cook with the ingredients from the Farm – they truly understand the diverse flavours.

Does your program have links to the wider community?

Karen: Other schools come to visit the Farm and kitchen regularly because they see our school as a successful model. They will pop in to ask for advice on how to start their own garden and to speak to Trudy about recipe ideas.

Sherrida: Our volunteers help Karen and Trudy and make it possible for me to run the lookalike program for the younger students. They help me with things that may sound simple but that are no easy task – like getting kids to wear gloves. Trying to get all their fingers in is hard work. Now they are even better at it than the bigger kids. The wider community is involved in the program too. There is local fruit tree specialist Chris Nathaniel who helps with the 60 fruit trees, local irrigation company Water Dynamic have donated materials, US marines have helped at working bees, Ark Veterinary Clinic provide free care to the chooks and more. Driver Primary School receives donations such as: pots from landscaping companies; cuttings and potting mix from parents; and frangipani cuttings from the Darwin Botanic Gardens to grow and sell.

Do you pursue any fundraising or promotional activities for the program?

Karen: We sell banana and tomato plants, galangal, dried turmeric, soap and eggs – anything that comes from the garden and kitchen – on election days, at market stalls and from the front office. We are running a logo design competition for labels for the produce – it is a good way to ensure the kids are involved in the fundraising and it increases their sense of ownership of the produce they grow. We communicate with parents and promote the program via the school's fortnightly newsletter. There is a regular section where we share news.

How do the parents of your students feel about the program?

Sherrida: Students take what we teach them home. I hear from parents that their kids have started cooking for the whole family and that they have been adapting recipes for healthier lunches. Parents will say things like, 'It's amazing – they would never touch vegetables before!'

Trudy: I organised a 'Mummy & Me' day where kids cook afternoon tea and drink Rosella Cordial with their mums. Sessions were booked out for two days. If parents have the time they love to be involved.

Karen: Parents often tell me that their kids now beg them for plants to grow at home – a lot of them have tomato plants. They will force trips to Bunnings[3] on the weekend.

What do the kids enjoy most about the program?

Sherrida: When the kids engage with nature there is a clear calming effect. When they are out there checking buds they are very absorbed. Students like to spend time at the Farm at lunch and recess. If they are playing up at lunch or recess they will come up to the Farm with me and be given duties – feeding the chickens or weeding – it is not a punishment per se but a way to redirect their attention and encourage them to do something positive. I will then have the challenge of trying to kick them out when the bell rings.

Karen: Students with major learning difficulties are some of my most devoted gardeners. I will find them at the Farm before school starts at 7.30am ready to help just because they love it.

Trudy: Overall, the kids are more game to try new things. They will watch other kids try and then feel inspired to as well.

Proof the programme works

The benefits are phenomenal. It fits into the curriculum very nicely. All the interpersonal skills are covered – teamwork, cooperation, relating to each other – in ways that cannot be replicated in a classroom.

– *Principal, Nunawading Primary School*

University of Wollongong evaluation

A Department of Health and Ageing funded evaluation of the Stephanie Alexander Kitchen Garden Program was undertaken between 2011 and 2012 by the Centre for Health Service Development at the Australian Health Services Research Institute, University of Wollongong.

The evaluation confirmed the positive impacts of the program, with key findings as below (Yeatman et al., 2013).

- 97% of teachers responded positively to how the programme supported classroom learning. They reported that students found the hands-on activities engaging and that the activities aided in learning across other subject areas, commenting that the programme 'forms an intrinsic part of our students' learning'.
- Students in programme schools were more likely to report that they would always try new foods as compared to students in comparison schools. The proportion was higher if the students had grown or cooked the foods themselves.
- More children are taking up cooking at home and starting backyard veggie gardens after participating in the programme.
- Participating students, staff, and school communities all reported that the programme had made positive impacts on the school and students.
- Students found the activities of the programme to be a positive context for learning across multiple subject areas.
- Teachers and parents reported improvements in students' social behaviours, with 86% of teachers reporting improvements in students' teamwork skills and 50% of parents reporting improvements across a range of student behaviours, including modifying previous bullying behaviour, managing difficult behaviour, interacting with people of many ages, leadership skill development, and sense of pride in the school.

In particular, teachers commented that the programme's hands-on approach to learning gave students from a range of socio-cultural groups and with differing levels of ability the chance to participate equally and to improve. Teachers reported the following changes in students at risk of social exclusion:

- healthier eating habits
- more likely to try new and healthy foods
- increased participation, engagement and attendance
- improved self-esteem and confidence
- increased opportunities to learn differently
- advancement in different areas
- further developed life skills
- improved social skills and communication

Parents shared that as a result of the programme:

- children always tried new foods if they had grown or cooked them
- children liked cooking more and helped with cooking more often at home
- children asked parents to cook the foods from the programme
- parents prepared more meals at home
- children exhibited greater confidence with garden activities
- students reported that they learned new things in the garden
- parents reported they worked more in their home garden with their children

University of Melbourne/Deakin University evaluation

An evaluation of the Stephanie Alexander Kitchen Garden Program was undertaken between 2007 and 2009, by a joint research team from the Faculty of Health, Medicine, Nursing & Behavioural Sciences, Deakin University and the McCaughey Centre: VicHealth Centre for the Promotion of Mental Health and Community Wellbeing, University of Melbourne. The findings were extremely positive and demonstrated that the Kitchen Garden Program is encouraging positive health behaviour change in participating children. The evaluation also showcased the transfer of benefits to the home and the broader community.

The key findings of the evaluation are as follows (Block et al., 2009):

- There was strong evidence of increased child willingness to try new foods including a significant difference between programme and comparison schools.
- There was evidence of statistically significant increases in child knowledge, confidence, and skills in cooking and gardening.
- The kitchen classes were greatly enjoyed by children, and the children at programme schools were significantly more likely than children from comparison schools to report that they liked cooking 'a lot'.
- Children's competent use of knives in the kitchen appeared to be particularly valued by all stakeholders as evidence of skill but also as a symbol of trust.
- The programme was considered particularly effective at engaging 'non-academic learners' and children with challenging behaviours.
- The programme helped to create links between schools and the community. This was often noted as one of the programme's most important outcomes.
- Transfer of programme benefits to the home environment was not one of the goals of the programme but is emerging as a flow-on benefit.
- The programme is associated with substantial financial cost and even greater community investment in terms of the resources of time and materials used.
- Programme schools on average generated $1.93 of additional resources for every $1 of government funding invested in the programme.

A study looking at the long-term impacts on young adults who participated in the programme at primary school is being undertaken in 2018–2019 by the

Jack Brockhoff Child Health & Wellbeing Program, Centre for Health Equity, University of Melbourne.

For more information please visit www.kitchengardenfoundation.org.au.

Notes

1 This is an extract of content from 'Kitchen Garden Cooking with Kids' by Stephanie Alexander with Anna Dollard, Penguin Group (Australia), 2006, revised 2012.
2 View all schools and centres in the kitchen garden community at www.kitchengardenfoundation.org.au/content/kitchen-garden-community.
3 Australian warehouse that sells garden supplies.

References

Block, K., Johnson, B., Gibbs, L., Staiger, P., Townsend, M., Macfarlane, S., Gold, L., Long, C., Kulas, J., Okoumunne, O.C. and Waters, E. (2009) 'Evaluation of the Stephanie Alexander Kitchen Garden Program: Final Report', Melbourne: McCaughey Centre. Full report available: https://mspgh.unimelb.edu.au/centres-institutes/centre-for-health-equity/research-group/jack-brockhoff-child-health-wellbeing-program/research/physical-health-and-wellbeing/evaluation-of-the-stephanie-alexander-kitchen-garden-program.

Yeatman, H., Quinsey, K., Dawber, J., Nielsen, W., Condon-Paoloni, D., Eckermann, S., Morris, D., Grootemaat, P. and Fildes, D. (2013) 'Stephanie Alexander Kitchen Garden National Program Evaluation: Final Report', Centre for Health Service Development, Australian Health Services Research Institute, University of Wollongong. Full report available: http://ahsri.uow.edu.au/content/groups/public/@web/@chsd/documents/doc/uow145163.pdf.

CASE STUDY 2
REVIVING LOCAL FOOD SYSTEMS IN HAWAI'I

Nancy Redfeather and Elizabeth Cole

School gardens, nutrition education, and farm to school initiatives are orienting palates and diets towards traditionally available foods, diversifying agriculture and increasing locally produced school snacks and lunches while circulating income throughout local farming communities in the Hawaiian Islands.

The problem

Self-sufficient for centuries, the colonial legacy of deforestation, plantation agriculture, and the current focus on tourism and military development has left the Hawaiian Islands more than 85% dependent on imported, primarily processed food (Page et al., 2007). The islands' distance from supply chains results in little opportunity to establish a sustainable economic trading base, while heavy reliance on processed foods from the continental United States is promoting poor diets that lack diversity and adequate nutrition. Furthermore, it is expensive to farm on Hawai'i as all farm inputs and fuel must be imported to the island, which require logistics that are both complicated and expensive, resulting in high food prices for even locally produced food. Being so dependent on foreign produce also makes the Hawaiian food system vulnerable to disruptions in the shipping chain, extreme weather, and fluctuating prices of food products, as well as higher prices for agricultural inputs such as fodder and fertilizer (Loke and Leung, 2013).

Native Hawaiian and Other Pacific Island (NHOPI) populations show very low consumption of fruits and vegetables, which stems from low-income employment, and leads to disproportionately high rates of obesity and related chronic diseases (Moy et al., 2010). This can also be detected among children where almost 1 in 3 entering kindergarten are overweight (Trogdon et al., 2012). The majority of Hawai'i's youth receive more than half their daily calories from school meals during the academic year. School gardening and local food procurement is needed to improve students' nutrient intake, strengthen local food security, and keep income circulating throughout local communities.

The project

Following the Island of Hawai'i food system report prepared by the Rocky Mountain Institute in 2007, the Kohala Center established the Hawai'i Island School Garden Network (HISGN) to develop and promote school gardens as an initiative to build a strong local food economy while providing youth with increased nutrition. With an emphasis on native Hawaiian plants and practices, the HISGN has since expanded to work with 60 elementary and secondary schools by assisting garden leaders, school faculty, and administrators in the creation and implementation of gardening and agricultural programmes.

The Kū 'Āina Pā teacher training programme focusses on deepening students' connection between ancestral knowledge of agriculture and agrobiodiversity, the ahupua'a systems management of natural resources on Hawaiian land, the preparation of food from the 'āina (land), and traditional Hawaiian values, protocols, and language. 'Ai pono (righteous food) engages students in growing and processing traditional food. The programme also gives classroom teachers the skills and knowledge they need to integrate garden-based learning into their core curriculum (Figure C2.1).

The Hawai'i School Garden Curriculum Map was created by teachers for busy teachers who may not be gardeners themselves but intuitively understand the

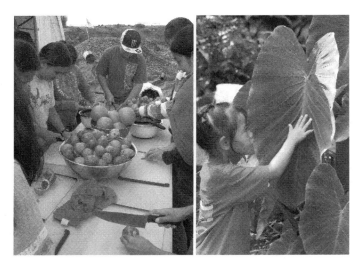

FIGURE C2.1 Students at the Māla'ai Culinary Garden cutting morning snack (right) and girls studying a taro leaf (Kalo i ke Kumu).
Source: Nancy Redfeater and Clare Loprinzi.

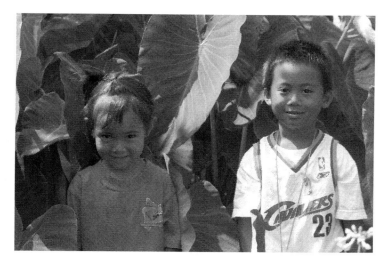

FIGURE C2.2 Some of the youngest participants in the loʻi (taro patch).
Source: Clare Loprinzi.

benefits of inquiry-based, place-based, project-based learning for their students. The School Garden Curriculum Map is a pathway that connects core curriculum in the classroom with opportunities for extending learning in the real world, the basis of both Common Core and Next Generation Science. The curriculum is divided into four sections providing traditional, theoretical and practical learning which strengthen children's connection to the land, nature and native foods. *The Four Big Ideas* begin with *A Sense of Place*, move to the all-important *Living Soil and Living Plant*, on to *Nourishment*, and finally *Nature's Design*, encompassing the science-based cycles, patterns, biodiversity and systems of the natural world.

The HISGN began by asking the question: What do students need to know about good food, the environment, sustainability, and nature's systems by eighth grade? Based on the findings, they created garden themes, topics, and learning outcomes and linked them to suggested garden activities and classroom extension. The activities were then included in the curriculum in alignment with Common Core, Next Generation Science Standards, and Hawaiʻi State Health Standards.

The HISGN today continue to offer five-day Summer Intensive courses on different Islands for teachers to dive deeply into the rich knowledge and biodiversity of Hawaiʻi and learn to connect this engaging content to their core curriculum (Figure C2.2).

Agrobiodiversity and Hawaiʻian culture

Climate change is impacting us all, and it is imperative at this time that we understand the natural world that surrounds us and how to work with that world in order to thrive as an isolated Island society.

Reviving tropical agriculture allows youth to reconnect with the food choices that provided high quality nutrition to their Hawaiian ancestors.

Traditional foods grown in school gardens include:

- kalo (*Colocasia esculenta*) or taro root and leaves, used to make the traditional dishes poi and lū'au
- 'ulu (*Artocarpus altilis*) or breadfruit, prized for its productivity in Pacific Island environments
- 'uala (*Ipomoea batatas*), also known as sweet potato
- mai'a (*Musa acuminata*), an edible banana species
- kō (*Saccharum officinarum*) or sugar cane
- niu (*Cocos nucifera*) or coconut milk and cream, used to make kūlolo and lū'au dishes

Served in schools as snacks and meals along with tropical fruits such as papaya, mango, pineapple, and liliko'i (passion fruit), these plants collectively provide:

- digestible fibre, potassium, calcium, and iron
- vitamin C and vitamin B-complex
- anti-oxidants and important trace elements

Additional indigenous plant species continue to improve the nutritional value of the Hawaiian diet, though not necessarily from direct consumption. Kaula (cordage or rope) is hand-crafted from various hardy plant materials and can be used for nets, traps, and fishing line. Valuable animal protein sources as well as the opportunity to diversify diets locally are made available thanks to this customary practice (Figure C2.3).

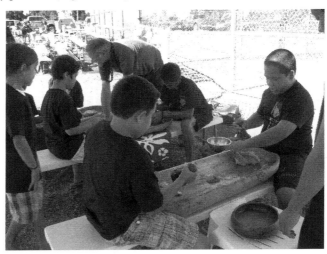

FIGURE C2.3 Students at Ke Kula 'o 'Ehunuikaimalino Public Charter School ku'i the kalo into poi.

Photo: Nancy Redfeather.

BOX C2.1

A recent study from Kamehameha Schools, University of Hawai'i at Mānoa, and the U.S. Geological Survey shows evidence that Hawai'i's traditional agroecosystems that existed in the past could have met the production levels necessary for the consumption demand today. In addition, it suggests that by restoring indigenous agriculture on 70% of the land that are not covered by development and still today zoned for agriculture, it would be possible to feed the Hawaiian population in the future, which is especially relevant as a response to climate change scenarios (Kurashima et al., 2019).

In the summer of 2019, the Hawaiian Voyaging Canoe Makali'i sailed to the Northwest Hawai'ian Islands provisioned with foods grown and prepared by the school gardens of Hawai'i Island. This programme was seven years in the making, and both navigators and community recognize the importance of an 'ai pono diet for the voyagers.

Scaling up

The HISGN supported and led programme expansion in 2012 into a multi-island initiative, the Hawai'i Farm to School and School Garden Hui, which now supports more than 217 school gardens on five islands, and has a diverse group of members including Island Networks, State Agencies, non-profit organizations, and institutional partners. A grant from the United States Department of Agriculture (USDA) Fresh Fruit and Vegetable Program will support and strengthen the capacity and impact of these initiatives. In addition HISGN is the host organization for FoodCorps Hawai'i, part of a federally funded programme which places 9 full-time emerging leaders at school garden sites in Hawai'i.

In 2015, the Hawai'i Farm to School Hui helped to pass the Hawai'i Farm to School Bill (Act 218) establishing a programme in the Department of Agriculture with a coordinator position. In 2018, the 'Aina Pono Farm to School Program moved to the Department of Education, which is currently being implemented in two pilot schools. In 2019, the Farm to School Hui has started working with the Hawai'i Department of Education-School Food Services Branch and has recently launched the first Garden to Cafeteria Program. Another new programme will involve the creation of School Peace Gardens and the implementation of a sustainability curriculum in pilot schools.

The primary barriers to programme scaling and full implementation are insufficient financial resources due to strains on educational and health system budgets, inadequate IT and accountability systems, a resistance to increasing aggregation and distribution points, institutional resistance to incorporating garden-based learning into the core curriculum, and resistance to the transition from industrialized agriculture to biodiverse agroecological production systems. Increasing curriculum integration and meaningful support for schools with learning gardens, which today includes 85% of all public schools, is still a challenge, but new opportunities are beginning to emerge.

Stakeholder and policy maker involvement

Activities and platforms for public engagement created by HISGN include sustained positive media attention, school gardening resource sharing on the HISGN website, regular workshops for teachers; garden and culinary events for community members; and yearly multi-stakeholder conferences to sustain garden and farm to school movement.

One of the keys to success has been HISGN's state-wide coalition, the Hawai'i Farm to School Hui. Members of the Hawai'i Farm to School Hui are actively working with representatives from the Hawai'i State Legislature and the Hawai'i Departments of Education, Health, and Agriculture to change institutional procurement policies. The aim is to foster increases in the purchase and preparation of fresh, locally produced food, as well as to provide resources for school gardening programmes. The coalition meet quarterly in Honolulu, funded by the Department of Health, and holds monthly Steering Committee Meetings and sub-committees. Today they are ready to celebrate a decade of collaborative work together, and for a diverse group of people and interests that are separated by a vast ocean, that is something to celebrate!

Impact

- 85% of Hawai'i Island schools have learning gardens which corresponds to 217 schools
- 830 teachers have been engaged in garden activities
- 21,577 students have received garden-based education
- 30 acres of land are devoted to school gardens
- 13,600 kg of food are produced annually in school gardens (Figure C2.4)

Read more

Hawai'i Island School Garden Network (HISGN): https://kohalacenter.org/hisgn

Hawai'i School Garden Curriculum Map: https://kohalacenter.org/hisgn/curriculum-map

Hawai'i Farm to School Hui: www.hiphi.org/farmtoschool

Polynesian Voyaging Society: the Hōkūle'a's World Wide Voyage: http://archive.hokulea.com/holokai/wwv/wwv_mission.html

Hawai'i Seed Growers Network: www.hawaiiseedgrowersnetwork.com

Reviving local food systems in Hawai'i **177**

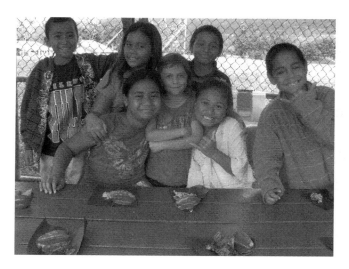

FIGURE C2.4 Students at Hōnaunau Elementary School Garden appreciating their morning snack of fruit and cassava, and each other!
Photo: Nancy Redfeather.

References

Kurashima, N., Fortini, L. and Ticktin, T. (2019) 'The potential of indigenous agricultural food production under climate change in Hawai'i', *Nature Sustainability* 2:191–199, doi:10.1038/s41893-019-0226-1.

Loke, M.K. and Leung, P.S. (2013) 'Hawai'i's food consumption and supply sources: benchmark estimates and measurement issues', *Agricultural and Food Economics* 1:10, doi:10.1186/2193-7532-1-10.

Moy, K.L., Sallis, J.F. and David, K.J. (2010) 'Health indicators of native Hawaiian and Pacific Islanders in the United States', *Journal of Community Health* 35(1):81–92, doi:10.1007/s10900-009-9194-0.

Page, C., Bony, L., and Schewel, L. (2007) 'Island of Hawai'i whole system project phase I report', Rocky Mountain Institute, Boulder, CO.

Trogdon, J.G., Finkelstein, E.A., Feagan, C.W. et al. (2012) 'State- and Payer-specific estimates of annual medical expenditures attributable to obesity', *Obesity* 20(1): 214–220, doi:10.1038/oby.2011.169.

CASE STUDY 3
FOOD PLANT SOLUTIONS
School gardens in Vietnam

Karalyn Hingston and Natalie Ching

Background

In recent decades, Vietnam has made great strides in ameliorating childhood malnutrition, as reflected in reductions in the prevalence of underweight and stunted children (GoV, 2012). However, Vietnam remains a country with one of the highest stunting rates in Southeast Asia, and nutritional deficiencies are still pervasive, especially among children. Many school-age children in Vietnam suffer from iodine, iron, zinc, and vitamin A deficiencies, posing a significant concern for public health (Chaparro et al., 2014).

In Quang Nam Province in Central Vietnam, a Vietnamese non-profit organization (AOG World Relief Vietnam) partnered with an Australian-based Rotarian Action Group (Food Plant Solutions) to improve the nutritional status of children and their wider communities in the communes of Dai Hung and Tam Phu. In these communities, most households are reliant on small-scale farming as a source of livelihood, with an estimated annual income of between 8 million and 12 million VND (USD $350–$550), close to the poverty line established by the Vietnamese government (Kozel, 2014). Many families cannot afford basic necessities and lack financial and physical access to nutritious foods. Moreover, access to nutritious foods is also impeded by the lack of nutrition information and education. Many farming families are unaware of the nutritional value contained in different plants and parts of plants – for example, cassava in this area is mostly grown for its roots and its leaves are commonly fed to pigs. Cassava leaves contain high concentrations of vitamins. A cassava root weighing 100 g contains about 15 mg of vitamin C, while the same weight of leaves contains about 275 mg of vitamin C.

As a result of these financial and social barriers to quality nutritious foods, these communities experience many negative health and nutritional outcomes, which is perpetuated in the poverty cycle. Parents in these two communes were found to be predisposed to conditions such as respiratory illness, high blood pressure, stomach upset, and multiple nutrient deficiencies, and 11.1% and 19.8% of kindergarten-age children were found to be malnourished in Tam Phu and Dai Hung, respectively. Adequate nutrition during childhood is crucial for physical growth and development, but also for cognitive and social development. Childhood malnutrition affects the ability to attend, focus, and learn in school as well as participate in community life. The damage caused by malnutrition (stunting) is life-long and irreversible. As adults these children will earn less than their peers and be more prone to non-communicable diseases. Mothers affected by under-nutrition are more likely to have children who suffer from stunting or wasting, perpetuating the cycle of poverty and under-nutrition (Ozaltin et al., 2010). Well-nourished children are 33 percent more likely to escape poverty as adults (Horton and Steckel, 2013).

Moreover, similar to households in the community, schools in the area also face financial limitations, which impacts upon their ability to provide nutritious school meals for their students. As a result, many parents elect for their children to return home for lunch due to the perceived poor quality of school meals, which greatly impacts on both the working time of parents and learning time of children.

The project

In response to the high rates of malnutrition and the lack of access to affordable and nutritious foods in these communities, AOG World Relief Vietnam and Food Plant Solutions implemented school garden programmes in the communes of Tam Phu and Dai Hung. This partnership originally began with one pilot garden at a primary school in 2012, and the initiative has since expanded to 14 school gardens in 2018 to include over 3,000 students and 320 staff members.

This school garden project focusses on participatory approaches to empower the communities of Tam Phu and Dai Hung, striving to work collaboratively with community members to develop action plans, mobilize local assets and resources, and ultimately to empower them to determine and sustain their own future development. The objectives of implementing school gardens include not only addressing the nutritional needs of children and ensuring year-round access to nutritious school meals but also empowering them with nutritional and agricultural knowledge to share with their families and to utilize in the future.

Implementation of a thriving school garden begins with the training of teachers and educators using a field guide and picture guide, created by Food Plant Solutions Technical Team experts. Both were translated, a key component in the process. The field guide is a technical publication and used by the headmaster and trainers to train the staff; this publication requires a high degree of literacy. The picture guide contains many colourful photos of the various local species and diagrams depicting the nutritional content of different plants. Both

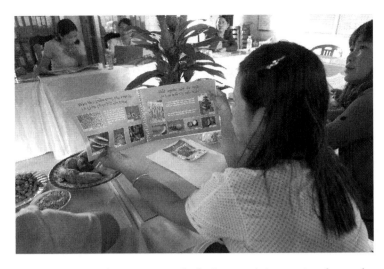

FIGURE C3.1 Exploring the picture guide during a training session for teachers.

publications provide information to teachers about how to establish and maintain their school garden, how to care for the plants, how to use the plants, as well as about how these plants relate to health and nutrition. The picture guides also explain what nutritional food is and why our bodies need it, which is critical information that many people do not know or understand. It was observed that the visually engaging format of the pictures and in-depth information about the nutrient content of the different plants increased teacher involvement in the project (Figure C3.1).

After this period of training, it is then the task of the teachers to share and disseminate this information with their students by incorporating the knowledge into interactive lessons. Through these lessons, students learn practical skills such as how to create garden beds, how to recognize different soil conditions, how to identify different type of plants, and how to utilize sustainable methods to maintain their gardens. These practical skills are complemented by educational programming about nutrition and the importance of eating nutrient-rich foods for healthy bodies. Moreover, the students are also involved in the preparation of the nutritious meals that they consume during the school day and are encouraged to bring seeds from school to plant with their families at home.

The role of agrobiodiversity

From the field guide created by Food Plant Solutions, initially four vegetable species were selected and prioritized to be included in the school garden and nutrition education programme in Tam Phu and Dai Hung. These plants include *rau muong* or water spinach (*Ipomoea aquatica*) that contains high amounts of vitamin A, iron, zinc, and plant-derived proteins; *rau mong toi* or Malabar

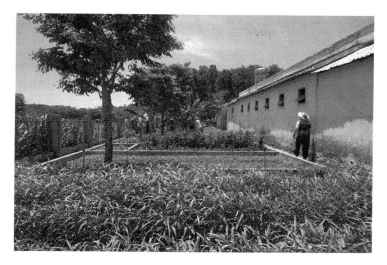

FIGURE C3.2 An example of one of the school gardens.

spinach (*Basella alba*), which contains high levels of vitamin C and iron, moderate amounts of vitamin A and plant-derived protein; *rau den* (*Amaranthus tricolor*), which contains high levels of vitamin A and moderate amounts of vitamin C, iron, zinc, and plant derived protein; and *bi dao* or winter melon (*Benincasa hispida*), which contains Vitamin C, iron, zinc, and plant-derived protein. Within the field guide, there is detailed information about the optimal growing conditions and methods for these plants, how and when to cultivate them, and how to utilize them in cooking. Plants in the field guide were selected because of their suitability for the local environment and their particular nutritional qualities. In addition, these plants are also easy to prepare at the schools, and importantly, well-liked by students as an ingredient in soups or rice porridges (an essential staple food for children in Vietnam) (Figure C3.2).

Impacts

The implementation of school learning gardens in the two communes of Tam Phu and Dai Hung resulted in dramatic improvements in health outcomes for the students. In Dai Hung, 50 students at the beginning of the 2016 school year were classified as malnourished and 22 in Tam Phu. By the end of the school year, only 10 students were classified as malnourished in Dai Hung, and just one in Tam Phu, a reduction in malnutrition of 80% and 95% respectively.

In 2018, across the eight schools that measured results the rates of malnutrition were reduced by an average of 50% (as measured by height) and 64% (as measured by weight) in one year.

However, the impacts of this project extend far beyond improvements in the students' health. Since the implementation of school gardens, student enrolment

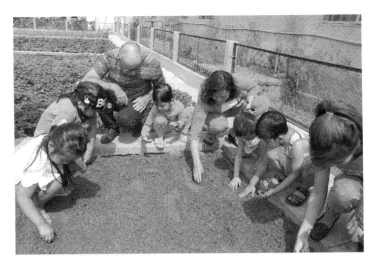

FIGURE C3.3 Students examining the soil.

in some schools increased dramatically due to the improved quality of school meals. The ability to use produce grown from the on-site gardens in school meals greatly reduced the financial strain on school budgets and as a result, schools could spend the saved money on other school necessities. In Dai Hung, schools were able to save 1.5 million VDN (USD $65) per month on food purchases.

Moreover, this project generated much interest and enthusiasm from schools and teachers from neighbouring communities. The project schools hosted interested teachers from other schools who wanted to observe and implement a similar programme at their schools. In addition, the school learning gardens helped to engage the parents of these students, as students were encouraged to share knowledge that they gained during the school day about agriculture and nutrition with their families. The schools reported very positive responses and reactions from parents, and widespread adoption of home gardening in these communities. This in turn contributes to enhanced food security for students outside of the school setting, as well as for their parents and wider communities. As a result, families can also save money by harvesting their own produce and to put it to use for other necessities (Figure C3.3).

Scaling up

The successful expansion of the programme from one pilot project in 2012 to fourteen in 2018 was not solely due to the work of AOG World Relief Vietnam to establish more gardens, but the initiative taken by the local community members. Exposed to and inspired by the Food Plant Solutions model and witnessing the nutritional and economic benefits of the programme, many parents and community members created similar gardens in their homes and many teachers from surrounding communities replicated the programme in their respective schools.

One challenge was noted, a primary school with a functioning learning garden was not able to harvest all of the benefits of the gardens because they did not have adequate kitchen facilities to prepare the fresh produce. It is therefore critical that to ensure the successful implementation of this programme, a school has an equipped, functioning school kitchen, and dedicated funding to initiate and to maintain the school garden education programmes.

Stakeholder and policy maker involvement

Given the unique governance system in Vietnam, not only do clear mandates need to be decided upon and followed, but project monitoring also occurs regularly throughout the intervention. AOG World Relief Vietnam is assigned a partner from a governmental department, the Department of Labour, Invalids, and Social Affairs (DOLISA), which works alongside them and guides their activities such as the selection and contact of appropriate stakeholders and community members. In addition, AOG World Relief Vietnam also liaises with the People's Committee (the main governing body of Vietnam) and the Department of Education at the district and commune level as required. In addition to working closely with the governmental partners, other primary stakeholders crucial to the success of the programme include the relevant schools, their committees of educators and administrators, and of course, the parents and students.

And, there is the partnership between AOG World Relief Vietnam and Food Plant Solutions who created the publications from which AOG World Relief Vietnam work and use as their guide in the schools. Such partnerships between the organizations, multiple levels and multiple sectors of government, and other local and external bodies are characteristic of project implementation in Vietnam, and are also what ensures effective programme outcome.

At the local level in the schools, there were specific protocols that contributed to the successful adoption of the school gardens project. As Vietnamese society is shaped by hierarchical relations and a top-down structure, the placement of the school principal and other lead staff members as 'champions' of the project is crucial. The role of these 'champions' were crucial in achieving recognition in the community of the value of the programme and in encouraging participation from other staff members and students. Moreover, as most of the school teachers in these communes are female, and mothers themselves, the school staff members were keenly aware of the importance of providing the children with healthy and nutritious foods and had a stake in adopting the strategies needed to transform the school meals and educational programmes. The participation; investment; and, above all, enthusiasm on the part of the teachers were a vital component that ensured the successful adoption and sustainability of this school garden initiative.

Key lessons learned

Physical factors that were crucial to the success of the programme include well-functioning and well-equipped kitchens on school premises and a designated cook to transform the harvested produce into nutritious meals. In terms of relations with local and governmental partners, ensuring all stakeholders fully comprehend the specific expectations and are equipped to fulfil the responsibilities required to sustain the programme in the respective schools is important to the programme's continuation and growth. This is also supported by selecting strong leadership, encouraging long-term commitment, and continued passion for the project.

In Tam Phu, the primary lesson learned was the necessity to balance the trade-off between scale and economic viability. One kindergarten in this commune had adequate funding, but did not have a sufficient amount of land to adequately grow food to feed and nourish the student population, whereas another kindergarten in the area possessed viable land for such a project but did not have adequate capital to implement it. Thus, future endeavours may involve coordinated programmes that create mutually beneficial collaborations between schools, given a close physical proximity.

Further information

Additional information on this case study can be found at www.b4fn.org/case-studies/case-studies/food-plant-solutions-school-gardens-in-vietnam/.

References

Chaparro, C., Oot, L. and Sethuraman, K. (2014) 'Vietnam nutrition profile', Washington, DC: FHI 360/FANTA.

GoV (2012) 'National Nutrition Strategy. For 2011–2020, with a Vision toward 2030', *Medicinal Publishing House*. Government of Vietnam, Hanoi, Vietnam, https://extranet.who.int/nutrition/gina/sites/default/files/VNM%202011%202.%20National%20Nutrition%20%20Strategy%202011-2020.pdf.

Horton, S. and R.H. Steckel (2013) 'Malnutrition: global economic losses attributable to malnutrition 1900–2000 and projections to 2050', in B. Lomborg (ed.), 'How much have global problems cost the world?', Cambridge: Cambridge University Press, doi:10.1017/CBO9781139225793.010.

Kozel, V. (2014) 'Well begun but not yet done: progress and emerging challenges for poverty reduction in Vietnam (English)', Washington, DC: World Bank Group, doi:10.1596/978-0-4648-0006-1.

Ozaltin, E., Hill, K. and Subramanian, S.V. (2010) 'Association of maternal stature with offspring mortality, underweight, and stunting in low- to middle-income countries', *JAMA: The Journal of the American Medical Association* 303, 1507–1516, doi:10.1001/jama.2010.450.

CASE STUDY 4

PRESERVING LOCAL CULTURAL HERITAGE THROUGH CAPACITY BUILDING FOR GIRLS IN THE MOROCCAN HIGH ATLAS

Pommelien Da Silva Cosme

Background

The High Atlas Mountains, rich in biodiversity and cultural heritage, have been shaped by a long history of close human-environment relationships, and the traditional landscape management practices of rural communities. These practices include traditional water management systems, seasonal short-distance transhumance, communal management of high-elevation pasturelands, maintenance of culturally managed trees, soil conservation through terracing, and smallholder agriculture and agroforestry. Additionally, local communities harvest medicinal and aromatic plants from the wild, a practice which is traditionally important to sustain local livelihoods. All these living traditions contribute to a diversified use of High Atlas landscapes, flora and ecosystems. Today, these traditional practices are under threat as a result of multiple drivers including climate change, overgrazing, desertification, rapid socio-economic change, and lack of supportive policies (Klik et al., 2002; GDF, 2019).

The High Atlas Mountains are inhabited by Amazigh (or Berber) communities – an ethnic group indigenous to North Africa. The Amazigh diet, known for its rich diversity, is suffering from culinary erosion as a result of socio-economic changes (e.g. food imports, rural exodus, and the industrialization of agriculture) (Barrow and Hicham, 2000), which contributes to the homogenization of diets and loss of food diversity. Wild edibles are often the first food component to be left out of the diet, despite being traditionally important in the local cuisine (Belahsen et al., 2018). Traditional plant knowledge and horticultural practices are an important part of well-being in High Atlas Amazigh communities. However, when children leave the region to attend public schools for higher education, they often lose the opportunity to learn about agriculture, gardens, and wild plant use. Traditional knowledge is also at risk of disappearing due to other factors, such as the younger generation moving away to neighbouring cities to find employment. Therefore, knowledge transmission to younger members of these communities is increasingly important for the preservation of traditional practices for future generations (Montanari, 2014).

Access to education after primary school remains a challenge in rural areas, especially for girls who live in remote villages in the High Atlas Mountains. In these areas, secondary schools are commonly located too far away for girls to travel back and forth to every day, and families often lack the resources to accommodate them near a school (Slawson, 2016). Due to poor opportunities for further education, illiteracy rates for women and girls in Morocco are up to 90% in rural areas such as the High Atlas, where only 26% of girls enrol in secondary school (World Bank, 2019). Dar Taliba, which means 'house of the female student' in Arabic, is an innovative boarding school system in Morocco, enabling girl students to pursue their secondary education and overcome challenges such as distance and lack of public transport. Through a collaborative ethnobotanical school garden project at a Dar Taliba in Ourika, Global Diversity Foundation supports girls' education beyond primary school while educating students about traditional plant knowledge and conservation of endemic, threatened, and valuable plant species.

The project

In 2015, Global Diversity Foundation established a model ethnobotanical school garden at Dar Taliba Ourika, a boarding house for girls created in 1999 to welcome students from remote villages of the Ourika Valley in the Moroccan High Atlas. An average of 130 girls enrol in the Dar Taliba boarding house annually. Over the past years, Dar Taliba students have been involved in the process of designing and developing the garden and participating in its everyday management in collaboration with a local team. The garden's main purpose is to educate the students in residence and help them learn about Amazigh indigenous plant knowledge, which has its origins in their communities located in the High Atlas Mountains. The project works to increase awareness and strengthen knowledge about traditional practices to support the conservation of the unique biodiversity and practices of the communities that have managed and maintained High Atlas landscapes for millennia (Figure C4.1).

In 2017, in collaboration with partners Moroccan Biodiversity and Livelihoods Association (MBLA) and Radiant Design, Global Diversity Foundation started organizing weekly permaculture trainings to teach the girls in residence agricultural practices such as seed saving, mulching, compost-making, enrichment planting and organic fertilizer production. These trainings help the students understand how to protect soil and local biodiversity through sustainable practices that combine traditional land and resource use with innovative approaches and enhance local economies.

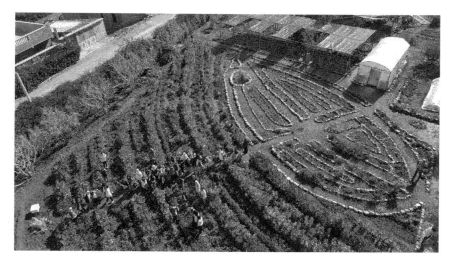

FIGURE C4.1 The Dar Taliba ethnobotanical school garden design from above.
Source: Fabien Touran

The ethnobotanical school garden now encompasses an area of 6,000 m^2 (almost one and a half acres), which is organized into different sections, including:

- A plant nursery and greenhouse for cultivation and production from seeds of wild species and traditional crops;
- An ethnobotanical garden to help students learn about the local flora and the diverse High Atlas landscapes;
- A vegetable garden to grow produce on site for school meals;
- An aromatic and medicinal garden to grow useful, valuable, and threatened species such as lavender, thyme, and sage;
- A demonstration garden for recreation, enjoyment and training for students.

Over the years, the garden has become multifunctional. It now holds great capacity to accommodate the students' outdoor trainings and garden activities, while also providing a space to read and study for their exams.

The benefits of agricultural biodiversity

Conserving local species and bringing back knowledge to the community

Over the past two years, the Dar Taliba girls have been actively engaged with local biodiversity conservation efforts while rediscovering local cultural heritage related to plants, a knowledge base which is rapidly falling into disuse and must be maintained for future generations. The ethnobotanical garden, for example, has been designed to educate the girls about local plants endemic to the regions they originally come from. The girls learn about the ecological diversity found in the High Atlas and their own cultural heritage while learning from each other about traditional practices and cuisine.

The cultivation of healthy crops in local communities is increasingly threatened by drought, lack of quality seeds, and the use of chemical fertilizers. During the garden trainings, students are learning different techniques and practical skills such as seed saving, making organic fertilizer and creating smart irrigation systems. Students share and transfer this practical knowledge to their families and communities back home, where agriculture is an important economic activity. Furthermore, the girls are cultivating threatened medicinal and aromatic plant species that have economic value such as lavender, thyme, and sage. Once the seedlings are strong enough, these valuable plants are distributed to the students, who take them to their families and plant them in their home gardens. A small number of the plants are kept for the demonstration garden within the school grounds (Figure C4.2).

Documenting traditional plant knowledge

Throughout their educational programme, the Dar Taliba students are encouraged to bring seeds and cuttings of useful plants from their villages to enrich the ethnobotanical school garden while sharing important plant knowledge from their communities. To valorize this traditional knowledge, the Dar Taliba girls worked with their families to document Amazigh names of plants, their various uses, traditional classification and associated beliefs about the natural world. The

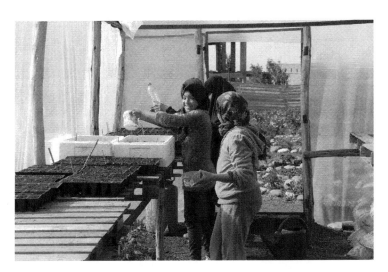

FIGURE C4.2 Dar Taliba students planting seedlings in the greenhouse.
Source: Pommelien Da Silva.

result of this joint project with other schools in the region is a plant booklet for children, which the Dar Taliba students have shared with their families. The booklet includes a selection of medicinal plants traditionally used by Amazigh communities, including:

- **Azuka** (*Tetraclinis articulata*), a small tree in the cypress family from which you can make powder useful during Ramadan fasting to avoid thirst and nausea. When its leaves are dried and burned, they can be used as a headache reliever.
- **Mkhinza** (*Dysphania ambrosoides*), a herb in the spinach subfamily that grows in the shade and humid habitats. Juice extracted from its leaves mixed with orange juice is used to treat fever.
- **Tafleyout** (*Mentha gatefossei*), an herb in the mint family that grows in fragile areas, is threatened by overgrazing. The leaves have a pleasant scent and are commonly used to prepare tea.
- **Aghdmi** (*Armeria alliacea*), a herb also known as sea pink, or thrift, grows in mountainous environments. The red roots of the plant are used to treat colds, either as an infusion or as a powder which can be added to food.
- **Tarubi** (*Rubia peregrina*), a vine in the madder or coffee family, the roots of which are used to treat anaemia. The infusion of these roots is red as blood.

Self-sufficiency and organic food production

- The students and local staff are currently growing a wide variety of plants in the school garden, such as the nitrogen producing species lucerne (*Medicago sativa*), and berseem clover (*Trifolium alexandrinum*). These are grown and used to produce organic fertilizer to stimulate the cultivation of vegetable crops such as turnip, eggplant, cucumber, tomatoes, zucchini, lettuce and green beans. In addition to the cultivation of these vegetables, the garden is surrounded by a selection of different fruit trees, including pomegranate, lemon, fig and quince. The vegetables, fruits and herbs produced in the garden are harvested during weekly garden trainings and used by the Dar Taliba kitchen staff to provide healthy and nutritious school meals for the girls and local team. The olive trees surrounding the Dar Taliba grounds provide an annual supply of olive oil, which lasts throughout the school year. This is also true of the onions, potatoes, and garlic, and fresh herbs such as parsley and coriander, which are grown in a separate small garden next to the kitchen. These are all staple ingredients in traditional Moroccan cuisine and support the school's self-sufficiency in organic food production. The Dar Taliba students and gardeners all agree the organic vegetables and fruits they grow themselves taste much better than those bought in the local market or 'souk'. When the girls leave for school breaks, vegetables, herbs, and medicinal plants are distributed to encourage the girls to share the fruits of their work with their families and to avoid any food waste (Figure C4.3).

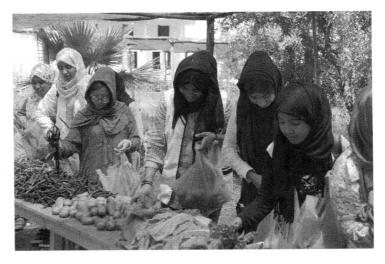

FIGURE C4.3 Students during a plant and vegetable distribution.
Source: Pommelien Da Silva.

Impact

So far, 700 Moroccan girls have benefited from the school garden training programme. Through this project, Global Diversity Foundation is not only supporting girls' access to further education, it is providing healthy outdoor activities and nutritious food for the students in residence, while offering opportunities to learn about traditional agriculture and wild plant use.

The current director at Dar Taliba was a student at the boarding house herself almost 17 years ago and benefited from the opportunity to pursue her studies after primary school at the boarding house. In her role as director, she has experienced the benefits of involving students in the running of the garden, especially cultivating and harvesting their own food, which they find to be very rewarding work. She is currently conducting a survey in collaboration with Global Diversity Foundation to understand how the experience in the boarding house has impacted the lives of alumnae who were previously in residence.

This school programme has already inspired several girls to pursue higher education in agriculture. The Dar Taliba team hopes this programme will encourage the rising generation to support their communities with new knowledge and techniques.

Future

First developed in 2015, the Dar Taliba garden project is now well established and has garnered interest from neighbouring schools in the Ourika Valley who have reached out to visit the garden to learn more about the project. These visits, from both primary and secondary students, have encouraged the team to think about partnering with other schools in the region to establish school gardens and educational programmes similar to the model at Dar Taliba.

Furthermore, the project will continue to nurture existing and new partnerships that help sustain and further develop the garden and the educational programme provided to all the students in residence.

Key lessons learned

Clear and regular communication between the boarding house, the school, local team, and project partners has been key to ensure the success and smooth running of this project. Furthermore, the active involvement of local community members and the students themselves, throughout the creation of the garden and educational programme has been instrumental in establishing this model project. Another key lesson is the benefit of reaching out to local experts – who later became important project partners – to support the development of the school garden, which was designed based on permaculture principles and further expanded with an innovative drip irrigation system to ensure a stable water supply throughout the year. Finally, it is very important to carry out regular evaluations of the functioning of the garden, as well as the educational programme and activities provided to the students, with all partners involved.

Acknowledgements

Projects like these are impossible without the commitment and passion of a local team and project partners and this project is no exception. The Dar Taliba students, local team, project partners, community members, local authorities, and project funders have all played an important part in creating this green space where students can learn about traditional plant use and agricultural practices, and share the knowledge and skills learned with their communities in the High Atlas Mountains. Finally, this project would not be possible without the generous and ongoing support of the MAVA Foundation, Darwin Initiative and private donors.

Read more

- The Dar Taliba school garden: www.global-diversity.org/programmes/mediterranean/preserving-local-cultural-heritage-through-capacity-building-for-girls/
- Global Diversity Foundation: www.global-diversity.org/
- High Atlas Cultural Landscapes: www.global-diversity.org/programmes/mediterranean/school-gardens-project-in-morocco/
- Medicinal plants in Imegdal – a book for children www.global-diversity.org/wp-content/uploads/2015/03/Medicinal-Plants-in-Imegdale.pdf

References

Barrow, C.J. and Hicham, H. (2000) 'Two complementary and integrated land uses of the western High Atlas Mountains, Morocco: the potential for sustainable rural livelihoods'. *Applied Geography*, Vol 20 (4): 369–394, doi:10.1016/S0143-6228(00)00010-2.

Belahsen, R., Naciri, K. and Ibrahimi, A.E. (2018) 'Food security and women's roles in Moroccan Berber (Amazigh) society today'. *Maternal; Child Nutrition*, Vol 13 (S3), doi:10.1111/mcn.12562.

GDF (2019) 'Enhancing the resilience of High Atlas agroecosystems in Morocco'. Global Diversity Foundation. Accessed 24 April 2019: https://www.global-diversity.org/programmes/mediterranean/enhancing-the-resilience-of-high-atlas-agroecosystems-in-morocco/.

Klik, A., Kaitua, R. and Badraoui, M. (2002). 'Desertification hazard in the Mountainous Ecosystem in the High Atlas region, Morocco'. 12th ISCO Conference.

Montanari, B. (2014) 'Aromatic, Medicinal Plants and Vulnerability of Traditional Herbal Knowledge in a Berber Community of the High Atlas Mountains of Morocco'. *Chinese Academy of Science/Plant Diversity and Resources*, Vol 36 (3): 388–402, doi:10.7677/ynzwyj201413160.

Slawson, N. (2016) 'In Morocco's Atlas Mountains, Berber girls find the way out of rural poverty: an education', The Guardian, 19 Jun 2016.

World Bank (2019) 'Databank – Education Statistics'. Accessed 24 April 2019: https://databank.worldbank.org/data/reports.aspx?source=Education%20Statistics.

CASE STUDY 5

LEARNING GARDENS CULTIVATING HEALTH AND WELL-BEING – STORIES FROM AUSTRALIA

Peter Dawe, Anthea Fawcett, and Torres Webb

Introduction

The multi-functional benefits of traditional food gardens in school and learning settings

Biodiverse gardens that marry traditional food plants with introduced fruits and vegetables at school and other learning settings help to promote better health and well-being and support the transmission of traditional knowledge in a variety of ways in Australia. Indigenous youth participation and learning outcomes are demonstrably strengthened when elders and community members provide input to the design and delivery of learning activities both at school and on country in the greater garden.

This case study presents the story of three approaches that utilise food gardens, traditional knowledge and strengths-based learning to engage indigenous youth and older generations in learning together to foster better health, nutrition and emotional well-being. Torres Webb, an indigenous man and educator from the Torres Strait, shares insights from his experiences with school and community gardening initiatives in northern Australia. Peter Dawe from the Royal Botanic Garden's Youth Community Greening (YCG) program describes the process and benefits of an innovative Aboriginal learning space and garden where Elders provide cultural learning, connections, and support to youth in juvenile detention. Third, a brief story about EduGrow, a modest strengths-based gardening awards programme that was conducted in East Arnhem Land for several years to encourage students to learn about growing and enjoying healthy food in enjoyable, culturally relevant ways.

Each story speaks to its time and place, and offers insights about different types of strength-based leadership and garden benefits. Traditional knowledge

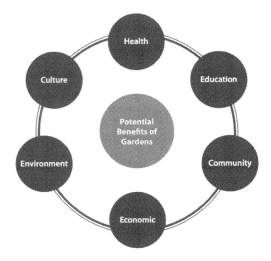

FIGURE C5.1 Potential benefits of gardens.
Source: Anthea Fawcett.

about food and plants is integral to each story albeit in different ways. All share the understanding that school and learning based gardens offer diverse and multifunctional benefits and that these are best realised in partnership and consultation with local leaders, community organizations and parents. Learning about nutritious foods and healthy lifestyles through garden-based programmes are executed in a variety of ways across mainstream Australia.[1] The stories shared in this case study offer additional perspectives on well-being benefits that garden based activities may offer Indigenous youth and communities in less mainstream contexts, as the following schematic suggests (Figure C5.1).

Setting the scene

Connection to country, caring for and drawing from the greater garden of traditional food and healing plants, animals and ecosystems that make up Australia's rich and diverse landscapes are integral to the languages and cultural knowledges and practices of Australia's Aboriginal and Torres Strait Islanders. For over 60,000 years Australia's First Peoples have lived and prospered with the land, practising food and land management practices that nurture country, culture and people with respect and a view to the health and well-being of future generations and of mother earth who nurtures and is home to all.

The layered traumas of European colonization have contributed to complex, adverse inter-generational biopsychosocial health impacts[2] that resound today and are the subject of ongoing Close the Gap and National Reconciliation efforts. As Australia approaches and reflects upon 230 years of European settlement and its legacies, growing numbers of people are taking action to address food sovereignty, food security, food justice, and help build healthier, more diverse and resilient food systems. In this environment, the creativity and resilience of Australia's First Peoples abounds, and Indigenous professionals and community leaders are at the forefront of healing their communities that face disproportionate levels of preventable chronic disease, incarceration, youth suicide and socio-economic disadvantage.

Indigenous researchers and writers are helping all Australians to recast modernist (economic and ontological) ways of thinking and being with mother earth ('we are all indigenous to the earth') (Arabena, 2015). Since publication in 2014, Bruce Pascoe's *Dark Emu: Black Seeds: Agriculture or Accident?* has not only recast Australian history as one radically 'other' to past simplistic views of First Peoples as nomadic 'hunter-gatherers' but is helping drive a dramatic reimagination of 'new-but-"innovatively"-old' prospective food futures. By revealing the sophisticated food systems, agricultural and productive land management practices of First Australians, Pascoe's groundbreaking work is generating active reflection, debate and new potential pathways to propagate healthier landscape and agricultural plantings for healthier people, environments and more biodiverse food futures.

The United Nation's International Year of Indigenous Languages (2019) issues a call to amplify efforts to protect and preserve traditional knowledges and support the generation, transmission and protection of language/s that can capture and transfer cultural world views and values that often entail intimate, sacred, traditional healing and food plant knowledge. Not 'all' people – actually – are entitled to access this knowledge if we truly wish to respect the preservation of traditional culture and knowledge by those who own it and or rightly should first prosper from it. As attention turns to the potential of cultivating indigenous plant species as food crops, it is important to not again appropriate indigenous knowledge and practices for the benefit of others rather than Aboriginal people (Larsen et al., 2019).

Agrobiodiversity initiatives[3] recognise and aim to promote the value of more people accessing more traditional foods to add diversity to diets and agricultural production systems, to alleviate hunger and help redress the legacies of mono-agriculture; environmental degradation; and the growth in preventable chronic disease associated with high-fat, high-carbohydrate, low-nutrition, modern, highly processed foods and diets that especially contribute to high levels of preventable chronic disease.

In Australia, as elsewhere, the transition from traditional diets to high-fat, high-sugar, highly processed poor nutrition foods has been very damaging and has resulted in an escalation of preventable diet-related chronic diseases. These dilemmas are well recognised. Over the past decade these health and related food system challenges have been tackled by the efforts of research initiatives such as those led by Dr Julie Brimblecome at the Menzies School of Health Research, and now at Monash University, and Close the Gap healthy and active lifestyle health promotion initiatives. The efforts of diverse NGO and community-based programs that promote better awareness of healthy foods and the importance of good nutrition and healthy and active lifestyles are helping to improve Indigenous health and well-being. Indigenous lead school garden and learning on country initiatives play powerful roles to reconnect students with culture, healthy life skills, and healthy 'fusion' diets that include traditional foods alongside introduced fruit and vegetables – approaches that combine cultivated gardens with traditional food knowledge and land management practices of tending the greater garden landscape.

European colonisation resulted in wide-ranging dislocation and dispossession of First Peoples from their traditional lands and the right and ability to continue cultural practices on country and to sustain uninterrupted transmission of traditional food and health knowledge. The Mission era required many first contact First Peoples to disavow traditional (healthy!) food traditions of lean bush meats and high antioxidant and complex fibre bush plants in favour of tea, sugar and flour. These severances coincided with further familial and emotional traumas of the Stolen Generations era that saw many children dispossessed from their families and country. Australia is a very culturally, historically and topographically diverse continent – with wide-ranging growing conditions, food traditions and colonial alienation experiences. Australia was once home to more than 250 Indigenous Australian languages including 800 dialectical varieties. Today, only 13 traditional Indigenous languages are still acquired by children and approximately another 100 or so are spoken to various degrees by older generations, with many of these languages at risk as Elders pass away.[4]

Australia's First Peoples and their lived experiences are as diverse as the breadth of language groups suggest. This diversity is amplified by the different experiences of dispossession from family and country that colonization delivered in different parts of Australia. Some First Peoples have retained relatively uninterrupted connection to country, cultural knowledge and land management practices while many in regions that were more intensely settled by European settlers and where First People were more fully dispossessed from country and/or stolen from family now often seek ways to reconnect with and engage with family, country, and culture. Each story speaks a different and nuanced type of trauma and healing process. All experiences speak to the diversity, resilience, and sophistication of Australia's First Peoples, who often straddle two worlds and may live and move between remote, rural, and urban Australia.[5] In 2016 the majority (81%) of Aboriginal people lived in cities and non-remote areas, and only a quarter lived in remote (7%) and very remote (12%) areas. That said, in the Northern Territory, where 30% of the population are Aboriginal, 81% live in remote communities, and these populations are growing.

So with this diversity to mind, we turn to three contemporary school and learning environment garden models that share stories drawn from the diversity of Australia's First Peoples' experiences in remote, rural, and urban Australia.

Championing growing our own food for the future

Torres Webb

I am a proud Australian Indigenous man from the Torres Strait, Erub (Darnley Island). I am of the Samsep Clan and one of my key totems is the Nam (Green Turtle).

My heritage and ancient culture hail from the beautiful picturesque volcanic soil islands of the eastern Torres Strait and is based around the importance of sustainability with the garden, planting and growing our own at the centre. Our ancient sacred lore and rule (*Malo ra Gelar*) which can be likened to something like the commandments from the bible have always been a guide for myself and family throughout my life passed on from generation to generation.

Our lore *Malo ra Gelar* states the following:

Malo tag mauki mauki:	*Malo keeps his hands to himself; he does not touch what is not his.*
Teter mauki mauki:	*He does not permit his feet to carry him towards another man's property.*
Wali aritarit, sem aritarit:	*Malo plants everywhere – under wali (a creeping vine) and sem the yellow flowered hibiscus.*
Eburlem, esmaolem:	*Let it drop and rot on the ground.*

Having grown up and being grounded in my cultural lore and customs, I have always had a strong affiliation, understanding, and connection to the importance of 'growing our own', gardening and planting for a sustainable future to not only provide for ourselves in the present but to also think of future generations and the importance of leaving a positive legacy for a sustainable and hopeful future.

Stewardship of our natural environment through sustainable planting and gardening practices is instilled from birth. One of our ancient traditional customs that has been practised for thousands of years is that once a child is born the afterbirth is saved and buried in a special place of cultural custodianship, where a tree is then planted to link, from birth, the child to the planet with a sense of belonging, a sense of identity, a sense of responsibility, and a sense of pride. These foundations on which our culture is based have inspired me and spurred me on throughout my life to actively preserve and protect our culture.

I have worked in various natural resource management roles throughout my career and experienced many challenges as to the implementation of sustainable management practices through Indigenous ways of seeing, being, and living in the world. I have learned, and know, that it is only through education that we could have the biggest impact in creating positive, equitable and sustainable change into the future.

Moving into a role working within the education system in Queensland as a community engagement project officer, I was tasked with the job of assisting school communities in Far North Queensland to strengthen learning relationships between school, family, and community. With education systems already having a myriad of frameworks, strategies, and operational plans in place, I knew that the key first step was to ask the parents, families, and communities what was most important to them to not only improve student achievement but to also foster improved student well-being and life-chances into the future. In doing so, I drew from research (West-Burnham et al., 2007) and my work as an associate to the Centre for Relational Learning.[6] This knowledge clearly indicates that only 20% of a child's achievement and success in life lies within the school gate and 80% of potential achievement and success sits within the social and personal, family and community – *it takes a village to raise a child*. Otero and others have documented research to show that over 80% of the factors that determine achievement, well-being and success in life lie outside the gates of the school house.[7] Personal and social factors such as family, poverty, ways of knowing, language, history, motivation, ability, resilience and strong relationships all influence learning and therefore achievement. These personal and social factors are all heightened when the culture of the school is not reflective or responsive to the culture of the community which that school serves.

Knowing this, I organized and facilitated many community conversations (similar to a yarning circle) based around three key questions. Who are we? What's worth learning? How can we learn best together? These community conversations provided a space where people felt safe and equal to share their feelings, thoughts and ideas in a trusting, mutually respectful environment. In this space, parents and community were in partnership with the school and felt valued about their strengths, aspirations, and abilities to contribute. It was then possible to develop a shared vision and to articulate key priorities and shared expectations, and to collectively identify and develop key priorities. Priorities commonly identified were to be leaders, to build strong community and culture – and to be able to confidently walk in both worlds. From these co-designed key commitments one of the key actions which frequently followed was the importance of *growing our own* food to improve work towards self-sufficiency. This included not only bush tucker native plants but also garden-based vegetables (sweet potato, watermelon, and corn) and beautiful exotic tropical fruit trees (Rambutan, chempadek, durian, sapote, etc.) which grow very well in the tropical environment of Far North Queensland.

There are many great examples of successful projects one of which the below photograph depicts working with the Tagai State College School Community in the Torres Strait where our students have not only have had the opportunity to learn from Elders passing on intricate knowledge of gardening and planting techniques but also an opportunity to take the lead in contributing to the community planting not only within the school grounds but also in local community garden spaces (Figure C5.2).

These activities demonstratively build a real sense of pride, ownership and leadership not only within students themselves but also the wider community. Through dialogue forums and discussions with parents, families, children, youth,

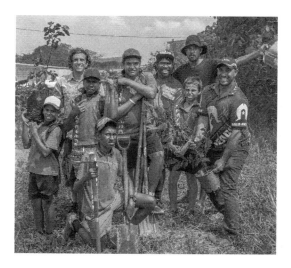

FIGURE C5.2 Torres (right) with students from Tagai State College School Community in the Torres Strait.
Source: Chris La Rosa.

school, and community, many benefits were discussed as to the importance of our 'growing our own' project to inspire self-sufficiency within our communities. The added benefits noticed and noted were:

- Financial: Less strain on the household income as food could be harvested free from the garden. Exorbitant prices for food – particularly in the more remote parts of Queensland
- Nutritional: Due to the tyranny of distance and the vast transportation mileage. Much of the food that does arrive into our communities is often quite old; bruised; or, in some cases, close to rotten. Growing food locally not only tastes better but also improves nutrition leading to improved health especially with the high rates of chronic disease being so prevalent in our Indigenous communities.
- Well-being: A sense of pride and respect, sense of belonging, and a sense of responsibility. These were all named as important benefits, foundational to a positive sense of identity, contribution, and achievement. Noticeable behavioural improvements of students were noted when they were given an opportunity to take the lead on a project through the development of a sense of ownership.

Now currently working with one of Australia's science organizations, I lead a project around embedding the ancient (non-secret/non-sacred) Indigenous science knowledges and wisdoms within the school curriculum through an inquiry-based learning approach. I have noticed that not only have our Indigenous students' STEM (science, technology, engineering, mathematics) engagement and achievement improved, but so too has the performance of non-indigenous students. I find these outcomes extremely powerful and rewarding, as they illustrate not only the benefits of improving educational outcomes but also the benefits of cultural bridging and building reconciliation for the future. These multiple benefits are being realized by taking a strengths-based approach by focussing on what's strong rather than what's wrong.

Wiridjiribin Nura within the Reiby Juvenile Justice Centre

Peter Dawe

The Royal Botanic Garden Sydney's Youth Community Greening (YCG) programme is an environmental education programme targeting disadvantaged urban and regional youth from pre-school to young adults across NSW. One of the numerous sites that the programme works with is Dorchester School, within the Reiby Juvenile Justice Centre.

The Reiby Juvenile Justice Centre is located on Dharawal Country in Airds near Campbelltown in Sydney and has the capacity to detain and house up to 55 young people, with females up to the age of 20 and young males under the age of 16.

Since 2014 YCG has been heavily involved with the Centre's school – Dorchester School, in the garden programme and has been part of the Reiby Aboriginal Community Consultative Committee (RACCC). It was this committee's decision to create the Aboriginal learning space, Wiridjiribin Nura, (Lyrebird Country), within the centre, having identified the need for a space appropriate for young Aboriginal people to engage culture and connect to country and gain a stronger sense of identity.

Committee members include Reiby Juvenile Justice and Dorchester School staff, Tharawal Aboriginal Corporation, local Aboriginal Elders, Campbelltown Police, National Parks and Wildlife, and various community service providers.

All members of the RACCC and some selected students from Dorchester School were involved in the entire process including design, preparation, and implementation and ongoing maintenance. Throughout the design and development of the learning circle, Uncle Ivan Wellington (local Elder) and Uncle Dean Kelly (NPWS) had significant involvement providing guidance and wisdom.

The design incorporated three paths throughout the garden, connecting the different spaces. These paths are significant in Aboriginal culture representing teaching disciplines. They are 'respect', 'patience', and 'observation' and before entering into the space for ceremony, all are reminded of these values (Figure C5.3).

The Centre's youth were involved in most aspects of the garden development. Even when contractors were used for breaking existing concrete and creating the paths, they were assisted where possible by the students from the school/centre.

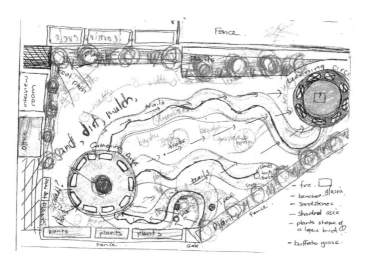

FIGURE C5.3 The Aboriginal learning space and garden. Illustration: Luciano Valeo.

Plants were either purchased through grants or donated by nurseries to the YCG programme. Every plant within the space had a traditional use to the Aboriginal people, from bush tucker to plants used for tools, weapons, and medicine. During the extensive planting process, which continues today, the youth have been engaged in learning about Aboriginal culture and practice by connecting and caring for the environment.

In the five years since conception, the space has continued to evolve. Particularly since the female detainees were relocated to Reiby in 2016. An extensive water feature was added as well as more weaving and fruiting plants. The dance area is regularly used for cultural dance workshops and performances by both the school and the centre. Counsellors use the green space to work with the youth and mentors regularly access the learning circle.

YCG works closely with Dorchester School within the Centre and is involved in garden programmes on a fortnightly basis. Several gardens and activities are included in this programme; however, Wiridjiribin Nura is certainly the most rewarding aspect of the programme. As part of the Dorchester School programme, each detainee learns about the cultural significance of the plants in the garden and many are used in cooking and weaving activities. The youth also take pride in maintaining the space by pruning and weeding and often by suggesting additional plants which they know of from their country.

With the involvement of the Tharawal Aboriginal Corporation and local Elders from the outset, their knowledge and participation continue to play a vital role in the cultural education of the youth within the centre. Uncle Ivan, in particular, regularly visits and talks to the detainees, connecting them to their culture. Aboriginal Education Officers from the Australian Museum also visit

202 Peter Dawe et al.

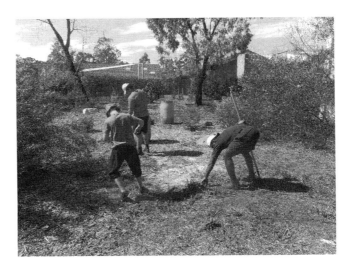

FIGURE C5.4 Cultural learning, gardening and leadership in action at Wiridjiribin Nura.
Source: Peter Dawe.

providing lessons on Aboriginal culture. All these lessons and talks take place around the inviting and tranquil learning circle.

During NAIDOC and other significant cultural events, Wiridjiribin Nura is the focal point for celebrations and the young detainees showcase their cultural knowledge and respect. Uncle Dean Kelly will often talk at these events emphasizing the three paths – respect, patience, and observation and instilling in the young people a deep pride in their culture and an understanding of the importance to connect with it.

The school garden programme is one of the longest running and most successful programmes within the centre. It provides young people from all cultural backgrounds the opportunity to connect with the earth and enjoy all the benefits of this. YCG will continue to support and guide this programme as it has helped so many of the incarcerated youth mentally, physically, and spiritually for the last five years (Figure C5.4).

The EduGrow School Garden Awards – East Arnhem Land

Anthea Fawcett

The EduGrow School Garden Awards were created to encourage and provide support to teachers, students and school community members who live and learn together in some of Australia's most remote, small northern communities to create and to sustain school food gardens that could provide a safe, fun and engaging third space for gardening, cooking and diverse cross-curricula learning activities that might include maths and literacy, enterprise development, art, local plant knowledge, science, and language.

Food insecurity, poor student health, nutrition, and low participation rates associated with the challenges of students being required to learn in English, a second (if not third or fourth) language in potentially intimidating school environments were some of the contextual drivers for the creation of the EduGrow Awards. The award categories and the pathways to enter were designed to be fun and flexible, and were open to schools of all sizes, with students of all ages. The programme ran over one to two school terms each year from 2012 to 2015.[8] Participating schools ranged from small, isolated Homelands schools, with perhaps 15–30 students of all ages, to schools located in larger remote indigenous communities whose student numbers ranged from 200 to 700 students from preschool to final year high school.

All of these schools are in communities located in tropical, cyclone areas and in direct proximity to country, the greater garden, where educational activities for older students about land conservation and management is conducted by schools and Ranger groups. Accordingly that is where many bush foods and plants are studied, cared for, and cultivated or collected. These schools and their communities regularly experience wet seasons and can be cut off by road from larger centres for many weeks. This means that local food stores are critical to the provision of a regular, accessible supply of food staples and play an important role in the community. Tropical conditions also mean that it is possible (with the right skills and knowledge) to grow food at school, at home and in the community for most of the year and can contribute to food resilience.

A celebratory, strengths-based programme

EduGrow's overarching theme was to encourage growing 'good food, good learning and good times' at school in the spirit of 'food, family and community' and to do so in ways that invited and encouraged the two-way sharing of knowledge and the involvement of different generations in learning and sharing knowledge about traditional and introduced healthy foods and lifestyles.

Although structured as an awards programme (students and schools appeared to enjoy the dynamics of friendly local competition and award ceremonies in their communities!) the program was designed as a celebratory, strengths-based recognition programme in which 'everyone' was winner. The programme was initiated by and run by the Remote Indigenous Gardens Network, a small programme based in Sydney who approached and received in principle encouragement and some sponsorship support from the Arnhem Land Progress Aboriginal Corporation Aboriginal (ALPA) to develop and conduct the awards. With a small budget, a strong and highly respected local partner organization, and in response to challenges posed by remoteness, the programme was delivered mainly via on-line, email, and phone communications. On-ground support was also provided by respected local community partners and nurseries who provided gardening supplies and other practical support to participating schools. Modest cash incentives to help initiate gardens, along with cash and book prizes and 'many' Award Certificates encouraged participation and provided recognition at the conclusion of the awards each year.

Flexible categories and an appreciative judging process ensured that every school and school project who participated were recognized as winners and were awarded for their particular efforts and achievements that were then celebrated and shared via an awards ceremony in a participating community, newsletters, and programme communications.

Each year the awards invitation and entry process invited schools to submit entries that told the story about their school garden and the activities undertaken to plan and develop it; how the school garden was used as a learning place; and how the school garden and associated cooking, healthy lifestyle or enterprising activities were used to invite and involve elders, parents, and community members in inter-generational learning and school community building. Optional special themes or topics were also suggested and schools were welcome to elect to focus upon one or more as might best suit opportunities to link with other activities underway at their school and in their community.

Themes such as 'Healthy soil for healthy food and people' generated wonderful entries about worm farms, composting and learning about how to use local materials and permaculture techniques to enrich local soils and create small nurseries at school. Wicking garden beds developed and created in a variety of ways and often decorated with artwork from students of different ages were popular in this theme and as an important way to create and sustain productive food gardens – something especially challenging in areas with often sandy, ancient depleted soils.

Other themes such as 'Planning and making special places', 'Special visitors and teamwork' and 'Local leaders and legends' provided opportunities to celebrate the achievements of Elders, students, and Indigenous educators and teacher aides who worked together to create special projects. Highlights in this area included entries that featured stories about special cultural and healing spaces and places that were designed by students and community members and involved artwork and placemaking within the school grounds and drew on local, special knowledge and historical memories of Elders. Small bush-tucker nursery beds and growing activities led by Elders who worked with children with behavioural issues in special classes illustrated the transmission of traditional knowledge as did entries that featured parents and grandparents participating in reading and story-telling classes in language to share knowledge about bush plants and popular traditional foods.

'Healthy food enterprise projects' was a popular theme across a number of locations. During the years the awards ran, a wide-ranging number of entries featured garden produce market days and student and family cook-up days that utilized garden produce. Others featured monthly school 'café' days at which healthy foods and gardening inputs were shared with and sold to the community. Numerous school entries shared stories about cooking classes and student efforts to prepare and then sell garden produce, cooked foods including jams, cordials, and cakes (often featuring tomatoes, eggplant, 'rosella', and other bush plant inputs) along with worm-juice, propagated plants and seedlings grown by students. These garden-based and healthy food activities demonstrate how schools used their garden programmes to provide engaging curricula and life-skills learning, along with providing students with the opportunity to enjoy developing and putting into practice planning, team work and enterprise skills while also generating some funds that were used to further develop their school gardens.

Linked-up skills for healthy food and good nutrition grow on

EduGrow was a modest awards programme that ran successfully for a number of years in Arnhem Land and northern Australia. For a variety of reasons, since 2015 the programme has changed focus and now offers informal advice, networking, and support, on request, to teachers at schools in remote and rural areas.

In November 2014 the EduGrow Awards ceremony was a large joyful and well-attended event that was held at Shepherdson College, at Galiwin'ku, on Elcho Island. Shepherdson College's garden was much loved, productive and beautiful. In just a few short years the garden had grown to encompass many areas of the large school grounds, provided a learning place for students of all ages, was home to diverse garden installations, wicking bed play areas and artworks, a much loved permaculture-based chicken coop whose chickens were even more deeply loved and cared for by primary school-age students. At those awards, Shepherdson College once again received many awards and an Elder from ALPA's Board presided over the presentations. Parents and community members were invited to tour the garden before the awards ceremony and to receive a mulberry tree propagated by students. According to some, the school received the greatest number of family

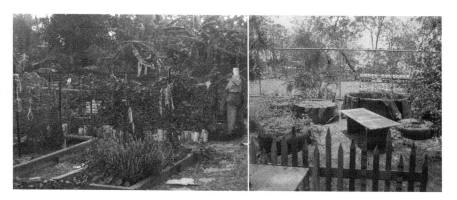

FIGURE C5.5 Diverse tropical planting garden (left) and Shepherdson College's Award winning 'Water-wise' food garden and play area (right). Both from Nov 2014.

Source: Anthea Fawcett.

and community visitors that day – they were rightly proud of their school garden and what their children and grand-children had achieved in it (Figure C5.5).

Early in 2015 two devastating cyclones struck Arnhem Land with devastating effects on Galiwin'ku and the coastal and island communities of Arnhem Land. Buildings and landscapes were flattened and the much-loved large trees of Galiwin'ku lost – as was much of Shepherdson College's garden and the gardens of other schools who participated in EduGrow.

The resilient people of Galinwin'ku and elsewhere in Arnhem Land continue to rebuild their communities and ALPA grows from strength to strength in the delivery of Aboriginal lead training, social, economic, and community development programmes, and in the management and operation of their community food stores. These stores, such as the one at Galiwin'ku, often include a nursery and gardening supplies. These inputs – along with those from the greater garden and the skills, ingenuity and resilience of people who know how to grow their own food continue to grow on.

Notes

1. The Stephanie Alexander Kitchen Garden programme provides gardening and cooking resources and support to hundreds of Australian schools in urban, regional, and some remote locations. In remote northern Australia, the EON Foundation partners with community leaders to establish edible gardens at school or in the community in order to secure a supply of fresh food that is coupled with practical gardening, nutrition, cooking and hygiene education to promote healthy lifestyles and help prevent disease. See https://www.kitchengardenfoundation.org.au and https://eon.org.au (cited June 2019).
2. See A Contributing Life: the 2013 National Report Card on Mental Health and Suicide Prevention, Australian Government, National Mental Health Commission for elaboration of the biopsychosocial model of health and as it especially relates to inter-generational health challenges experienced by Australia's First Peoples.
3. See Summary Experts Report – United Nations Decade of Action on Nutrition 2016–2015, High-Level Expert Seminar on Indigenous Food Systems, building on traditional knowledge to achieve Zero Hunger, Final report, FAO Headquarters, Rome, Red Room A121.
4. https://aiatsis.gov.au/explore/articles/indigenous-australian-languages – cited 15 June 2019.
5. In 2016 the majority (81%) of Aboriginal people lived in cities and non-remote areas, up from 75% in 2006. 37% lived in major cities, 24% in inner regional areas, and 20% in outer regional areas. Contrary to what is commonly believed, only a quarter lived in remote (7%) and very remote (12%) areas. That said, in the Northern Territory, where 30% of the population are Aboriginal, 81% live in remote communities; see www.creativespirits.info/aboriginalculture/people/aboriginal-population-in-australia#toc0.
6. http://relationalearning.com/about-crl/associates/.
7. For example, Dr George Otero, Centre for Relational Learning, Santa-Fe, New Mexico; see www.education.sa.gov.au/teaching/teaching-effective-learning/project-colleagues-teaching-effective-learning/dr-george-otero.
8. The EduGrow Awards began in 2012 and were initiated to support community activities conducted by the Arnhem Land Progress Aboriginal Corporation Aboriginal (ALPA) to celebrate their 40th Anniversary. In 2012 the awards were open to all schools in ALPA's five original member communities. From In 2013 and 2014 the

awards were promoted and open to all schools in Arnhem Land and in 2015 to those across remote Australia. ALPA is an outstanding Aboriginal owned and controlled organization who own and/or operate food stores in the Northern Territory, Cape York, and the Torres Strait Islands as well as running diverse social and economic community development programmes and services in their member communities. ALPA has a deep commitment to health and nutrition education and to the promotion of healthy food. Numerous initiatives deliver this, via their Health and Nutrition Policy. These include consumer support such as the Nutrition Checklist App, community-based food basket, and healthy food systems research that they have partnered with Menzie's School of Health Research on and sustained commitment to in-store healthy food promotion activities that have included collaboration with the Jimmy Little Foundation's 'Thumbs Up! Good Tucker – Long Life' programme to provide culturally engaging, in-store healthy food labelling and information. To learn more about ALPA, visit https://www.alpa.asn.au.

References

Arabena, K. (2015) 'Becoming Indigenous to the Universe: Reflections on Living Systems, Indigeneity and Citizenship', Australian Scholarly Publishing, ISBN:9781925333060.

Larsen, K., Sheridan, J. and Hill, S. (2019) 'Sustainable Food Systems', Australian Environmental Grantmakers Network Philanthropy, Briefing, March 2019, https://www.aegn.org.au/2019/03/sustainable-food-systems/, accessed June 2019.

West-Burnham, J., Farrar, M. and Otero, G. (2007) 'Schools and communities – working together to transform children's lives', Network Continuum Education, ISBN:9781855395213.

CASE STUDY 6

AFRICAN LEAFY VEGETABLES GO BACK TO SCHOOL

Farm to school networks embrace biodiversity for food and nutrition in Kenya

Aurillia Manjella, Alessandra Grasso, and Victor Wasike[1]

School gardens that supply or complement school feeding programmes have been identified as a best practice for mobilizing biodiversity and improving dietary diversity in schoolchildren by the Biodiversity for Food and Nutrition (BFN) project. In Kenya, school gardens are especially important to provide nutritious meals to growing children and adolescents, who may otherwise go hungry.

Background

Kenya is constantly struggling with severe droughts and water shortages, challenging food production in rural areas where 80% of the population live (Langinger, 2011). Other factors contributing to food insecurity include high costs of domestic food production due to high costs of inputs, high food prices and high levels of poverty (IFPRI, 2019). As a result, it is estimated that 10 million people today live in food insecurity corresponding to 20% of the population in Kenya. For children the numbers look even worse with 26% suffering from chronic under-nutrition (IFPRI, 2016). In many rural areas the percentages are substantially higher.

Through the governmental school feeding programmes, simple, unvaried meals are served to students, which are comprised of maize-based gruel or maize-bean mixtures and are, at best, supplemented by meat, kale, or cabbage, depending on seasonality. The school budget is limited and thus many nutrient-rich foods are out of a schools' price range. Instead cheaper, but often less nutritious, alternatives are prioritized for the school meals (Hunter et al., 2017). A simple meal is far better than no meal, yet children are still suffering from nutritional stress – the stress that is caused by nutrient deficiency. This is a significant educational problem in Kenya influencing the attendance and performance negatively in the schools (Mukudi, 2003).

School gardening, or school farming as often referred to in a Kenyan context, has been practiced as part of education in Kenya for many years, especially in rural areas where it goes back to colonial times (Foeken et al., 2007). Today, farming activities in schools are usually organized through the 4-K clubs[2] or other youth clubs, through agricultural classes or the school itself. The species that are grown in the school gardens (*shambas* in Swahili) are usually maize, beans, banana, and other staple crops. These are healthy and important, but they do not cover all the necessary vitamins and mineral intake for a balanced, healthy diet.

In conclusion, traditional, highly nutritious, and biodiverse foods are simply not finding their way to the plates of Kenyan students, despite the capacity that lies in this unused resource.

The project

In Busia county in western Kenya, the Biodiversity for Food and Nutrition (BFN) project is changing this by giving children opportunities to acquire agricultural skills with attention to the cultivation of nutrient-rich African leafy vegetables (ALVs) and their contribution to improved nutrition amongst rural children. Funded by the Global Environment Facility (GEF) and the Australian Centre for International Agricultural Research (ACIAR), garden demonstration plots were established in seven primary and secondary schools. This was done in collaboration with the Department of Education, along with a local community-based organization Sustainable Income Generating Investment Group (Kenya) (SINGI) and Departments of Agriculture and Health.

Teachers from the selected schools took part in Training of Trainers (ToTs) workshops, where they learned the importance and practice of school gardening to improve child and adolescent nutrition. The newly trained staff were then able to take their own unique approach to introduce and implement the BFN gardens at their schools. Now equipped with local trainers, schools in Busia's seven sub-counties broke ground and planted various local ALVs such as spider plant, amaranth, vine spinach, jute mallow, slender leaf, black nightshade, African kales, and pumpkin leaves and fruit trees such as guava, gooseberry, avocado, jackfruit, and passion fruit (Figure C6.1).

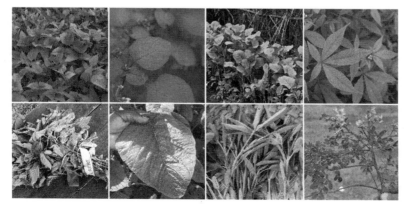

FIGURE C6.1 A selection of ALVs in Kenya. From the left corner: cowpea leaves (*Vigna unguiculata*), African nightshade (*Solanum nigrum*), Ethiopian kale (*Brassica carinata*), spider plant (*Cleome gynandra*), jute mallow (*Corchorus olitorius*), amaranth (*Amaranthus*), slender leaf (*Crotalaria brevidens*), and moringa (*Moringa oleifera*).

> **BOX C6.1: THE POTENTIAL OF ALVS IN AFRICA**
>
> Kenya is home to more than 200 ALVs that could be helpful in strengthening the nutritional status of the population. ALVs have traditionally formed an important component in diets for both the rural and urban population in Kenya, but people have lost interest in consuming these vegetables. However, ALVs offer easy access to important nutrients, especially to vitamin A and iron from which many Kenyan children suffer deficiencies. These nutrients are largely missing in the predominantly simplified modern diets, often containing many processed and imported foods. ALVs are resilient crops that are able to grow in poor soils and extreme climate such as drought. On top of that they do not require the same extent of inputs as other exotic crops do, making them more affordable to grow and buy, while reducing impacts on health and the environment. Their weedy nature is also a reason why the crops are not as appreciated as more manageable horticultural crops. ALVs are also not considered suitable for the market and are often stigmatized as being food for the poor or elderly and thus young people in particular do not want to be associated with them. Not only consumers but also researchers have been neglecting these species for decades, which is the reason why there has been limited promotion of improved varieties and cultivation methods.
>
> Source: Guarino, 1997; Abukutsa-Onyango, 2007; Bioversity International, 2013

The multiple opportunities of school gardens

Currently, about 600 pupils are involved in preparing, planting, maintaining and harvesting their school garden, simultaneously learning about sustainable agricultural practices, climate-smart technologies and methods, and the nutritional value of diverse, locally available foods. Given the diversity of Busia's landscapes, cultures, and food, as well as assets and challenges, each school is taking its own approach to adopting the practice of gardening. For instance, Burumba Secondary School partnered with a neighbouring farmer to gain access to more fertile land for cultivation. The determination, commitment, and creativity of students, teachers, and staff drive the progress and success of their gardens. Here students have turned what used to be flowerbeds into vegetable plots where they grow ALVs. When the vegetables are ready, they are sent directly to the school kitchen to top up and complement the lunch menu.

In Samia sub-County, Malanga Primary students and staff have been harvesting and eating seasonal ALVs from their garden only a month and a half after the rains started. The school principal is leading the efforts to establish a school garden by engaging parents, pupils, and staff in the process of procuring seed, preparing garden beds, planting, maintaining, and harvesting nutritious vegetables.

At Amagoro Primary School in Teso North sub-county, an enterprising young teacher trained by the BFN project engaged parents, students and staff to work in the school's new garden. Harvest from the garden is being sold to community members, particularly parents of the students, and profits are being used to buy additional garden inputs and to pay school fees for the most hardworking students. The garden has grown two-fold in a matter of just three months, promising to provide enough produce to start a fully fledged school meal programme and to sell to the wider community.

Busia County is prone to long periods of drought and has inadequate or non-existent irrigation systems. Therefore, preservation of ALVs is an important activity that can enhance household food security. In Bunyala sub-county, St. Anne's Girls Secondary School started not only harvesting, but drying and preserving leafy vegetables using traditional methods. Drying adds value to leafy vegetables, since it lengthens shelf-life while preserving their nutritional value. Trained staff from all seven project-supported schools are emphasizing the nutritional value of traditional leafy vegetables, including the BFN garden at Igera Primary School in Nambale sub-county that displays a diversity of leafy vegetables and highlights their nutritional value on plant labels.

Another school, the Mundika Special Needs School for deaf children have now solved the problem of not having enough vegetables to eat during the dry season by establishing a school garden and integrating ALVs in their garden without any extra cost for the parents or the school. During holidays they sell their vegetables and use the profits to buy seeds and other materials. The garden skills help the children earn money for their basic needs and gain independence, particularly important for children with disabilities to be prepared for the future (Figure C6.2).

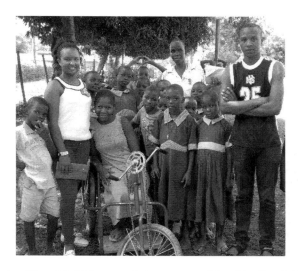

FIGURE C6.2 Aurillia with Nakayo and classmates at Mundika Special School.

In a nearby primary school, a BFN-trained instructor is using the existing 4 K-club to convert flowerbeds into a multi-storey vegetable plot. The school has been successful in engaging both parents and students in nutrition education activities during which they learn about optimal nutrition, the benefits and uses of local nutritious crops – such as amaranth, slender leaf, cowpea, Ethiopian kale, African nightshade, and spider plant – and recipes for their preparation. A cooking demonstration was organized by both parents and students. Mothers and fathers alike learned about the different food groups, the importance of feeding their children a balanced diet and were trained in the preparation of different dishes using their own school-grown vegetables. Dishes included brown porridge using millet, sweet potato flour and soya flour, mashed sweet potato and beans, local vegetables, fish, and pumpkin, which together contribute to the recommended daily requirements of energy, protein, essential fats, and micronutrients such as iron and vitamin.

Getting rich on 'food for the poor'

Through the school garden projects the students are changing the negative perceptions linked to indigenous vegetables, which are often perceived as earlier mentioned 'food for the poor' and even backward. Increased interest in the nutritional properties of indigenous vegetables means that pupils are able to sell any surplus production to teachers and other school staff and make extra pocket money, learning that agriculture can be a profitable business when markets exist (Figure C6.3).

For instance, in Mundika Girls primary school, students have become so keen on farming they have started their own small-scale agribusiness. With an initial investment of 5 Ksh to buy seeds, which they planted in the school compound,

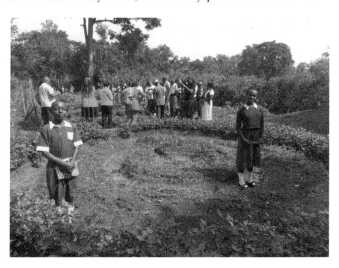

FIGURE C6.3 Students in Busia proudly showing their mandala garden.

they made a profit of 50 Ksh from selling the harvest. With the help of BFN, the girls are now cultivating local vegetables in a larger area including the school greenhouse with the aim of supplying the school kitchen and the staff. The students are also keeping local chicken. Such entrepreneurial exercises build up a skill set that is highly useful for the student's future independence, particular important for girls in the country.

Scaling up

The BFN Project plans to further develop the initiative to integrate general nutrition education, cooking classes, and value addition into garden activities. Only a few seasons into the project, the schools and pupils are aware of the nutritional value of biodiversity and are determined to share their knowledge and experience with their families and the broader community to enhance the nutrition and well-being of Busia County residents.

Notes

1 This case study is based on already published material on the BFN website. Find them here:
    - http://www.b4fn.org/from-the-field/stories/school-gardening-in-busia-county-kenya/
    - http://www.b4fn.org/from-the-field/stories/disability-is-not-inability-growing-indigenous-vegetables-at-mundika-special-school-for-the-deaf/
    - http://www.b4fn.org/from-the-field/stories/once-were-flowerbeds-home-grown-school-feeding-and-nutrition-education-enhances-indigenous-vegetabl/

2 A counter concept to the American 4H. In Kenya the 4-K clubs were established to teach youth improved farming methods, to increase the appreciation and respect for farming as a profession, to increase the production of food for consumption and sale within families and to develop leadership skills among youth.

References

Abukutsa-Onyango, M. (2007) 'The diversity of cultivated African leafy vegetables in three communities in western Kenya', *African Journal of Food, Agriculture, Nutrition and Development* 7.

Bioversity International. (2013) 'African leafy vegetables come out of the shade', EIARD, Bioversity International, Rome, Italy.

Foeken, D.W.J., Owuor, S.O. and Mwangi, A.M. (2007) 'School farming and school feeding in Nakuru town, Kenya – Practice and potential', *African Studies Center Working Paper* 76 / 2007.

Guarino, L. (ed) (1997) 'Traditional African Vegetables. Promoting the conservation and use of underutilized and neglected crops', 16, Proceedings of the IPGRI International Workshop on Genetic Resources of Traditional Vegetables in Africa: Conservation and Use, 29–31 August 1995, ICRAF-HQ, Nairobi, Kenya. Institute of Plant Genetics and Crop Plant Research, Gatersleben/International Plant Genetic Resources Institute, Rome, Italy.

Hunter, D., Giyose, B., Pologalante, A., Tartanac, F., Bundy, D., Mitchell, A., Moleah, T., Friedrich, J., Alderman, H., Drake, L., Kupka, R., Marshall, Q., Engesveen, K. and Oenema, S. (2017) 'Schools as a system to improve nutrition: A new statement for school-based food and nutrition interventions', United Nations System Standing Committee on Nutrition (UNSCN). Discussion Paper. Sept 2017.

IFPRI. (2016) 'Global nutrition report 2016: From Promise to Impact. Ending Malnutrition by 2030', Washington D.C.

IFPRI. (2019) 'Policy Responses to Food Crisis in Kenya', Food Security Report (Prepared by Kenya Agricultural Research Institute), http://www.foodsecurityportal.org/kenya/food-security-report-prepared-kenya-agricultural-research-institute, accessed 15 March 2019.

Langinger, N. (2011) 'School Feeding Programs in Kenya: Transitioning to a Homegrown Approach'. *Stanford Journal of International Relations*.

Mukudi, E. (2003) 'Nutrition status, education participation, and school achievement among Kenyan middle-school children', *Nutrition Volume* 19, Issues 7–8, July–August 2003, pp 612–616. https://www.sciencedirect.com/science/article/pii/S0899907003000376.

CASE STUDY 7

GROW TO LEARN – LEARNING GARDENS FOR SYRIAN CHILDREN AND YOUTH IN LEBANON

Nina Lauridsen[1]

Background

Nine years into the war in Syria, Lebanon remains at the forefront of one of the largest humanitarian, political, and developmental challenges of our time. The Government of Lebanon estimates that the country hosts 1.5 million of the 6.3 million Syrians who have fled the conflict since 2011. The Syrian refugee population in Lebanon remains the fourth-largest refugee population in the world and the largest concentration of refugees per capita (UNHCR, 2019). As the war and conflicts in Syria continue, an estimated 80% of the refugees lack legal status, leaving them unable to meet survival needs of food, health and shelter as well as being restricted in their access to education and healthcare. The crisis, brought by the war, continues to have an enormous social and economic impact on the host countries, with many local, municipal, and national services such as health, education, and water under severe strain (Halldorsson, 2017; UNHCR, 2019). Despite the support provided and recent improvements in school and training enrolment, displaced Syrians in the region are becoming increasingly vulnerable and more than half of the displaced Syrian children are still out of school (UNHCR, 2019). Efforts are needed in order to increase school enrolments, increase participation in alternative education systems and improve employment opportunities for displaced Syrian youth. On top of this, many of the refugee households, especially in the eastern part of Lebanon in Bekaa Valley, are severely food insecure (Diab El Harake et al., 2018). Children in food insecure households may suffer from nutrient deficiencies, increased illnesses, poor general health, and increased cognitive and behavioural problems that can affect not only their educational attainment but also their economic productivity later in life (Schmeer and Piperata, 2017).

The project

Since 2016 the Danish NGO, Zaher – Grow to Learn, together with the Lebanese NGOs SOILS – Permaculture Association, Buzuruna Juzuruna, and Food Heritage Foundation, has been working with Syrian communities displaced as refugees in Lebanon. Zaher aims to facilitate a platform where NGOs with expertise in permaculture, organic gardening and in the education of stigmatized Lebanese and Syrians can come together to support and engage marginalized children and youth. A key component to this work is to transform unused patches of land into functioning learning gardens that can accommodate garden education programmes. These programmes contribute to enhancing the environmental, social, and economic sustainability of the communities by promoting the use of organic or permaculture practices. By offering new educational spaces and alternative learning opportunities, they strengthen the education and involvement of the participating children and youth, to develop their knowledge of nature and to increase their livelihood resilience through the learning garden activities. They further ensure preservation of traditional gardening knowledge, increase the availability of and access to healthy food, and promote social cohesion.

Participants attend weekly workshops in the learning gardens, receiving education on subjects related to gardening such as plant life, water, insects, soil, compost, cultivation techniques, and much more. Each workshop consists of a theoretical and practical part. Inside the classroom or underneath the canvas, a local trainer introduces a subject and the theory behind. Afterwards, outside in the garden, the knowledge is put into practice. The lessons taught are rich in principles of permaculture, organic gardening and traditional Middle Eastern agricultural practices. The preparation takes place in the spring, and during the planting season, participants are invited to take part in all steps of creating the gardens: From preparing the soil, planting the seeds, maintaining the crops, and finally harvesting the greens. At the end of each season a harvest celebration takes place together with the participating children and youth. At the celebration, crops from the gardens are harvested and either consumed directly or turned into preserves (Figure C7.1).

One of these learning gardens was established in the backyard of the Baraem El Moustaqbal education centre in Bar Elias, Beqaa Valley. The garden was managed by the local NGO *Sawa for Development and Aid* (SDAID) in collaboration with SOILS. The students, all with Syrian background, created a sustainable blooming garden through a series of six educational workshops that provided both theoretical and practical knowledge about permaculture (Figure C7.2). Starting with the creation of an organic compost station, students designed the garden to grow plants for a variety of purposes, for food as well as for medicinal use and aesthetic reasons. By the end of the workshops, the learning garden boasted evergreens, fruit-bearing trees, and nine vegetable beds with a variety of plants including fava beans, chicory, and beetroot, and flowering perennials such as callistemon, verbena, and night-blooming jasmine. To ensure the continuation of the learning garden, dedicated student leaders were trained to care for the garden after the conclusion of the workshops.

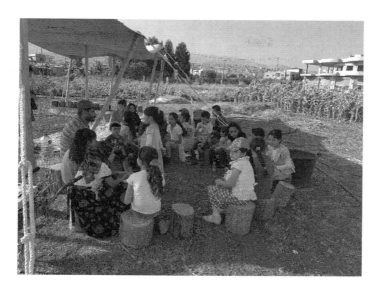

FIGURE C7.1 The theoretical part of the workshop in Sa'adnayel takes place in the outdoor classroom under a tent canvas where the participants and the trainer can seek cover from the sun while exchanging knowledge (2018).

Source: Zaher – Grow to Learn.

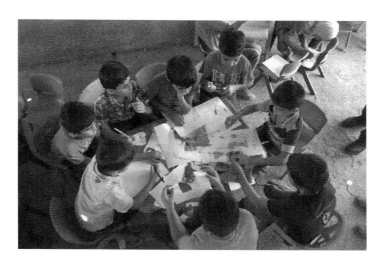

FIGURE C7.2 Learning garden pre-workshop for children and youth from the local community in Bar Elias, Beqaa Valley. Placed in groups around tables with pens and papers, the attendees had to draw their hopes and dreams for the upcoming garden, which later came to frame the design for this garden (2016).

Source: Zaher – Grow to Learn.

> **BOX C7.1: PLANT AND SEED SELECTION**
>
> While vegetable seeds and some of the annual flowers for the gardens were sourced from Buzuruna Juzuruna's organic farming school, the perennials, trees and some flowers were sourced from a common nursery. Ghassan al Salman from SOILS Permaculture Association explains about the plant selection for the garden in Bar Elias: 'We tried to give the participants the broader perspective of agriculture, focussing on all the many benefits and synergies of plants and the ecosystems they support. Garden designs are based on what the participants want in their garden. We revised the list of plants, and then removed the incompatible crops, such as bananas (the garden was in a semi-arid climate at an altitude of 1000 m). Many children wanted crops that made them nostalgic of home, such as jasmines, roses, and grapes. We integrated permanent vegetable beds with fruit and trees, as well as some aromatics, flowers, and ornamentals. A willow tree, two poplars and a cypress can serve as a windbreak and bird habitat as well as produce wood. Callistemons, trumpet vines, and jasmines cover concrete surfaces and create a cool microclimate as well as offer shelter and/or forage for small animals and insects. Rose, verbena, and oleaster are good vegetable companions and can be consumed for their medicinal values. The vegetable varieties we planted were peasant varieties for the sake of seed production and garden sustainability'.

In collaboration with the local NGO Buzuruna Juzuruna, Zaher is also facilitating a space for another learning garden at the organization's organic farming school. The local biodynamic farm has dedicated a piece of land to a learning garden for Syrian children from neighbouring refugee camps. Every Friday children are picked up by a bus and taken to the garden that simulates an outdoor classroom. Here children receive education in the various school subjects based on the elements that can be found in the garden to compensate for their inadequate schooling.

The value of learning gardens for stigmatized and displaced children and youth

As the agricultural sector was a source of livelihood for half of the Syrian population before the conflict (Tull, 2017), an additional aim of the learning garden project is to ensure the continuation of traditional agricultural knowledge and practices and thereby improving employment prospects for Syrian youth. Furthermore, it allows the young people to prepare themselves for rebuilding their home country when and if they will be able return. By adding extra-curricular learning opportunities to the daily life, the aim is also to support the student

BOX C7.2: FOOD AID IN LEBANESE REFUGEE CAMPS

Most of the Syrians in Lebanon living in refugee camps rely on food aid programmes to secure their food. E-cards distributed by the World Food Program are one example; these are loaded with money at the end of every month and used to purchase food from contracted shops around the country. Another form of food assistance is provided through community kitchens where Lebanese and Syrian women cook together and hot meals are distributed to families in the camps as well as vulnerable Lebanese families. The kitchens are run by either women cooperatives or local NGOs and are financially supported by international organizations. The Food Heritage Foundation has been involved in upgrading several kitchens and building the capacity of the ladies working there. Nevertheless, inadequate diets are still a huge challenge in the refugee camps with one third being severely of moderately food insecure (UNHCR, UNICEF, and WFP, 2018). The main food groups consumed in the camps are sugar, fats, bread, pasta and dairy while, according to the UN, fruits and vegetables on average are only eaten 2–3 times per week. This explains the high deficiencies especially for iron and vitamin A (ibid.) and emphasizes the importance of increasing the accessibility to fruits and vegetables.

to build their capacities and facilitate new perspectives on their possibilities and self-capabilities. At the same time, engaged children and youth obtain skills that can inspire and enable them to create agricultural spaces in their homes and camps in Lebanon. This is particularly valuable since food is the biggest household expense taking up almost half of the budget for the average refugee household. As the local youth attend the workshops they get to add layers of knowledge to what they already know about gardening, which eventually enable them to become trained learning garden specialists and teachers.

Scaling-up

The project aims to expand its reach to involve more children and youth. Through its activities it will build a strong platform of knowledge that will support local partners to advocate for a learning garden movement in Lebanon. In 2019, the project received a large grant from the Civil Society in Development (CISU) – an association of Danish civil society organizations – to open four new school gardens together with the local partners, Buzuruna Juzuruna, Food Heritage Foundation, Action Aid Arab Region, and Malaak, in collaboration with groups of local stigmatized youth and children – primarily from Syria. With time the aim is to promote learning gardens at Lebanese public schools as well so that Lebanese kids can acquire the same skills as their Syrian counterparts (Figure C7.3).

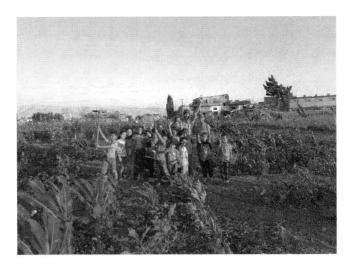

FIGURE C7.3 The participants and local trainer, Walid, wrapping up a day of hard work in Sa'adanyel after nursing and cultivating their blooming garden (2018).

Source: Zaher – Grow to Learn.

Lessons learned

The success of these projects is solely based on local anchoring. Each garden design and content need to be formed in a close collaboration between the local partners and local participants to ensure that the learning gardens can be of value to the vulnerable communities within the local context. Transparency, good coordination, and consistent communication between the different stakeholders are crucial.

Using local trainers and inviting volunteers, parents, teachers, or janitors to be part of the project has contributed to success. This ensures that the projects align with local needs and local sustainability while contributing to community cohesion and a longer life span of the gardens.

The lack of accessible land to be converted into productive gardens as well as the lack of sufficient funding are two very essential challenges that Zaher is facing in the Bekaa Valley. Some of the young adults in the camps are also difficult to engage as their families are highly dependent on the income they get from their daily labour. In addition, displaced families live a very unstable life and are often in a state of limbo without knowing how long they will stay in the same camp. Sometimes they have to leave to move to another camp during the project phase thus disrupting the kids' learning process and connection to the garden.

Note

1 This text was developed by Nina Lauridsen based on material and inputs from Mabelle Chedid (The Food Heritage Foundation), Ghassan al Salman (SOILS), and the founders of Zaher – Grow to Learn.

References

Diab El Harake, M. Kharroubi, S., Hamadeh, S.K. and Jomaa, L. (2018) 'Impact of a pilot school-based nutrition intervention on dietary knowledge, attitudes, behavior and nutritional status of Syrian refugee children in the Bekaa, Lebanon' *Nutrients* 10, 913, doi:10.3390/ nu10070913.

Halldorsson, D. (2017) 'Syrian refugee children in Lebanon at risk of child labour, missing out on education', UNICEF, accessed 4 Mar, 2019: https://www.unicef.org/stories/syrian-refugee-children-lebanon-at-risk-of-child-labour.

Schmeer, K.K. and Piperata, B.A. (2017) 'Household food insecurity and child health', *Maternal & Child Nutrition* 2017, 13, doi:10.1111/mcn.12301.

Tull, K. (2017) 'Agriculture in Syria', K4D Helpdesk Report 133, Brighton, UK: Institute of Development Studies.

UNHCR (2019) 'Syria regional refugee response. Operational portal – refugee situations', last updated 28 Feb 2019, The United Nations Refugee Agency, accessed 4 Mar, 2019: https://data2.unhcr.org/en/situations/syria/location/71.

UNHCR, UNICEF and WFP (2018) 'VASyR 2018- Vulnerability Assessment of Syrian Refugees in Lebanon'.

CASE STUDY 8
SCHOOL GARDENS (*MĀRA*)
Today's learning spaces for Māori

Nick Roskruge

In recent years, there has been a resurgence of interest in growing food sustainably and locally at all levels of society. The rapid urbanization of Māori following the Second World War has meant successive generations of young Māori have missed considerable opportunity to experience growing their own foods, or learning with their parents and grandparents how to interact and gain from working their own whenua or land. The resurgence for Māori is part of a phenomenon across New Zealand generally, where intergenerational activities are being applied to introduce our younger generations to growing and utilizing foods. These activities are now many-fold, with a myriad of promotional names: paddock to plate, plant to plate, spud in a bucket, and more. This case study will introduce the 'Spud in a bucket' project promoted to schools through the National Māori Horticultural Collective known as Tahuri Whenua.[1]

Background and context

The term *Māra* in Māori alludes to land under cultivation, for whatever purpose. *Māra kai* is that land under cultivation for the production of food. There are several parts to what constitutes a māra. First, the location and history of the land under cultivation. Second, the selection of crops to suit both the location and the intended users of the produce once harvested. Thirdly the tikanga or traditional processes/inputs used in the production system and lastly, the learning experience which is socialized throughout the life of the *māra*. So any *māra kai* activity contributes positively to all those involved in its evolution and application.

School gardens (*māra*)

From times past, pre-colonial society through to the depression of the 1930s and following decades, until the 1970s, Māori had *māra* of all types to support their *whānau* or families and the wider community, especially at tribal (*iwi*) and sub-tribal (*hapū*) gatherings. Important occasions were catered for from local production, trade or exchange. All *whānau* had generational experience to draw from to support their garden activities, but post-war urbanization, rapid technical adaptation, and the new fast-paced lifestyles interrupted this type of activity with the nuclear Māori family becoming more dependent on supermarkets than on their fresh fruits and vegetables and other food types.

It is from this scenario that the genesis of *māra kai* for schools came, and many Māori with broad horticultural experience have come together in a collective to support the establishment of māra in schools. The collective this case study follows is known as *Tahuri Whenua*, literally meaning 'to turn back to the land'. In 2009 *Tahuri Whenua* were early innovators in working together to create an opportunity for Māori children to return to the land, get their hands 'dirty' and experience growing their own food. This aligns well with an old *whakataukī* (or proverb) – *he kai kei aku ringaringa* – literally meaning 'I can grow food with my own hands'. The proverb reminds us of the role of self-sufficiency and sustainability to achieve survival. Yet the concept of school gardens is not entirely new. As an example (see picture from 1915 below), Waihi (later known as Motunui) School in North Taranaki (North Island, New Zealand) involved their students in practical gardening: boys growing vegetables and girls growing flowers (Figure C8.1).[2]

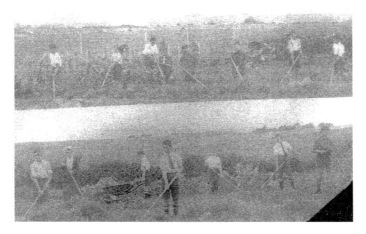

FIGURE C8.1 Waihi (later Motunui) School (*Rohe o Ngāti Rahiri*) Taranaki. 1915.
Source: Nick Roskruge.

From a Māori perspective, *māra* or gardens are not just about growing food products but are important contributors to providing an experience that contributes to the well-being of those involved, children and adults alike. We understand the physical sustenance that food products contribute, but we also know that complete sustenance is only achieved when our holistic well-being is achieved. This requires meeting the spiritual, social, and intellectual needs of humankind alongside the physical needs.

I TE AO MĀORI

In terms of *whakapapa* (cultural expression of genealogy) and through our mythology, we as Māori recognize a relationship of all of the plant kingdom to mankind as all are descendants of Papatūānuku the Earth mother. The role of plants is primarily to adorn Papatūānuku in the nakedness which she found herself in following her separation from Ranginui, her husband and the 'sky father' to our mortal *whakapapa*. All plants with or without edible portions are contributors to Papatūānuku and mankind's survival and good health.

Papatūānuku promised all her descendants that she would provide for their sustenance, hence the food value of many plants. But sustenance is more than just nutritional value. Those other realms which support us also need to be sustained. Therefore, gardens and garden produce contribute to our medicinal needs, physical demands such as in building materials, social needs through the collective approaches taken at all stages of the *māra*; planning through to harvest and consumption, and in the intellectual and sensual experiences through stimulation of all five senses. Plants of the *māra* or garden contribute to all of those senses. For example:

- hearing because our history tells us of the relationship each of the plants has to us as mankind;
- sight in the appearance of the garden, of individual plants and of the final produce, and the similarities between plants or crops;
- touch as in the need to work with Papatūānuku during production, harvest, and food preparation among other things and including biodiversity driven activities;
- smell as in the aroma in the *māra* or in the meal being cooked;
- and lastly taste, because the complete experience is found when the meal is consumed. If our senses are collectively imbued with the values and outcomes of the garden then we all benefit positively.

Herein lies a *kinaki* or relish for us, something that will give cause to remember the experience of the production and harvest of plants to create a meal. This is a contribution to mana or status of mankind in its highest realm (Figure C8.2).

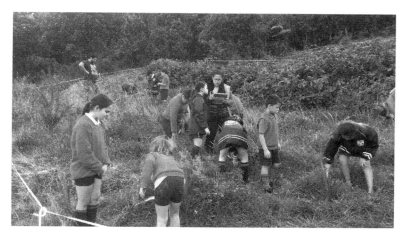

FIGURE C8.2 *Kura Kaupapa* children assisting with planting native plants around a māra near Whanganui (Putiki). An example of biodiversity in the garden.
Source: Moari Bailey, Putiki.

The Tahuri Whenua māra initiative

The first project established by Tahuri Whenua in 2008 was called Spud-in-a-bucket and promoted to all schools, but Māori immersion schools in particular. The concept was to resource these schools with information including the traditional lunar calendar (*maramataka* in Māori) and seed *taewa* or Māori potatoes to be grown either outdoors in-ground or in a bucket and a range of activities were aligned to this activity to contribute to the children's learning. This was well before the current raft of programmes which have arisen: plant to plant, paddock to plate, etc. The initiative was trialled at over 20 Māori immersion schools or *kura* throughout New Zealand. Base materials including the seed *taewa*, buckets (where requested), and potting mix were supplied. The reason for the promotion of container gardening was because of the summer break schools undertake each year which coincides with the peak growing period for most crops (Figure C8.3). During the summer the staff and students are absent from many schools so any crops planted are generally ignored and therefore poorly managed. Through container gardening the *taewa* or Māori potato could be planted earlier, strategically placed or moved for best environmental conditions in the spring and harvested before the end of the school year. The kura or schools all had the option of planting their *taewa* seed in-ground or in-buckets. *Taewa* were the chosen crop at the early stage of the project because of their historical and cultural relationship to Māori communities. This was an opportunity for all generations, students, parents, teachers, and wider *whānau* or family, to experience growing one of the foods our forebears grew as a staple food. The renaissance of Māori culture and

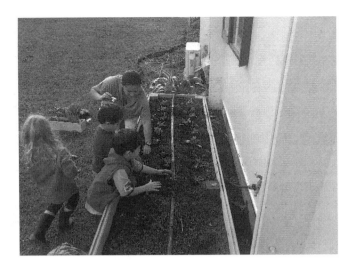

FIGURE C8.3 Māori Pre-School known as *Kohanga Reo* (language nest) establishing their version of a container garden.
Source: Mellany Albert, Te Uru Karaka, Manawatū.

Māori foods in particular, was a key driver in the establishment of the project. From its inception the project was extended to include all other vegetables and some fruits as well as nursery activities, especially for native plants, and the sharing of plants and resources locally, that is, beyond the school gates.

The project was highly successful. Schools took it upon themselves to be creative in how they gained the involvement of their students. Many utilized the *maramataka* or lunar calendar to support when and how they undertook key activities. Harvest time or *hauhake* allowed for unique extension of garden work. Some schools took a competitive approach to the harvest (e.g. number or yield weights). Another used police as a community representative to oversee the weighing process. In another case, a potato lunch with a range of dishes prepared by groups of students was undertaken. And in yet another case, the schools of a region came together to collectively celebrate the successful garden through sports, food, and community activities.

The importance of the initiative

The horticulture activities and resulting gardens, both in-ground and in-bucket, have highlighted the loss of experience and knowledge about our foods within the current generations. The older generations regularly lament the loss of knowledge and lack of experience in the garden for the younger generation. Urban drift, new food choices and availability, busy lives and new technologies have exposed this generation to many things but often the practical and so-called mundane activities are ignored. Gardening is seen by many as labouring for food rather than the satisfaction of growing for sustenance. This programme has shown that most of our children have an innate interest in getting their hands dirty in the garden and the opportunity to actually experience the food as an end result is a bonus. It has also drawn together generations of *whānau* to share experiences. The older generation are happy to pass on what they know of the crops or local growing opportunities, and the younger generations are building on their love of technology and social media to make the experience more enjoyable.

The initiative also benefits through the incorporation of elements of agrobiodiversity in the *māra*. The children learn to recognize and name the various other biological interests in and among their crops: birds and browsing animals (and humans!), insects and invertebrates, pathogens and weeds. The Māori perspective is to understand the māra from a holistic perspective and value all elements for how they support the plants, which provide the food source for us. While many biological elements are considered as a negative component of the gardens, we respect that they all have a role to play, even if it is to compete with the crop as ultimately, they pay back something to the production system.

Outcomes and impacts

Several benefits can be recognized from the *māra kai* or gardens programme. From a selfishly Māori perspective, this has been a very positive and interactive activity. In particular, it has helped to restore and enhance *Mana*; that unique cultural value which recognizes the contribution to the status of Māori within society. Mana acknowledges the association to the various realms of Māori society and more especially the support of the spiritual realm through valuing elements important to the role of cultural deities, ultimately through which success can be guaranteed. The māra kai therefore contributes to cultural and individual well-being. In line with traditional thought, if the activity has a positive impact on the collective whole then it is also a source well-being for individuals.

Second, it contributes to a broader renaissance of cultural being. *Mātauranga Māori* or traditional knowledge supports historical discourse, *whakapapa* and learned experience which in turn supports the physical well-being of those involved. Our *tamariki* or children are being exposed to their culture in a more practical way and learning from their Elders in a culturally supportive environment. The education system itself also benefits as it is exposed to intergenerational learning within a cultural environment. Recent decades have seen the accelerating loss of traditional knowledge with the passing of those generations with a first-hand association to the old-world Māori. We cannot replicate what they knew or experienced – and we cannot underestimate the volume of knowledge lost. But programmes such as the 'Spud-in-a-bucket' and *māra kai* contribute to the learning of the emerging generations, ever so incrementally, and that in itself helps build confidence in how we contribute into the contemporary world our children will know.

Most importantly, this programme is about food – or *kai* as it is known in *te reo Māori* (Māori language). Food is what sustains us and many of our young people are now removed from the origins of the foods they consume so take for granted what is available or eaten. This activity is hands-on food production and the produce is available for preparation and consumption. In a Māori context food for physical well-being is supported by other inputs for a more complete benefit, social well-being through communal interactions, intellectual well-being through learning, and spiritual well-being through the direct association to spiritual benefactors achieved through cultural means (*karakia* or incantations/prayers; *whakapapa* or mythology that aligns to the spirit world).

Relationship to policy

Policy is the driver for the future and education is the key for the future. Both have moved towards a more embracing approach to exposing our children to the activities of horticulture and other practical areas. Two distinct policy drivers support this initiative and are also informed by this and other similar initiatives.

Within Māori society there is a drive for *Rangatiratanga* or 'self-determination' status. This term refers to Māori being in charge of their own destiny through the process of being the drivers of policy and other processes that affect their future. The conception and implementation of this programme helps contribute to that status through supporting the broader Māori community role in contributing to their emerging generation in a culturally acceptable way.

The New Zealand Ministry of Education has a current policy known as *Ka Hikitia*[3] which includes an approach to Māori education and future development. This policy *Ka Hikitia* showcases the critical role parents, *whānau* and communities play in helping their children to learn. It illustrates that Māori educational success can be achieved when communities, iwi, schools, early learning centres or the Ministry work in collaboration – *mahi tahi* or working as one, is the term they use to capture this ideology. Māra such as this activity in schools has a clear alignment to this policy.

Efforts to replicate/scale-up

Since the 'Spud in a bucket' project was initiated several other like-minded projects have arisen within the wider community[4] and across all levels of schools in New Zealand and including community gardens. This has broadened the opportunity for all schools and some of the more recent programmes are well funded and resourced. The *Tahuri Whenua* project was always limited in resource and cash funding so was kept within a cluster of schools with a particular Māori emphasis to meet the objectives of the collective. So scaling up has been achieved through the accessibility of alternative programmes which have in effect replicated the original concept. What remains for *Tahuri Whenua*, however, is the ongoing relationship between members and local schools, in particular *Kaupapa Māori* or culturally centric learning environments. The early *māra* or garden activities have morphed into a broader range of activities with ownership retained by the communities and families involved. This well exceeds what was anticipated by *Tahuri Whenua* at the project inception.

Key outcomes and where to go from here

The establishment of a working relationship between our Māori community and schools through the establishment of *māra* has been a very positive activity. All contributors gain in some form and the early project has progressed to a wide range of māra type initiatives including nursery work with traditional plants, both food and non-food types. As with any Māori-centric initiative, the aim is always to achieve a culturally appropriate space which is owned by those who will gain from it. The community at large, whether it be *iwi* (tribal), *hapū* (sub-tribal), *whānau* (family), or *pan-iwi/tauiwi* (multiple interests), is key to the education of our children, and this project has allowed them to contribute with their experience and knowledge of gardening in a setting that continually works.

From here it remains for *Tahuri Whenua* to continue to support these types of initiatives through the collection and sharing of knowledge. As a collective they promote these activities through published information and regular regional and national hui or gatherings. Schools have been empowered through the relationships and sharing of knowledge that has ensued. *Tahuri Whenua* contribute to this through ongoing resource sharing such as information brochures, seeds as available and advice.

We further recognize that our children are the future knowledge bearers and land managers who deserve the opportunity to experience the relationship they have to Papatūānuku and Ranginui, our primal parents, and what that means for future generations (Figure C8.4).

Here the *whakataukī* (or proverb) applies: *He manu hou ahau, he pī ka rere* – I am a young bird, a chick just learning to fly!

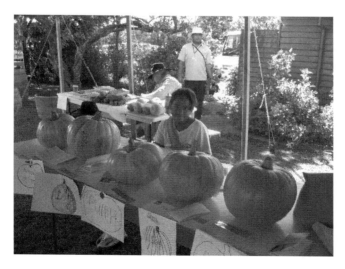

FIGURE C8.4 Māra kai produce (and Sarah Puha), Hauiti marae hui, Uawa/Tolaga Bay, East Coast, North Island, New Zealand.
Source: Nick Roskruge.

Notes

1 See www.tahuriwhenua.org – Tahuri Whenua Inc. Soc. The National Māori Horticulture Collective. Any communications to: tahuriwhenua@gmail.com
2 Commentary and photo supplied by *Kaumātua* (elders) of Ngāti Rahiri, Taranaki.
3 *Ka Hikitia*; accelerating success 12013-2017 (2013) Te Tāhuhu o te Mātauranga (Ministry of Education).
4 See for example the *Tui* initiative (www.tuigarden.co.nz/ideas-and-inspiration/spring-projects-in-the-school-garden/) or Enviroschools programme (http://enviroschools.org.nz/in_your_region/manawatu-whanganui), both New Zealand initiatives.

CASE STUDY 9

INTERGENERATIONAL TRANSFER OF KNOWLEDGE AND MINDSET CHANGE THROUGH SCHOOL GARDENS AMONG INDIGENOUS CHILDREN IN MEGHALAYA, NORTH EAST INDIA

Melari Shisha Nongrum

Background

Indigenous peoples all across the globe have been the custodians of the rich biodiversity that still exists today. The North Eastern Region of India is considered one of the biodiversity hotspots of the world of which Meghalaya, a state in the region contributes to this rich biodiversity. Meghalaya is one of the states in the North Eastern Region of India and shares an international border with Bangladesh on its southern side. According to the State Biodiversity Board, Meghalaya represents an important part of the Indo Burma biodiversity hotspot which is one of the 4 biodiversity hotspots in India and 34 in the world. Seventy percent of the state is under forest cover. A large proportion of 90% of the forest area of the state is outside direct government control and is owned by the indigenous clans and their communities. The forests are a source of food, medicine and also commercially viable products such as non-timber forest produce (NTFP) which is a source of income for the communities. Wild edibles sourced from the forests are also an integral part of the traditional food of the indigenous communities. These include green leafy vegetables, fruits, tubers, shoots, nuts and seeds, fodder, and dyes. There have been a number of studies that have identified a large number of wild edibles in the state (Agrahar-Murugkar and Subbulakshmi, 2005; Agrahar-Murugkar, 2006; Kayang, 2007; Hynniewta and Kumar, 2010). For instance, in one study, 249 species of wild edibles have been identified (Sawian et al., 2007). Moreover, in a recent study conducted by the North East Slow Food and Agrobiodiversity Society (NESFAS) in 32 villages, it was found that there is a rich agrobiodiversity in the participating villages of the NESFAS programme. It was found that the average number of plant food available in a village is 202. This included green leafy vegetables, starchy staples, nuts and seeds, fruits, orange fleshed fruits, other vegetables, and pulses throughout the year.

Nestled in the hills and biodiversity of Meghalaya are three main matriarchal indigenous communities, Khasi, Jaintia, and Garo communities which inhabit the state. They constitute 86% of the population of the state. The larger proportion (80%) of the indigenous peoples resides in the rural areas and agriculture is their main livelihood activity, although today people have various sources of income but mostly related to agrobiodiversity. Though a large proportion of the communities live amidst a diversity of micronutrient rich species, it is astonishing to see the poor indices of health of children and women. A study conducted by McGill University and NESFAS in West Khasi Hills District of Meghalaya (Chyne et al., 2017) revealed that there were high rates of anaemia (68%) and micronutrient deficiency (59% vitamin A Deficiency) among children (1–5 years) and 83% of women had anaemia. Similarly, according to a national study, the National Family Health Survey 2015–2016, it was found that 56.2% of women (15–45 years) are anaemic, 48% of children (6–59 months) are anaemic and 43 of children (below the age of 5 years) are stunted which indicate that they were undernourished (Ministry of Health & Family Welfare, 2015–2016). Moreover, NESFAS had conducted a dietary diversity survey in 32 villages based on the 10 food groups promoted by FAO. The minimum diversity for food intake is to consume at least five food groups in a day. It was found that the average dietary diversity score is 4 and the missing food groups from the diets of the people are mainly green leafy vegetables, orange fleshed vegetables and fruits, pulses, nuts and seeds, fruits, eggs, and dairy.

In terms of education, the literacy rate in the state is 74.43% (Census 2011, 2019). Formal education among the Khasi, Jaintia, and Garo people was initiated by the Christian missionaries in the 19th Century whereby they established schools in many areas. After India's independence in 1947, the church took upon itself the onus of establishing schools, therefore a large number of schools are managed by the churches. Subsequently, the government also established or supported the privately managed schools. In 2009, the Indian Parliament passed the Right of Children to Free and Compulsory Education Act which has led to an increase in the number of schools and enrolment of children. The existing education system in the state and country is quite theoretical in its approach and thereby draws the child away from knowing and understanding his/her own environment. There is no mention of the types of wild edibles or traditional vegetables found in the region. As a result, the children and adolescents lose their connection to mother earth and lose the traditional knowledge about their own environment. More often than not, adolescents who have completed high school or higher grades do not want to work in the agricultural sector. Their aspirations are to have a white-collar job in the urban centres.

Among indigenous peoples, traditional knowledge relating to flora and fauna, soil, water resources and nature at large forms the basis for their identity, culture and heritage, food and medicine systems etc. These communities have survived over the centuries on this traditional knowledge which has been passed orally from one generation to another. This traditional knowledge has also enabled the communities to sustainably use the resources. However, there are social changes that have taken place. The intergenerational transfer of traditional knowledge has also been reduced since as mentioned, the children are in school and the time spent with children in the fields has reduced. The loss of traditional knowledge will therefore affect the wellbeing of indigenous people, including consumption of indigenous food such as wild edibles in this part of the world.

The project

In this context, NESFAS, an organization working in 130 communities to raise awareness of traditional foods for food and nutritional security is promoting and initiating school gardens in its communities. The purpose of these school gardens is to enhance the connection of students to farming, enhance intergenerational transfer of knowledge and to increase dietary diversity in the mid-day meals of the children. NESFAS initially started to work with 3 school gardens in 2013 and now there are 22 school gardens which have been established. The approach adopted for the school gardens is agroecology where the adoption of using traditional ecological knowledge in the farming system is encouraged. However, the agroecological approach that is promoted is also intercultural where both traditional wisdom and modern science are integrated. For instance, in terms of seed storage and assessment of the moisture in seeds, a 'humidicator' paper is used. A unique aspect of our work is that a custodian farmer is identified as the facilitator for the students in terms of selection of traditional seeds, maintenance of soil health through intercropping and even pest management in the school gardens. Traditional seeds are used for growing different vegetables. The seeds are contributed by the custodian farmers who themselves are parents of the children. NESFAS focuses on planting the missing food groups, highlighted earlier, in the school gardens. The average number of plants cultivated in the school gardens is 10 vegetables. The highest number of plants cultivated is in the Khweng Lower Primary school garden with 22 types of vegetables including wild edibles but school gardens in Mawhiang and Khliehumstem are also planting 18 to 20 types of food plants at any one time. Wild edibles especially green leafy types are also planted in the school gardens as they serve as a regular source of food for salads served to the school children.

In terms of other inputs, the manure is either made in the school through composting or contributed by parents. The sowing of many plants commences in the month of February which also coincides with the commencement of the academic school year (Figure C9.1). Thus, once the custodian farmer(s), which also includes parents, have facilitated the selection of seeds and guided the school in maintenance of soil health, the school teachers and students take up the responsibility of maintenance which is included in the Socially Useful Productive Work (SUPW) course. It is worth noting that in many school gardens, the parents and community at large have contributed towards creation of a fence for the school gardens. Each school also has a seasonal calendar of plants to make it easy for students to understand the planting, harvesting, and availability of vegetables in the different seasons.

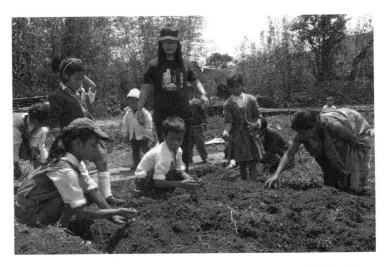

FIGURE C9.1 School Garden activity at Nongnah, South West Khasi Hills.
Source: NESFAS.

The Indigenous Food System Curriculum

In addition, NESFAS has facilitated the development of the Indigenous Food System (IFS) Curriculum which is aimed at enhancing the knowledge of students about their own environment and food system. The components included in this curriculum are soil, water, forests, seeds, pollinators, and markets. A participatory approach was adopted to develop the curriculum. NESFAS initiated discussions in 2018 about the possibility of having such a curriculum with a group of school teachers from 12 schools in Sohra region of East Khasi Hills District. The importance of having an experiential curriculum was unanimously agreed upon by the teachers. After a couple of meetings and discussions, a curriculum had been developed by the teachers along with NESFAS and eventually, seven schools are piloting the IFS curriculum in the academic year 2019. As indicated, the curriculum is experiential in nature where the learning happens outside the classroom, in the school garden or nearby forests and cultivated fields and any other suitable areas. Nevertheless, the scope of the curriculum is beyond the school gardens. For instance, as the students learn about trees and forests in the science course, an agrobiodiversity walk is conducted whereby a traditional knowledge holder(s) from the village facilitates the walk by explaining the different types of flora and its benefits (Figure C9.2). On their part, the students learn about and document the flora available in their villages. As indicated earlier since the existing school curriculum is quite theoretical, it is hoped that the IFS curriculum will enhance the knowledge of students about their own local environment and also enable them to appreciate their natural resources.

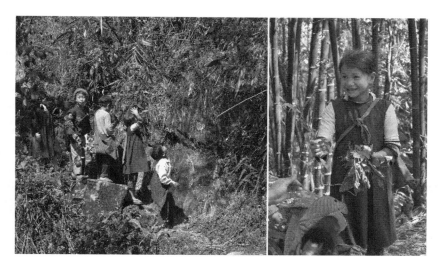

FIGURE C9.2 Agrobiodiversity walk at Nongtraw, East Khasi Hills, with the children (left) and Ibanjalis Rani explains about the wild edibles she has collected during the Agrobiodiversity walk at Nongtraw, East Khasi Hills (right).
Source: Alethea Kordor Lyngdoh, NESFAS.

Improving diets with vegetables and wild edible species

As a result of the school garden, it has been seen that the schools have started to harvest their produce. These vegetables supplement and increase the diversity of the mid-day meals which is often limited to three food groups as provided by the government, an initiative aimed at increasing enrolment and nutrition of children. NESFAS in working on this aspect has also trained the mid-day meal cooks on how to enrich the menu of the school meals through cooking demonstrations using local traditional plants. As the school gardens cannot be expected to meet the full need of vegetables for the mid-day meals, the schools have encouraged students to bring a bunch of wild edibles from their home kitchen gardens by rotation and therefore, the same children do not need to bring the wild edibles everyday but as per the roster. Through these initiatives and vegetables from the gardens, the diversity on the plate has also increased.

Assessing children's knowledge about indigenous food

In connection to the impact of school gardens, NESFAS wanted to assess the knowledge of students regarding the indigenous foods. There were 10 schools that participated, 4 of them had school gardens (villages which NESFAS worked since 2013) and 6 schools did not have school gardens. It was found that regardless of the availability of the school gardens, all the students had some knowledge on the source of their food which is forest, kitchen garden, shifting cultivation and other cultivation fields. The students with school gardens had 12% more knowledge on wild edibles, listed an average of 10 wild edibles as against 6 wild edibles listed by the students without a school garden. In terms of the students' perception of taste of wild edibles, 74% of the students with a school garden considered them to be tasty. Apart from wild edibles, the students with a school garden could list 34% more vegetables than the other students without a school garden. In terms of consumption of wild edibles and cultivated vegetables, the level of consumption was similar among all students.

This study has revealed some positive trends of having a school garden. The indicators of consumption of clean vegetables including wild edibles in the mid-day meals today, show that there has been an appreciation of the contribution that wild edibles can make towards the nutritional diversity of the children by the cooks, teachers, students, and parents.

A broader community impact

An important aspect that has emerged is that the school garden is also becoming a demonstration plot for the community by the inclusion of the missing food groups in the cultivation of vegetables and wild edibles in school gardens. This is made possible through the seed exchange that occurs between schools. The learning from the school gardens will also encourage the communities which have very few plants grown in their kitchen gardens to cultivate the missing food groups in their kitchen gardens. Through the intergenerational transfer of

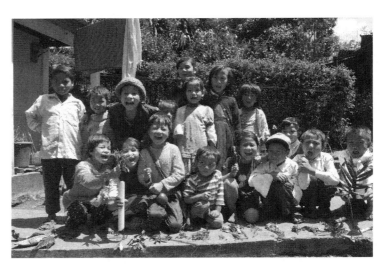

FIGURE C9.3 Children showcase wild edibles gathered during the agrobiodiversity walk at Nongtraw, East Khasi Hills.
Source: Alethea Kordor Lyngdoh, NESFAS.

knowledge that occurs through the school gardens, IFS curriculum coupled with the change of mindset towards indigenous food systems, the food diversity in the mid-day meals can be increased and sustainable use of natural resources can be ensured (Figure C9.3).

References

Agrahar-Murugkar, D. (2006) 'Interventions using wild edibles to improve the nutritional status of Khasi tribal women', *Human Ecology Special Issue*, (14), 83–88.

Agrahar-Murugkar, D. and Subbulakshmi, G. (2005) 'Ecology of food and nutrition nutritive values of wild edible fruits, berries, nuts, roots and spices consumed by the Khasi tribes of India', *Ecology of Food and Nutrition*, 44, 207–223.

Census 2011. (2019) What is literacy rate of Meghalaya? Census population 2019 Data. Available from: https://www.census2011.co.in/questions/23/state-literacy/literacy-rate-of-meghalaya-census-2011.html.

Chyne, D.A., Meshram, I.I., Rajendran, A., Kodali, V., Getti, N., Roy, P., Kuhnlein, H.V. and Longvah, T. (2017) 'Nutritional status, food insecurity, and biodiversity among the Khasi in Meghalaya, North-East India', *Wiley Maternal and Child Nutrition* 13(S3):e12557, doi:10.1111/mcn.12557.

Hynniewta, S.R. and Kumar, Y. (2010) 'The lesser-known medicine Ka Dawai Ñiangsohpet of the Khasis in Meghalaya, Northeast India', 9 (July), 475–479.

Kayang, H. (2007) 'Tribal knowledge on wild edible plants of Meghalaya, Northeast India', *Indian Journal of Traditional Knowledge*, 6(1), 177–181.

Ministry of Health & Family Welfare. (2015) 'National family health survey', Mumbai.

Sawian, J.T., Jeeva, S., Lyndem, F.G., Mishra, B.P., and Laloo, R.C. (2007) 'Wild edible plants of Meghalaya, North-East India', *Natural Product Radiance*, 6(5), 410–426.

CASE STUDY 10

LABORATORIOS PARA LA VIDA

Action research for agroecological scaling through food- and garden-based education

Bruce G. Ferguson and Helda Morales

Introduction

The *Laboratorios para la Vida* (LabVida[1]) action research team in Chiapas, Mexico trains educators to use school gardens and local food systems as venues for experiential learning. Our experience confirms the tremendous mobilizing potential of school gardens, as well as their efficacy for building bridges between academic and local knowledge, improving education in science and other fields, and promoting agroecology and conscientious eating based on regional agrobiodiversity. At the same time, we have identified a set of structural, organizational, and pedagogical challenges to implementation and continuity of garden programmes. In many ways, foodways can be a more straightforward starting-off point from which to approach many garden programme topics. Because educators often lack sufficient support in their immediate work environments, horizontal networks for exchange of knowledge, solidarity, and seeds contribute to strengthening, continuity, and growth of garden programmes.

Problem/context

The Food and Agriculture Organisation of United Nations (FAO) as well as many governments and civil society organizations now recognize agroecology as a necessary strategy for feeding the world's population while caring for the Earth.[2] A priority of agroecology as a science and a movement is to identify, analyze, and strengthen strategies for agroecological scaling (Mier y Terán Giménez Cacho et al., 2018). Teaching-learning processes that elucidate and promote agroecological processes and complexity are one key driver of scaling. These processes – phenomena such as soil fertility, pollination, and biological pest prevention – are all tightly linked to biodiversity in fields and landscapes.

Chiapas offers a complex and motivating scenario for the development of agroecological education. It is among the Mexican states with the worst indicators for education, health and marginalization. Food insecurity is a daily reality for many families. At the same time, agri-food system industrialization has been remarkably rapid. Rates of disease associated with metabolic syndrome – diabetes in particular – are soaring to an extent that has drawn international attention (e.g. Lopez and Jacobs, 2018).

Milpa (polycultures of corn, beans, squash and edible volunteers known in Chiapas as *verduritas* and in central Mexico as *quelites*, and often also including tree crops) and highly diverse home gardens are the foundation for traditional diets. These foodways, with variants pertaining to Maya, Zoque, and *mestizo* cultural groups and their adaptations to Chiapas' dramatic topography, persist today. However, this intertwined biological and cultural diversity is fast eroding in the face of urbanization, extractive industries, and expansion of industrial agriculture.

The education system and food and agriculture programmes typically disregard this diversity, and end up hastening its demise (e.g. Gutiérrez-Narváez, 2011). School separates children from their communities' food and farming traditions, and exposes them to junk food together with racist attitudes toward indigenous foodways. At the same time, various social movements, notably the Zapatista uprising and dissident teachers, have created a breeding ground for counter-hegemonic educational proposals.

LabVida's approach

Faced with these opportunities and challenges, and inspired by California's Life Lab programme,[3] we formed a team of natural and social scientists and project staff dedicated to participatory action research (Méndez et al., 2013) in constant dialogue with educators and their educational communities. Since 2009, we have promoted school gardens and local agrofood systems as teaching-learning environments (Meek et al., 2017; Ferguson et al., 2019).

We designed and implemented a pilot training programme (six four-hour workshops) and then four generations of a certificate programme (120–140 hours) that included modules on agroecology, conscientious eating, the scientific process, and school gardens and food as catalysts for horizontal dialogue between local and academic knowledge. Throughout the training, we modelled constructivist pedagogy and facilitated inquiry-based, experiential learning that educators could adapt to their specific contexts. Certificate programme participants were mostly primary- and middle-school teachers at public schools but also included educators working at the pre-school, high school, and university levels as well as in autonomous and private schools and non-governmental organizations. We documented educators' experiences within the programme through observations during trainings and school visits, surveys, interviews, and focus groups.

We touched on agrobiodiversity in relation to each of the training modules, as exemplified in Table C10.1. Clearly, however, assigning most of these activities to a single module is arbitrary. Experiments with companion planting, for example, allowed us to reinforce agroecological concepts around polyculture design, competition, and mutualism, and reflect on the ecological sophistication of the *milpa* as a manifestation of traditional knowledge, as well explore the scientific process. In one activity that turned out to be particularly engaging, we presented the latest science on healthy eating,[4] then asked participants to create a 'good food plate' using foods from the communities in which they work (Figure C10.1). We linked practically all of these activities to multiple curricular contents to help educators envision the multi-functionality of food and garden activities. Some key resources for learning

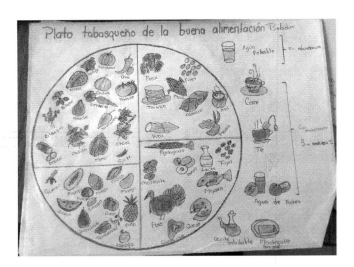

FIGURE C10.1 Good food plate created by Lupita Rivera Alcázar, a student in Juan Marcos Mendoza's science class at a preparatory school near the border of Chiapas and Tabasco.

TABLE C10.1 Examples of agrobiodiversity-related content in each of LabVida's main certificate programme modules

Module	Contents and activities related to agrobiodiversity
Agroecology	• the role of biodiversity at the plot and landscape scales in assuring agroecosystem functions such as pollination, regulation of herbivore populations, and maintenance of soil fertility • *milpa* and home garden functional diversity
Conscientious eating	• agrobiodiversity and *milpa* polycultures in particular as a foundation for healthy, culturally appropriate diets • cooking and eating wild edibles and insects and *verduritas* from the *milpa*
Scientific process	• companion planting experiments for learning principles of experimental design • transects to register wild edibles for learning sampling methodology
Knowledge dialogues	• creation of healthy eating plates based on local food traditions • food fairs celebrating ingredients, recipes, and related traditions from participants' cultural backgrounds

about agrobiodiversity included a special issue of *La Jornada del Campo* on *quelites*[5] and the documentary films *La Dieta Mesoamericana: Orígenes*[6] and *Seed: The Untold Story*.[7]

Snack and mealtimes were key moments for stimulating conversation around agrobiodiversity. Participants brought food from the communities where they lived or worked to share during our coffee breaks. We often asked local chefs to design lunch menus around themes we were studying on a given day, such as edible insects, the *milpa*, wild greens, amaranth (Figures C10.2a and b), and plant proteins.

(a)

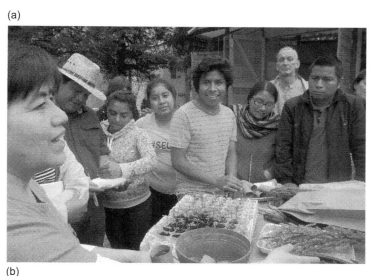

(b)

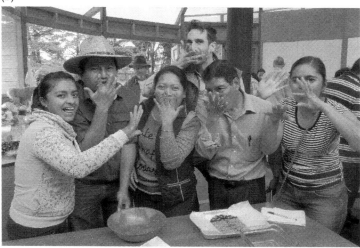

FIGURE C10.2 Educators in LabVida training learn to harvest (Figure C10.2a), plant, and cook with (Figure C10.2b) amaranth seed. Amaranth is a nutrient-dense pseudo-grain and vegetable historically grown in much of Mexico. The Spanish suppressed its use in the colonial era because of the religious significance of amaranth-seed figurines for the Aztecs.

Source: Helda Morales.

Early on, we realized that educators would need lasting support structures. In 2010, we organized an encounter of garden-based education programmes and created a network now named the *Red Internacional de Huertos Educativos* (RIHE).[8] As this network became more international in scope and began to hold its encounters in other states and countries, LabVida staff and trainees launched a state-level network, the *Red Chiapaneca de Huertos Educativos* (RCHE).[9] These networks have become important spaces for sharing ideas around garden-based learning, and for teachers to build relationships with like-minded colleagues. They have contributed to garden programme continuity and expanded the reach of LabVida's work.

What have we learned?

Interest in garden-based education is growing, and diverse initiatives are emerging throughout Latin America and the Caribbean. They vary widely in their objectives, but the majority incorporate elements of agroecology and healthy eating. This represents a great opportunity for agroecological scaling. Some programmes, however, lack an integrated approach, and tend to reduce agroecology to its technical-productive aspects. There is also the risk of co-optation, as some transnational agri-food corporations seek to whitewash their images by financing school garden initiatives.

Our certificate programme emphasized the diversity and complexity of interactions that undergird agroecological production. We proposed that agronomic challenges in school gardens are rich opportunities for inquiry through engagement with local knowledge and experimentation. However, we saw that the tendency to look for 'magic bullet' answers is deeply rooted in many people. We believe that developing a pedagogy of complexity is an urgent task for agroecological education (Ferguson et al., 2019).

Accordingly, although we originally organized the certificate programme based on the modules listed in Table C10.1, the second time we offered the training we integrated these topics in units based on the *milpa* and growing in small spaces (such as home gardens and many school gardens). This allowed us to develop sequences of activities that contributed to a holistic vision of food systems and agroecology.

Although school gardens are a compelling idea, and many of our trainees have established and maintained vibrant teaching gardens, we are increasingly convinced that gardens are not for every teacher or every school. Teachers face a host of hurdles – many of them structural – to successful garden programmes. These include: high teacher turnover, especially at rural schools; lack of space and schoolyards that are increasingly under pavement; the difficulty of matching garden growth with the curriculum calendar established at the national level; principals, supervisors, colleagues, and, sometimes, parents who fail to understand the educational value of gardens; and uncertainty inherent in garden management, particularly for teachers without much gardening experience.

We quickly learned that activities revolving around food bypass many of these hurdles and were more engaging for many participants than school garden work (Ferguson et al., 2019). Sharing food as well as knowledge and experience of food allows us to very quickly arrive at profound reflections with our trainees regarding the challenges in their schools and communities. Therefore, we organized the next two rounds of our certificate programme around action research in local food systems. Educators and their groups used tools including food diaries, transects and mapping, interviews, and focus groups to identify both positive and problematic aspects of their food environments. They organized the information and stimulated reflection among schoolmates, their families, and the broader community using puppet shows, radio plays, and artwork as well as more conventional reports and presentations. Based on collective reflection, they identified staring points for continued action research, including: workshops and recipe exchanges organized by and for families focussed on healthy school snacks; fairs and other celebrations of healthy, regional foods; agreements allowing consumption of healthy food and drinks in the classroom; inviting vendors of fruit and other healthy foods to sell at schools; and a proposal for a student-run shop selling healthy food at a high school. Many also established learning gardens, but with a clearer idea of how garden activities relate to their food environment.

A welcome outcome has been the extent to which action research around food has allowed teachers to learn from students and students' families. Teachers often perceive rural and indigenous communities in terms of poverty and deficit. For many, appraisals revealed local knowledge and resources that had been invisible to them. These new connections with local context helped them connect with their students. As a result, several reported that they had become better teachers.

We began the programme with the premise that one key function of school garden and food-system work must be to support teaching of the formal curriculum. We also thought that it would be easy for teachers to draw connections between the content of our training programme and the curriculum each was required to teach. Some were remarkably creative in developing garden- and food-based lesson plans, and some could adapt the activities we created to their own teaching contexts. However, for many, the task of creating lesson plans for experiential learning was novel and difficult. We ended up dedicating a substantial amount of training time to lesson plan development, and compiled some of these lesson plans in a guidebook for educators. This is available on our web page along with other learning materials we have developed.[10]

Sadly, we have seen that many talented educators, particularly those working in public schools, feel isolated, limited, or even harassed by the system of which they form a part. The certificate programme and school garden networks have particular significance for many educators as spaces in which they feel supported and can experiment confidently with new ideas and approaches. Teachers value our visits to their schools and continuing contact with our team and their peers through network activities and social media.

These learning communities are becoming catalysts for broader change. Both the RIHE and RCHE continue to grow in numbers, depth, and autonomy. The RIHE held its first meeting outside of Mexico (Montevideo, 2017) and will celebrate its 2019 gathering in Chile. The RCHE now has a coordinating committee and several active commissions focussed on pedagogy, seeds, and communication. It continues to hold bimonthly meetings in schools and training centres around the state and hosted a dynamic national gathering in 2018.

Agrobiodiversity is a recurring theme in network gatherings, most often in the form seed exchanges. These are of practical importance because lack of access to locally adapted, agroecologically produced seed is a frequent bottleneck for school garden establishment. However, seed also holds particular significance as an element of biocultural patrimony and resistance to the homogenizing pressure exerted by agroindustry. This manifests itself in the ceremonial nature of many seed exchanges and participation of RIHE members in national and international seed sovereignty movements.

Next steps

Although the networks and educational materials extend LabVida's reach in space and time, we recognize that there is continued need for training like that we have offered in our certificate programme. We are currently systematizing the structure and contents of the programme to facilitate replication of the training and its adaptation to other contexts. We are also exploring the possibility of offering training using distance learning technology.

We identify school food and distributed action research as areas of opportunity for continuation of this work. The farm-to-school movement is thriving in countries like Brazil and the United States as a win-win strategy for improving children's nutrition while creating local and regional markets for small and medium farmers. Few such programmes have been developed in Mexico, but areas like ours in which many small growers co-exist with many small schools present intriguing opportunities for farm to school. Combining LabVida's action research approach with sourcing of local food for schools could be a potent way to simultaneously promote health, education, and local economies.

The RCHE and our extended network of trainees present an opportunity for collective action research oriented toward needs and interests of educational communities. By identifying shared questions and concerns, developing concrete actions in response, and sharing results among themselves and more broadly, the networks could make concrete progress toward documenting and confronting challenges related to topics like school food, erosion of traditional knowledge and agrobiodiversity, pest prevention, and climate change.

Acknowledgements

We are grateful for the collaboration of LabVida's technical team, our advisors and students, and the educational communities that have participated in our training programme and networks. We thank the WK Kellogg Foundation for its support.

Notes

1 redhuertos.org/Labvida.
2 For example, www.fao.org/agroecology/home/en/.
3 lifelab.org.
4 www.hsph.harvard.edu/nutritionsource/.
5 www.jornada.com.mx/2017/11/18/delcampo.html.
6 www.cicy.mx/sitios/Dieta-mesoamericana-origenes/index.html.
7 www.seedthemovie.com/.
8 redhuertos.org, facebook.com/redhuertos/.
9 facebook.com/RedHuertosChiapas/.
10 redhuertos.org/Labvida/resenas-diplomado/materiales/.

References

Ferguson, B. G., Morales, H., Chung, K., Nigh, R., Ferguson, B. G., Morales, H., Chung, K., Nigh, R. and Ferguson, B. G. (2019) 'Scaling out agroecology from the school garden: the importance of culture, food, and place', *Agroecology and Sustainable Food Systems*, vol. 43, doi:10.1080/21683565.2019.1591565.

Gutiérrez-Narváez, R. (2011) 'Dos proyectos de sociedad en Los Altos de Chiapas: Escuelas secundarias oficial y autónoma entre los tsotsiles de San Andrés', in B. Barronet, M. Mora Bayo and R. Stahler-Sholk (eds.) 'Luchas "muy otras": Zaptismo y autonomía en las comunidades indígenas de Chiapas', Universidad Autónoma Metropolitana, Mexico City.

Lopez, O. and Jacobs, A. (2018) 'In town with little water, Coca-Cola is everywhere. So is diabetes', *The New York Times*, 14 Jul, 2018. Available from: https://www.nytimes.com/2018/07/14/world/americas/mexico-coca-cola-diabetes.html.

Meek, D., Bradley, K., Ferguson, B., Hoey, L., Morales, H., Rosset, P. and Tarlau, R. (2017) 'Food sovereignty education in the Americas: Multiple origins, converging movements', *Agriculture and Human Values*, doi:10.1007/s10460-017-9780-1.

Méndez, V. E., Bacon, C. M. and Cohen, R. (2013) 'Agroecology as a transdisciplinary, participatory, and action-oriented approach', *Agroecology and Sustainable Food Systems*, vol. 37, no. 1, 3–18.

Mier y Terán Giménez Cacho, M., Giraldo, O. F., Aldasoro, M., Morales, H., Ferguson, B. G., Rosset, P., Khadse, A. and Campos, C. (2018) 'Bringing agroecology to scale: Key drivers and emblematic cases', *Agroecology and Sustainable Food Systems*, vol. 42, no. 6, 637–665, doi:10.1080/21683565.2018.1443313.

CASE STUDY 11

AGROBIODIVERSITY EDUCATION

The inclusion of agrobiodiversity in primary school curricula in Xiengkhouang Province, the Lao People's Democratic Republic

Chinda Milayvong, Kevin Kamp, and Manivanh Aliyavong

Summary

Losses of biodiversity in Laos are happening in areas where sustainable rotational farming in mountainous landscapes has been practiced for generations. This is due to a number of factors including recent reductions in fallow periods, agriculture expansion into forest areas, a greater focus on commercial crops and unsustainable harvesting of non-timber forest products (NTFPs). Another factor is that traditional knowledge and appreciation of biodiversity in farming landscapes is lost in the transition between the older and younger generations. In Naxaithong Village, Khoun District, in Xiengkhouang Province, the Swiss Agency for Development and Cooperation-funded The Agro-Biodiversity Initiative (Lao PDR) (TABI)[1] supports the inclusion of 'agrobiodiversity' (ABD) knowledge in school curricula to ensure the transfer of indigenous knowledge and appreciation for ABD to future generations, and highlighting the importance of ABD for local livelihoods.

In Xiengkhouang Province (see Figure C11.1), TABI has benefited from the commitment and motivation of Mr Sounduean Simsamai, who has developed an ABD curriculum which was approved by provincial authorities in 2012. The curriculum was adopted by 30 primary schools in 4 districts in the province as well as 5 non-formal education schools that target out-of-school adults. It includes three components: ABD theory, developing collections of agrobiodiversity species, and establishing school gardens focussed on medicinal plants or local cultivars of edible plants. The ABD curricula has been well accepted by the communities and has been expanded into the neighbouring Houaphan Province.

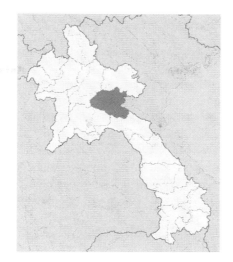

FIGURE C11.1 Xiengkhouang Province in Laos.
Source: Karte, NordNordWest, Lizenz/Wikimedia.

Introduction

Laos is recognized as having a very high diversity of plant and animals species and being a centre of origin for some cultivars, such as glutinous rice with over 2,400 varieties recorded.[2] The practice of shifting cultivation has ensured that a very high and unique diversity of wild plants and animals, referred to as 'agrobiodiversity' or ABD, inhabit fallow fields as populations of different species and biotic communities evolve over the rotation period. Farmers use a very high number of these species as food, medicine, construction materials, as sources of cash and for cultural/social purposes. Sadly, reductions in fallow periods, agriculture expansion into forest areas, a greater focus on commercial cash crops and unsustainable harvesting of NTFPs is reducing Lao PDR's ABD resources. In addition, a large number of cultivars also exist within these farming landscapes, including vegetable, rice and animal varieties which are often unique to Laos. Knowledge and the importance of local ABD resources is traditionally passed on from one generation to the next, but indigenous knowledge is fast disappearing due to changing lifestyles of both young and old and adoption of modern communication methods, such as smart phones, rather than traditional communication settings where indigenous knowledge is discussed. To regenerate and maintain this transfer of indigenous knowledge, and highlight the importance of agrobiodiversity for livelihoods, TABI supports the inclusion of ABD in school curricula. This directly supports the Ministry of Education and Sports strategy to integrate local knowledge into the formal curricula and support improvements in agriculture production via the education sector through mechanisms such as the establishment of school gardens, which also contribute to improved nutrition of students and as a source of medicinal plants.

The ABD curricula activity was built upon the successes and commitment of Mr Sounduean Simsamai, a very active staff member from the Xiengkhouang Provincial Office of Education and Sports (POES) who first developed a curriculum for silk worm feeding within the non-formal education system that received the winning prize from the Lao Ford Car Company on business innovations. In 2008, Mr Sounduean became interested in threatened ABD species and began investigating their habitats in the area. He had heard about the ABD curricula being used in Thailand in schools as well as a few other countries in the South East Asia region, supported by The Field Alliance (TFA). Based on seeing the TFA curricula, Mr. Sounduean moved forward to develop a unique curriculum for Xiengkhouang Province to use in the schools. A few schools began teaching it in 2009. After 5 years, Mr Sounduean submitted a proposal to the TABI project which included a revision of his original ABD curriculum. His proposal was accepted, the curriculum was updated and the Xiengkhouang Provincial Education and Sports Office (POES) revised curriculum was officially approved by the Ministry of Education. Teaching of the revised ABD curriculum in schools began in 2014 and today the POES goal is to integrate the ABD curriculum into the formal education system of at least 20% of schools by 2021. The curriculum uses experiential and participatory learning methodologies whereby students learn by documenting local agrobiodiversity.

> I am very concerned about the situation of biodiversity in Xiengkhuang, and if I may quote our former leader Mr. Kaisone Phoumvihan, *"Our Biodiversity is in the red light"*. That was very inspiring to me and I began thinking about the solution that would help preserve our biodiversity species via sustainable management. I wanted to start with raising awareness of children and ensure community ownership and empowerment
>
> – *Mr Sounduean, POES*

From 2009 until 2012, the curriculum was focussed on increasing children's awareness, knowledge, skills and recognition of the importance of ABD in local livelihoods. This was accomplished by collecting traditional knowledge and incorporating it into a curriculum that was made available to and used by schoolteachers and by encouraging community representatives to transfer this knowledge and skills to students. From 2012, the curriculum began to focus on the problems and importance of biodiversity and in 2014 the curriculum was further revised via a collaborative effort with the teachers, written in a more formal publication and printed. Since 2018 activities for raising awareness of the impact of agricultural chemicals on people's lives was added. Also added was a curriculum that focussed on concerns about nutrition and the benefits of consuming organic food. Community involvement was promoted further, including participation of community members in transferring their knowledge, teaching/training students, expanding the curricula and finally testing it in new schools. The project integrates two other components: the development of recipes using traditional medicine and forest foods to improve nutrition; and the collection of agrobiodiversity samples displayed in the school library to raise awareness about biodiversity.

ABD curriculum

At the beginning of the TABI project a workshop was executed engaging teachers from five schools in Khoun District (Ban Kheung, Ban Mein, Ban Poungmanh in Phoukoud District), the Village Education Promotion Committee as well as representatives from other relevant district offices. The main issues discussed included the importance of ADB and sustainable management which raised meeting participants' awareness about local vulnerable species and their sustainable management. This led to an action plan for the schools which included the collection of key species in their natural habitats in the areas of the schools including riparian habitats, forest habitats, rice fields and other agricultural fields. Many of these key species are now grown in the school gardens.

The participants from the schools distinguished between three main categories of species from their collection efforts: (1) edible species for human and animal consumption, (2) traditional medicines and (3) highly vulnerable species facing erosion. The teachers are using various techniques to preserve the specimens including drying and preserving in alcohol. The specimens continue to be displayed in the school library to raise awareness to students and community. Each year new species are added.

ABD curriculum development process and approval

The curriculum was developed during a workshop by the taskforce consisting of experienced teachers. The taskforce prioritized a number of main topics for educating the students and community including: ABD and associated habitats, changing of ABD populations, cause of ABD depletion, impact of ABD losses and conservation of ABD.

After a testing period of one semester and three writing workshops, the curriculum was finalized and sent to the Provincial Education and Sports for confirmation and the Provincial Governor for certification. After this the curriculum was presented to the Ministry of Education and Sports (MOES) where it was approved after 2 months (Figure C11.2).

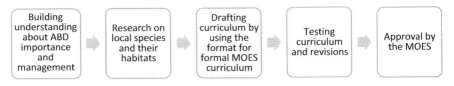

FIGURE C11.2 Schematic of the ABD curriculum development process and approval.

> We had good support on district level from the Education and Sports office and on the provincial level as well because we directly support the government strategy and have good relationship with related department. We also work in close cooperation with active teachers and communities
>
> *— Ms. Khankham, Task force member*

ABD curriculum activities

The ABD curriculum includes 3 main components: (1) ABD theory lessons (Figure C11.3), (2) agrobiodiversity samples collected and displayed in the school library, and (3) knowledge transfer through a school garden focussed on local food crops and/or medicinal plants.

The piloting of the new curriculum was useful to raise awareness about biodiversity, but the teachers realized that this did not fully support the improvement of livelihoods, nutrition or culinary practices at home as expected. The teachers then decided to involve the community in raising awareness of student studies by

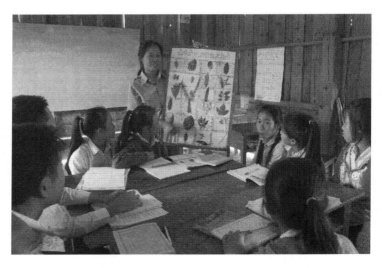

FIGURE C11.3 Ms Bouaphan is teaching on importance of ABD.
Source: TABI.

Agrobiodiversity education **251**

> **BOX C11.1: CHANGING PERSPECTIVES OF STUDENTS**
>
> - Awareness of ABD importance, sustainable management of agrobiodiversity, and detrimental practices such as the use of dynamite or electric shock to catch fish
> - Benefits of plants, animals, and medical plants for livelihoods
> - Greater concern about the harmful effects of chemicals in agriculture and deforestation
> - Family members at home are educated about ABD importance by students

introducing the activities of the students to the community. Each year the task force rewards model students and model families involved in the activities with a certificate of achievement.

Knowhow on local skills and food recipes

The curriculum includes classes on local skills. Building on this, teachers documented 6 stories of local skills from the community and use it for training/coaching of life skill to student 3–4 times per year and class on Lao food recipes 6 times per year. The community was further involved in raising awareness about handicrafts and Lao food which are dependent on ABD products and species, e.g. Lao cooking recipes, mat weaving, use of medicinal plants, etc (Figure C11.4).

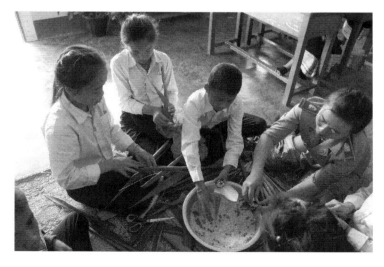

FIGURE C11.4 Students learning to make Lao sweet 'Khao Tom'.
Source: TABI.

BOX C11.2: LOCAL SKILLS TRANSFERRED FROM ELDERS TO YOUTH

- Local skills and recipes using ABD species are preserved and transferred to new generation.
- Students train other classes on mat weaving, pickled vegetables, spicy sauces and Lao sweets.
- Learning and sharing space between elders and youths was created.
- Students were trained in local skills by community members who then helped train other families in their communities.

ABD School garden and medicinal plants garden (Naxaithong Village School)

In Naxaithong Village School, for example, two gardens are located behind the school, covering approximately 640 square meters and including both edible and medicinal plants. Edible crops include local vegetable cultivars not available as seeds in the market such as maize, eggplant, and cucumber. Medicinal and herb species include varieties of mint and many other species. The teacher leads the students to understand agricultural practices including garden preparation, initial planting, management, and harvesting. The gardens cannot provide enough food to support the school nutrition programme, but it is useful as

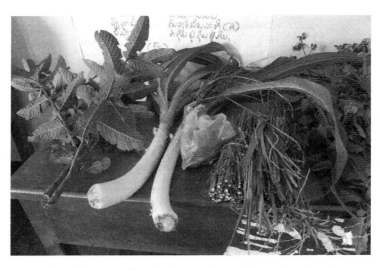

FIGURE C11.5 Traditional medicinal plants collected from school garden.
Source: TABI.

a demonstration garden in support of the ABD curriculum. The community participated in building the fences to protect the garden against domestic animals. Importantly, the community also uses the garden as a demonstration and supply of medicinal plants to raise awareness about local pharmacopeia species and how they are useful to cure frequent diseases.

The community uses some of the medicinal species grown in the garden to cure diseases such as diarrhoea, burns (from water and fire), or other injuries (Figure C11.5). The garden production is sometimes sold by students providing them with experience in marketing vegetables and raising school resources.

Promoting and expanding the ABD curriculum

A five-school event for Phoukoud District promoting agrobiodiversity was held in 2016 at the provincial level. Each school presented their own innovative ideas in terms of curriculum and student art performances related to promoting preservation of ABD. This was seen by thousands of residents of Xiengkhouang and important in disseminating messages on ABD and the value of teaching ABD in the schools.

Challenges and keys to success

- Xiengkhouang was the first province to develop and use this type of curriculum in its daily teaching. The process of getting the curriculum approved was a significant challenge that required substantial engagement until its approval by the Ministry of Education and Sports on 9 September 2012. The revisions to improve the curricula and quality printing have been important for upscaling.
- To date, the curriculum has been implemented in 30 primary schools and 5 non-formal education schools in 4 districts in Xiengkhouang Province and has reached approximately 15,000 students in the past 5 years with approximately 35 hours of education on ABD taught involving more than 500 teachers. About half of the teachers are directly involved in the ABD programme, while the other 50% also participate but to a lesser degree.

BOX C11.3: BEHAVIOUR CHANGES

- Reduction of illegal and unsustainable fishing techniques.
- Each school garden was established and maintained by students, teachers and community.
- Students actively supporting the family daily chores and household garden.

TABLE C11.1 Annual breakdown of schools, teachers, and students engaged in ABD learning

No.	District	2014 Schools	2014 Teachers	2014 Student	2015 Schools	2015 Teachers	2015 Student	2016 Schools	2016 Teachers	2016 Student	2017 Schools	2017 Teachers	2017 Student	2018 Schools	2018 Teachers	2018 Student
1	Phoukoud	8	53	826	8	72	908	8	72	908	16	157	1,921	16	157	1,921
2	Khoun	2	42	778	2	47	850	2	50	871	2	47	850	2	47	850
3	Kham	2	86	1,599	4	152	1,995	4	135	1,812	4	152	1,991	10	210	2,692
4	Peak				2	102	1,954	2	108	1,854	2	102	1,954	2	102	1,954
5	Non-formal Education															
6	Thathome	6	96	1,555										5	39	472
	Total	18	277	4,758	16	373	5,707	16	365	5,445	24	458	6,716	35	555	7,889

The table below (Table C11.1) provides an annual breakdown of schools, teachers, and students engaged in ABD learning. Note that each student receives 2 years of instruction.
- After the implementation of the ABD curriculum in schools, it is clear that a substantial amount of knowledge on ABD resides among the adult population, much more than what the current curricula covers. Engaging the local community is important. Village authorities and customary leaders are also very supportive.
- Getting good samples is important. The steps in sample collection concerning both animals and crops is challenging but the success is ensured by the dedication and the patience of the teachers.

Maximizing participation

- Conducting dissemination and awareness campaigns at community level should be timed according to the social and seasonal work calendar to avoid peak labour demand and select an appropriate time when villagers can fully participate by involving the community in determining the best timing.
- Mainstreaming ABD issues and problems into district development planning to ensure budget and technical support from the relevant divisions is important.
- Promotion of exchanges of lessons earned by welcoming other projects and communities to visit as per the example of visiting the Good Neighbours in Mok district in Vientiane Province.

Recommendations

- The Provincial Department of Education should use the curriculum in all of its schools, not just the schools which are supported by projects such as TABI. Very few materials are needed for implementing the curriculum hence it is not a significant expense for the schools.
- There needs to be continued development of the ABD curriculum – review and improve the current curriculum, make new topics and lessons, and make a textbook specifically for students.
- A greater number of copies of the curriculum for teachers is needed.
- Continual updating of teacher skills on the understanding and use of the curriculum, especially revised components, is necessary.

Opportunities for future development

- There is a need to organize sharing events both in central downtown and rural areas to gain support by parents, government, and other actors.
- Expand the garden component for medicinal plants and plant more species, as well as documenting medicinal plant using skills and knowledge available in the local community.

- Work with non-formal education departments to develop more topics and integrate the ABD curriculum into current student schedules with a focus on ABD-related livelihood skills.
- Expand the library spaces in the 30 schools that already implemented ABD curriculum or find ABD-dedicated space for specimens and learning.
- Include more focus on the dangers of agrochemical use on ABD species and local food and nutrition.

Notes

1 The Agro-Biodiversity Initiative (TABI), funded by Swiss Agency for Development and Cooperation, initiated its work in 2009, focussing on the conservation and promotion of agrobiodiversity in the highlands of three northern provinces in Laos. It does this via a thoughtful process of working closely together with communities and governmental bodies to identify important biodiversity issues in agricultural landscapes (agrobiodiversity); identify critical habitats and associated restoration and conservation needs for selected species; develop plans for management and marketing of selected species and associated products; support sound national policy development and make information on agrobiodiversity available to a wider audience.
2 Geographical Distribution of Glutinous Rice. P. Sattaka (www.tci-thaijo.org/index.php/mekongjournal/article/download/73311/59023/).

CASE STUDY 12

KATAKIN KŌMMAN JIKIN KALLIB ILO JIKUUL – REPUBLIC OF THE MARSHALL ISLANDS SCHOOL LEARNING GARDEN PROGRAM

Koh Ming Wei and Samuel Bikajle

Introduction

The Republic of the Marshall Islands (RMI) consists of over 2,000 small, low-lying coral islands and islets clustered in 29 atolls and 5 single islands on a table reef (Figure C12.1). These atolls and islands form two groups: the Ratak Chain and the Ralik Chain (meaning 'sunrise' and 'sunset') and lie just north of the equator and west of the international dateline. Land area totals only 182 Km^2 or 70 mi^2, and protected, shallower, and resources-rich atoll lagoons comprise 10,470 Km^2 or 4,040 mi^2. The population density in the Marshall Islands is 296 per Km^2 (766 people per mi^2). About 75% of the population is urban (40,224 people in 2019) (Worldometers, 2019).

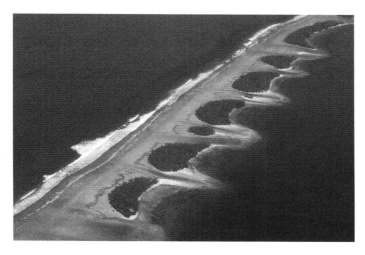

FIGURE C12.1 Aerial view of the reef and Islets.
Source: Island Research and Education Initiative.

In the Marshall Islands, society is structured hierarchically, with two classes of people: the *irooj* (chiefs, royalty) and the *kajoor* (commoners, literally meaning – 'the strength of the *irooj*'). A hierarchical structure is an effective way to make sure people accomplish what needs to be done. Under the direction of their leaders, everyone knows their roles and tasks, and there is no time wasted arguing over decisions or determining who will carry out which task. Everyone works together for the good of the community. This is what is known as *JERAMMAN*.

Jepilpilin ke ejukaan – Accomplishment through joint effort – *RMI Motto*

The problem

The diet of the Marshallese community has been disrupted and colonized since the First World War. The islands have the fertility to support the production of root crops such as taro (*Colocasia esculenta*), swamp taro (*Cyrtosperma chamissonis*), fruiting trees such as breadfruit (*Atrocarpus altilis*), banana (*Musa* sp.), papaya (*Carica papaya*), and citrus (*Citrus* sp.), and perennial greens such as bele (*Abelmoschus manihot*). Protein in the form of seafood such as fish, clams, shellfish, and crabs are generally abundant. Atoll dwellers learn from elders how to live in balance between exploiting and preserving natural resources. Unfortunately, event after event, from atomic fallout to mass migration from outer atolls to urban areas, to a shift to a cash economy, have subjected most residents to the convenience of canned goods, white rice, white flour, white sugar, salt, and fat (Culpin, 2017).

The consequence

Since the late 1980s, the UNICEF and the RMI Ministry of Health has been documenting junk food spreading malnutrition and stunted growth in the Pacific Islands. A recent study, 2017–2018, conducted in partnership by Canvasback Wellness Centre of Majuro and the Ministry of Health with the support of the Republic of China Taiwan Mission, showed little change in the percentage rate of stunting of teenagers, which is at an alarming 43% (Johnson, 2019).

Findings reveal that the risk factors of poor diet, lack of physical activity, and risky lifestyle behaviours are associated with overweight and obesity and subsequent non communicable diseases (NCDs) that are significant factors in the morbidity and mortality of the population. The leading causes of death include sepsis, cancer, diabetes-related deaths, pneumonia, and hypertension. Population-based surveys for the RMI show that 62.5% of the adults are overweight or obese and the prevalence of diabetes stands at 19.6% (Ichiho et al., 2013).

Furthermore, most of the Marshall Islands is regularly inundated by seawater as the sea level rises and the island nation is subject to more and more storm surges and King Tides. The inundation salinizes the soil, and if the event is followed by a drought or dry spell, the salt accumulates, affecting plant growth.

And it is hot in the Marshall Islands, with a daily average of 30°C, causing rapid transpiration from young plants. All these factors make the Marshall Islands a very interesting and somewhat challenging context for school learning gardens (Culpin, 2017).

The solution and research

Her Excellency President Dr Hilda C. Heine initiated the *Jikin kallib ilo jikuul* – RMI School Learning Garden Program in 2014 when she was minister of education. There were already other efforts in place for school gardens. However, these gardens were not integrated into the curriculum but were just stand-alone activities or after school activities. One of the first things she did was to hire a full-time learning garden coordinator, Samuel Bikajle, housed within the curriculum, instruction, and assessment department at the public school system (PSS), immediately institutionalizing the work. The research considers the impact and sustainability of school learning gardens when the activities and work in the garden are place-based, fully integrated into the daily curriculum, and supported institutionally.

The project

This case study focusses on the teacher development and curriculum integration aspects of school learning gardens. The RMI Learning Garden Program is designed in three phases. The first is the school garden teacher training and curriculum integration focus on Majuro, Kwajalein, Jaulit, and Wotje. These are atolls with both elementary and high schools. The second, overlapping phase, is the co-development of the RMI Learning Garden Curriculum Map and a train the trainers (ToT) capacity building initiative. The third phase is the expansion of the programme to outer islands/atolls.

Gardening as we know it in the West with orderly rows of annual vegetables is a rather alien concept in the low-lying atolls of the RMI. Atoll forests intercropped with coconut, bananas, and pandanus, with swamp taro pits in the middle of the islands, and arrowroot (*Tacca leontopetaloides*) fields on the outside are found in the *jikin kallib* – places reserved for planting. Thus, focussing on the learning garden as an outdoor lab to teach and learn in an interdisciplinary way opened up new ways of environmental education in the RMI. Composting for soil health and soil desalinization is the key practice taught repeatedly. Teachers are encouraged to integrate gardening with traditional Marshallese vegetables such as *bōb* – pandanus, *ni* – coconut, and *kieb* – spider lily as well as Marshallese 'windbreaker plants' like *kōññat* (*Scaevola taccada*), which is also an important medicinal plant, and *markinenjojo* (*Vigna marina*) a nitrogen fixer, excellent compost plant, and medicinal plant. Hereby the gardens support Marshallese language, arts, and science while promoting agrobiodiversity and food security (Figure C12.2).

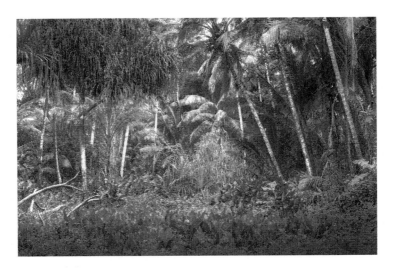

FIGURE C12.2 Atoll agroforest.
Source: Island Research and Education Initiative.

The RMI learning garden teacher training is adapted from *Kū ʻĀina Pā: Standing Firmly in Knowledge Upon the Land* (KAP) – a school garden teacher training and certification programme for Hawaiʻi's school learning garden and classroom educators. Since 2012 KAP has worked with seven cohorts comprised of 200 teachers from Hawaiʻi Island, Maui, Molokaʻi, Lānaʻi, and Oʻahu.[1] The co-author, Dr Koh Ming Wei, KAP designer, developer, and instructor worked with RMI PSS Science Specialists and other subject specialists and learning gardens coordinator, Samuel Bikajle, to adapt the course for the Marshall Islands. The four themes of

1. Cultivating a sense of place: Sustainable living is rooted in a deep knowledge of place and self;
2. The living soil, plants, and animals: We are all interconnected and related;
3. Nourishment: Feed the mind and body to stay healthy and flourish; and
4. Nature's design: Systems, cycles, patterns, and relationships, continues to be the backbone of both the Hawaii and the RMI school learning garden teacher trainings.

BOX C12.1: THE LEARNING GARDEN PROGRAM

The Learning Garden Program helps educate our students, teachers, parents, and community members to achieve a healthier lifestyle through learning to grow and prepare fresh fruits and vegetables in healthy soils, nourished by compost and place-based soil fertility practices. The Learning Garden Program's long-term vision is to educate our community to become:

i   Food Secure – and self-reliant
ii Healthy – decrease NCDs
iii Sustainable – decrease waste and increase soil health through composting

By integrating academics with learning gardens, students learn life skills as well as academic subjects. The learning garden also focusses on community building in terms of JERAMMAN.

Students learn science, numeracy, literacy, and our culture. Learning gardens help our students in science, math, social studies and literacy achievement, in both the Marshallese and English languages, by offering students year-round garden-based learning experiences. The Learning Garden Program focusses on building resiliency and sustainability through a deeper knowledge of interconnectedness and sense of place. Learning gardens support teachers to help students better explore and engage with essential questions around food, water, energy, and stewardship of their environment.

Statistically, we found that our island nation is highly challenged by increasing numbers of student dropping out after each school year ended. With this increasing range of drop out students, we found that our island nation is highly challenged with students 'academic status'. Another challenge that our island nation is trying to manoeuvre around are NCDs, the leading cause of death within our island nation which is diabetes causing 23% of registered deaths. Therefore, we believe the Learning Garden Program will be another source to help our teachers educate our students about healthier lifestyles and encouraging students to actively engage in exploring their environment.

Source: Samuel Bikaje

Findings, adaptations, and impacts

The first school learning garden teacher training for all Majuro schools was conducted in March 2015, proceeded by annual trainings in the summertime (starting in the summer of 2015) and follow-up site visits during the fall and spring semesters. The first important lesson we learned was to clearly differentiate between a compost pile (only organic, biodegradables) and a trash pit. The Marshallese keep their compounds very clean, raking leaves, pieces of plastic trash, and such everyday waste into piles along the edges of their property. While these piles eventually break down, the plastic is ubiquitous and could lead to toxicity. Also, due to generally eating canned foods, ramen noodles, and rice, when asked to bring meal leftovers to integrate into the compost system, teachers showed up with cans and plastic wrappers. The composting lesson for the training had to be modified to first explain what is biodegradable and what is not, which led to lessons in sorting and categorizing (mathematics integration). We also found the abundant free resource of copra cake – the leftover residue after the oil is extracted from the coconut flesh – as an excellent source of nitrogen. Tabolar Copra Processing Authority located in Majuro Atoll happily donates all the copra cake we can truck off and distribute to the schools. The copra cake attracts black soldier fly (*Hermetia illucens*) as an essential decomposer resulting in viable humus, which led to lessons about integrated pest management and the differences between insects and their functions (Figure C12.3).

The next big 'aha!' moment was during the spring of 2016, when a teacher proudly showed us the school garden's bumper crop of eggplants and said, 'We will sell all these vegetables and use the money for an ice-cream party'. We realized that most of the teachers had very little experience cooking the vegetables that did well in the atoll soils such as eggplant, yard-long beans (*Vigna unguiculata* subsp. *sesquipedalis* – a variety of cowpea), various bok choys (Chinese cabbage of sorts), and varieties of perennial greens – Malabar spinach (*Basella alba*), New Zealand Spinach (*Tetragonia tetragonioides*), and bele (*Abelmoschus manihot*). Learning to cook the vegetables raised became a priority in the teacher trainings. Cooking also provided a simple way to teach engineering design principles – to consider criteria and constraints – criteria such as health, tastiness, and reduced salt, and constraints such as time and limited tools. Engaging the teachers in the process in the form of a cooking competition proved to be fun and replicable. This summer (2019) several school principals reported that they conducted cooking competitions at their schools using learning garden produce and plans for an atoll-wide recipe book are in place (Figure C12.4).

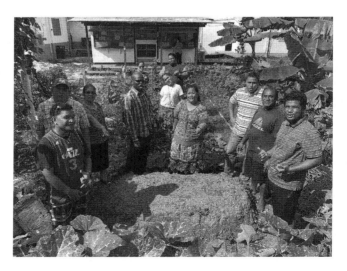

FIGURE C12.3 Compost pile with layer of copra cake.
Source: Koh Ming Wei.

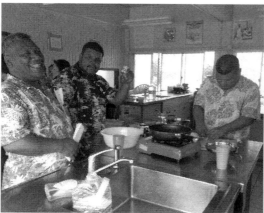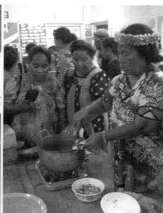

FIGURE C12.4 Teachers engaged in cooking.
Source: Koh Ming Wei.

Commitment and follow-up is the third key finding. It takes a while to build capacity and experience. Going from never gardening to managing 30 children working in a learning garden takes commitment, time, trial and error, and much support from the administration and community. It is no surprise that the schools with thriving learning gardens are the schools with engaged and supportive principals or vice-principals who see the value of an outdoor lab for learning, experimenting, and hard work. Visiting schools regularly and consistently is imperative; we developed a schedule for the learning gardens coordinator to visit every school in Majuro once a month, and the impact of those consistent visits is obvious.

Work on the RMI *Jikin kallib ilo jikuul* Curriculum Map (RMI Map) began in the summer 2017, with teachers and principals from various atolls, representing the urban and rural islands. Although the Hawaii School Garden Curriculum Map was the guiding document, the local epistemologies uncovered concepts that were not found in the Hawaii document. The most prominent was the continuity of *āne* (land, island) to *meto* (ocean), being on a low-lying atoll with no hills or mountains to block the view – wherever one is on an atoll, one can always see or hear the ocean. 'Reading' the ocean realm (*joormeto*) is just as decisive as reading the landscape (*joorāne*) when it comes to farming or gardening. Another unique element of the RMI Map is the specialized vocabulary afforded to certain central-to-life plants such as *bōb* (pandanus), *mā* (breadfruit), and *ni* (coconut). From propagation to cultivation to harvest to processing, each of these plants carried rich and colourful nouns, adjectives, verbs, adverbs, as well as spiritual and bio-cultural practices. These were not just food crops, but also a resource for timber, fishing materials, beverages, and medicines. The point here is – the learning that occurred for the teachers and principals when they had to develop the curriculum. Much of the knowledge mentioned above is getting lost, replaced by refrigerators and canned goods. By engaging the Marshallese educators in developing the RMI curriculum map, the traditional knowledge can be valued and perpetuated. Currently the RMI Map has three major overarching themes:

- *'Ijo Jikū* – Cultivating our sense of place in the living world;
- *Kabijikunen im Ekitōkmaroro* – The living soil, living plants, living islands – Connections and relationships; and
- *Mōñā ko Rōūne im Kaimourur* – Nourishment and healthy foods.

There is still much work left to do on this document including aligning the big ideas and topics to RMI National Curriculum standards and benchmarks.

The summer of 2019 was a *'Iokwe* summer' – *Iokwe* is both a greeting and a farewell, meanings include 'love', 'you are a rainbow', and 'goodbye'. This summer's teacher training was almost completely facilitated by the learning gardens coordinator, school garden/classroom lead teachers, and the PSS Science Specialist. This was the moment co-author Dr Ming Wei had been waiting for – enough capacity built and positive impact made for local ownership. The lead teachers took the other participating teachers on tours around their school learning gardens, sharing lessons learned and taught, challenges faced, and adaptations made including making fertilizer from *jipenpen* (sea cucumber, *Holothuria* sp.). The learning garden coordinator led the composting, transplanting, and garden cleaning work, and the Science Specialist ensured curriculum integration. Community members supported the cooking competition and the Taiwan Mission Farm supplemented the school garden produce with other freshly harvested vegetables.

Scaling up: the biggest challenge

The work has only just scratched the surface. Other than a handful of schools, we cannot yet see systemic change or impact. A transformation of palate is needed to change taste preferences conditioned to fat, salt and sugar back to whole foods such as breadfruit and fish. Lifestyle change, one of the most difficult things to do, is also necessary to shift from convenient fast food – canned goods and white rice to cooking from scratch. This will take concerted effort from all stakeholders. Even though the project has embraced many partners, there are still key organizations that do not know enough about the project and thus are yet to collaborate.

Two key challenges are at play – communication and transportation. Communication is best done face to face, which takes time and effort. Transportation affects communication. Often, folks do not show up for a meeting due to the lack of reliable transportation. Many residents do not drive, nor own a car. There is no public transportation system, only private taxis for hire. We managed to get a grant from Taiwan (Republic of China) to purchase a truck for the School Learning Garden Program; however, lack of fuel and maintenance plague the usability of the vehicle.

There are many requests from outer atoll principals and teachers to bring the Learning Garden Program to their atolls. Even though the teachers and principals have attended and participated in our trainings they still want us to come and launch the project – recall the societal structure here, a leader/expert must initiate. Transportation over great ocean distances is also a challenge. We have flown by small plane to various outer atolls, stuffing the cargo with tools, seeds, and plants. When we get there, we have to load up small boats to take the materials over to the schools. We have been stranded when the small planes cannot return to get us due to engine failure or bad weather. We've sailed to outer atolls, but this often triples or even quadruples the time needed to get from place to place.

Visiting outer atolls also demands a lot of logistics and communication. All stakeholders starting with traditional government to local government, and then on to schools, churches, and community are informed via radio calls. It is a time-consuming process for which a good sense of humour is essential. We go to the radio office with a call number and the signal goes out to that atoll, there's a long lag, often the person needed is not there and so you have to come back. Sometimes the signal needs to hop scotch from one atoll to another. The message is relayed to an atoll closer to Majuro, and they then relay the message to the intended atoll. It's often a miracle when we get out there and folks are ready for us. Most of the time, we show up and folks say, 'We didn't know you were coming. Why didn't you tell us?' All we can do is laugh and show them the tools and seedlings – *JERAMMAN*.

Note

1 The Kohala Center – Kū 'Āina Pā: Standing Firmly in Knowledge Upon the Land https://kohalacenter.org/kuainapa/kuainapa_archive.

References

Culpin, A. (2017) 'Child health and nutrition in the Marshall Islands'. Statistics for Development Division, Pacific Community (SPC), Development Bulletin 78.

Ichiho, H.M., deBrum, I., Kedi, S., Langidrik, J., and Aitaoto, N. (2013) 'An Assessment of Non-Communicable Diseases, Diabetes, and Related Risk Factors in the Republic of the Marshall Islands, Majuro Atoll: A Systems Perspective', Hawaii J Med Public Health, 72 (5 Suppl 1): 87–97.

Johnson, G. (2019) 'Stunted growth a major problem in Marshalls', Marianas Variety, http://www.mvariety.com/regional-news/113932-stunted-growth-a-major-problem-in-marshalls, accessed 22 July 2019.

Worldometers (2019) 'Marshall Islands Population', retrieved 22 July 2019 from https://www.worldometers.info/world-population/marshall-islands-population/.

Additional sources of information

Ahlgren, I.A. (2016) 'The meaning of MO: Place, Power, and Taboo in the Marshall Islands', Doctoral Dissertation, The Australian National University.

Koh, M.W. (2012) 'Discovering learning, discovering self: The effects of an interdisciplinary, standards-based school garden curriculum on elementary students in Hawai'i', Doctoral dissertation, Prescott College in Sustainable Education, ISBN-978-1-2674-1456-4.

Merlin, M., Capelle, A., Keene, T., Juvik, J., and Taborosi, D. (2018) 'Keinikkan im Ri-Aelōñ kein – Plants and people of the Marshall Islands', second revised edition, Island Research & Education Initiative, Palikir, Pohnpei, FM.

Walsh, J. (2012) 'Etto ñan Raan Kein: A Marshall Islands History'. Bess Press, Honolulu, HI.

CASE STUDY 13

WHERE THE WILD THINGS ARE

Ayfer Tan, Neşe Adanacioğlu, Saadet Tuğrul Ay, Malek Batal, Hala Ghattas, and Salma Talhouk[1]

Introduction

This book covers a vast range of examples of how the school garden becomes an extension of the classroom and a source of linking to the school curriculum and sometimes complementing school meals. Imagine removing the limitation of the school garden and letting the nature around the school – the wider school garden – form the extension of the classroom and the wild plants growing there serve as a basis for heathy and ecological learning. This is the reality for a number of schools in Turkey and Lebanon experimenting with consuming and cooking with wild edible species to overcome the challenges that are related to children's diets in both countries.

Problem

In Turkey and Lebanon, as in most other countries, dietary habits are changing along with cultural and social norms. In Turkey, wild edible plants have been an integral part of human diets since prehistoric times and are still today common in local Turkish cuisine. Yet traditional and essentially varied dishes are unpopular with the younger generations who prefer more Western-style foods (Tan et al., 2017). This modern diet often result in vitamin and mineral deficiencies and the rise in overweight and obesity, a condition which is becoming increasingly common both in adults and children in Turkey (Erem, 2015).

A similar pattern can be seen for Lebanon where traditional and inherently varied diets, often containing wild edible plants, today are perceived to be 'less prestigious' by younger generations. Traditional dishes are being replaced by a limited range of high calorie high sugar foods, many of which are imported (more than 70%), coupled with an increased consumption of red meat (Batal et al., 2012). This has a negative impact on health with an increasing prevalence of overweight and obesity, which today is 21.2% and 10.9% respectively, among children and young adults (6–19 yrs) (Nasreddine et al., 2012).

Both Turkey and Lebanon are located within the 'Fertile Crescent', where agriculture was first developed more than 10,000 years ago. Despite being exposed to agriculture for so long, many endemic plant species can still be found in the area – plenty of which are edible. Unfortunately, increasing urbanization, habitat loss, and overexploitation threaten the unique growing grounds of many of these species, with the disappearance of unique ecological systems all over these countries (Sekercioglu, et al., 2011; MoE/UNEP/GEF, 2016).

The traditional food production systems are also threatened by the loss of biodiversity, which is further emphasized by people moving from small-scale farming to commercial agriculture or abandoning their land for a life in the cities. On top of that, though ethno-botanic knowledge and use of wild edible species is still widespread, it is generally the older generations who hold this knowledge. Transition to the younger generation rarely happens and thus traditional knowledge erodes with time (Batal et al., 2012; Tan et al., 2017). Therefore, the continued conservation and use of wild edible species in traditional food systems in both Lebanon and Turkey relies on renewed interest and knowledge of their consumption as being practised in the following projects in these countries.

BOX C13.1: THE POTENTIAL OF WILD EDIBLE SPECIES

Since ancient times, wild edible plants have been essential to diets all over the world. Today, tribal people and small holder farmers are still dependent on wild edible plants (Heywood, 1999) while in the Western world a renewed interest in wild plants for modern haute cuisine is appearing (Łuczaj et al., 2012). Wild edible plants are known to be high in nutrients and can thus improve the quality and diversity of diets. Evidence from the BFN Project in Turkey shows that wild species and landraces can contribute considerably to requirements of dietary fibre, vitamin C and some minerals such as iron, potassium and phosphorus (Güzelsoy et al., 2017).[2] Research from Lebanon also suggests that dishes with wild edible species generally offer a healthier alternative to popular Western equivalents (Batal and Hunter, 2007).

Despite all the benefits and renewed interest in some countries, the overall use of wild edibles is in decline. It could be tempting to think that this has something to do with the abundance of easily accessible food that people are exposed to today, which is probably also true. However, the use is decreasing even in areas of food shortages as external impacts such as climate change, soil degradation, pollution and land use transformation are pushing people away from their traditional food systems (FAO, 2017). Nevertheless, wild edible species have great potential to provide income and improve nutrition, in particular for households that are unable to buy expensive food from the market and at the same time, are unable to grow enough food to feed their families (Batal et al., 2012).

The projects

The collection of wild edible species offers a cheap solution to boosting school meals with a variety of nutrients. In Lebanon, as part of a larger project funded by the International Development and Research Centre (IDRC) Ecohealth Program, two school feeding programmes were set up in 2010 involving a local women's cooperative – Healthy Kitchen – and two elementary schools in the arid region of Arsaal. Over a 6-month period, 135 children aged between 6 and 9 years were provided with a mid-morning snack that met 25% of their daily energy, protein and micro-nutrient requirements and reduced their intake of processed foods. The snacks were made based on traditional recipes optimized to contain wild edibles with high nutrient levels. School-feeding was complemented by a nutrition education module offered to participating students, families and teachers to encourage the consumption of wild edibles and locally grown foods, to renew interest in the local food culture and raise awareness of food as an ecosystem service, resulting in the improved management of key (and in some cases threatened) natural resources. The project was carried out in partnership with the Nature Conservation Center of the American University of Beirut, the University of Ottawa and the University of Montreal in Canada.

While the project in Lebanon targeted primary schoolchildren for increasing the consumption of wild edible species, the project in Turkey encourages young chefs to forage and integrate wild species into their cooking.

In 2017, the Aegean Team of the Biodiversity for Food and Nutrition (BFN) project in Turkey partnered with the Halim Foçali Anatolian Vocational and Technical College (Halim Foçali VTAH) to deliver a 3-day training to 16 student chefs. Through a series of lectures and handout materials, students learned about wild edible plant diversity, the variety of aromatic and medicinal plants existing in Turkey, their various uses, sustainable harvest techniques and production, the nutritional value of vegetables and wild edible plants and their importance in food-based approaches to tackle malnutrition (Figure C13.1).

Lectures were reinforced by practical activities and nature walks led by the BFN Team, schoolteachers, local foragers and research staff from the Foça District National Education Directorate. During the nature walks, students were trained to identify the species, collect and photograph the plants to start a school herbarium and use the plants in cooking demonstrations and practical sessions led by school staff for the preparation of traditional salads, roast dishes, pancakes, and omelettes.

During the Foça Science Education Festival, the students involved in the project set up an exhibition stand to deliver their new-found knowledge to teachers, students and parents visiting the event (Figure C13.2). The stand was called 'Training on the international Biodiversity for Food and Nutrition (BFN) Project: Students in Nature and in the Kitchen'. Posters and other information material on the species, including recipes for their preparation, were distributed to visitors.

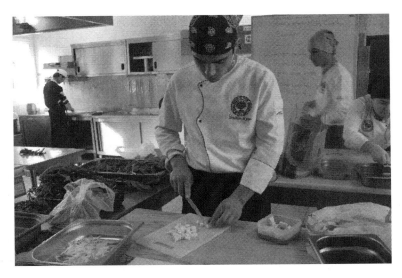

FIGURE C13.1 Student chefs cooking with wild edible plants.
Source: BFN Turkey.

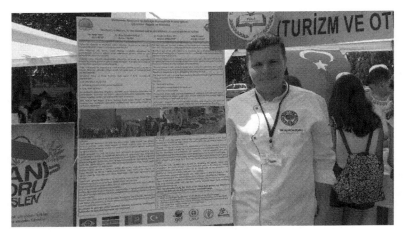

FIGURE C13.2 Student presenting a poster about wild edible plants at the Foça Science Education Festival.
Source: BFN Turkey.

Future plans at Halim Foçali VTAH include the establishment of an herb garden on school premises where wild edibles will be grown to be used in the kitchen during cooking classes.

BOX C13.2: WILD EDIBLES TO ENHANCE AGROBIODIVERSITY IN LEBANON

Wild edibles plants are the mainstay of traditional Lebanese cuisine, which is based on fresh and local ingredients. Fool's watercress (*Apium nodiflorum*), wild thyme (*Origanum syriacum*), mallow (*Malva sylvestris*), green purslane (*Portulaca oleracea*), salsify (*Tragopogon buthalmoides*), *Eryngium creticum*, tumbleweed (*Gundelia tournefortii*) and fennel (*Foeniculum vulgare*) are just some of the wild edibles commonly used in Lebanese cuisine. Rarely sold in conventional vegetable markets, these plants are informally collected by local communities (mostly women) from their wild habitats and generally perceived as improving dietary diversity and diet quality.

BOX C13.3: WILD EDIBLE SPECIES IN TURKEY

Turkey is home to three of the world's 34 identified global biodiversity hotspots, containing almost 12,000 known species and sub-species of seed plants, of which 34% are endemic and around 10% identified as edible (Guner et al., 2012; Ertug, 2014).

Wild edibles plants are equally important in traditional Turkish cuisine. Golden thistle (*Scolymus hispanicus*), Chicory (*Cichorium intybus*), Foxtail lily (*Eremurus spectabilis*), Wild Radish (*Raphanus raphanistrum*), Crown Daisy (*Glebionis coronaria*), Curly dock (*Rumex crispus*), Rush skeletonweed (*Chondrilla juncea*) and Eastern borage (*Trachystemon orientalis*) among many others are often weedy plants that are found growing on roadsides, in wastelands and natural habitats. Rich in macro- and micro-nutrients, they are collected from the wild by local residents and eaten raw, cooked, dried and pickled but also used for their medicinal and health properties. In the Aegean region they are still widely consumed in households as an inexpensive alternative to cultivated vegetables and continue to be served in traditional restaurants.

Impact of integration of wild edible species into schools and educational programmes

In Lebanon

- A significant decrease in anaemia prevalence among schoolchildren ($p<0.0001$) was recorded. In addition, eating habits improved at both schools with a significant decrease in number of children not consuming breakfast ($p<0.001$).

- Participating children demonstrated improved attitudes towards traditional diets and healthy lifestyle practices.
- The women's cooperative which produced the school food is generating income by using and promoting wild edibles (the cost of the snack was 0.40 USD per student per day).

In Turkey:

- Neighbouring schools took part in the Science Festival learning from their peers at Halim Foçali VTAH about the importance of wild edibles, their nutritional value and their importance in healthy diets.
- Within Halim Foçali VTAH, student chefs will start using wild edibles in their cooking classes, while BFN project staff will continue providing support in teaching students about traditional food plants.
- Encouraging awareness and motivation among youth to adopt environmentally friendly behaviour can ensure both long-term environmental protection and economic benefits, giving them a competitive advantage and employability.

Scaling up

As a result of the project in Lebanon, Healthy Kitchen cooperatives were set up in 3 villages and training provided to 25 women in the collection, processing and marketing of wild edibles. Women were also involved in documenting traditional recipes using these plants which have been collected in a food-safety manual in Arabic and the Healthy Kitchen cookbook containing over 40 local recipes, traditional knowledge and scientific information on the nutritional and health properties of 15 wild edible plants (Figure C13.3). Recipes are also being promoted in catering events, village cooking festivals and trade shows which have captured media attention and increased the visibility of traditional foods. The network has played a key role in promoting wild plants and ecosystem protection.

In Turkey the activities undertaken as part of this project have fostered interest from the National Education and Development Directorate of Foça to extend the programme to other schools and officially include traditional wild plants as part of the school curriculum. Furthermore, it has been assessed that the activities undertaken as part of this project can easily be integrated into:

- Technical and Vocational Education and Training (TVET) programmes in Turkey
- The Higher Education Strategy 2007–2025 (School curriculum)
- Action Plan for Strengthening the Link between Education and Employment (IMEIGEP).

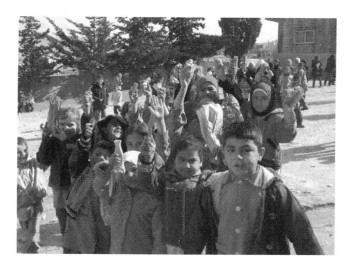

FIGURE C13.3 Children enjoying hummus sandwiches and fresh carrots prepared by community women.
Source: Rheam Abou-Ezze.

BOX C13.4: TESTIMONIALS FROM THE TURKISH BENEFICIARIES

- 'The students who took part in this course put learning into practice when foraging for wild herbs…. We want our students to be involved in activities where they can also learn examples of different biodiversity outside their regions'. – *Coşkun Coşkuner, Halim Foçali FVTAH Food and Beverage Services Field supervisor*
- 'Our horizons have broadened as a result of this project. We have seen the plants and herbs we studied in their natural environment, collected them with our own hands and turned them into a meal. I believe the project will have lasting effects on our professional life'. – *Ahmet Sezer Şanlioğlu, Halim Foçali FVTAH student*
- 'The course taught us that herbs are not just food but that they are also good for health'… 'We have learned to appreciate new tastes, new species, new ideas and new cultures. Furthermore, knowing which natural foods to pick can be very useful in times of need'. – *Sarp Doruk Erdem – Halim Foçali FVTAH student*

Further information

Batal, M., Ghattas, H. and Abou-Ezze, R. (2013) 'A school feeding program based on the Eco-Health approach: A case study from rural Lebanon'. *FASEB Journal* Vol. 27, No. 1
Country page for Turkey on BFN website: http://www.b4fn.org/countries/turkey/

Tan, A., Adanacioğlu, N., Karabak, S., Aykas, L., Tas, N. and Taylan, T. (2017) 'Biodiversity for Food and Nutrition: Edible Wild Plant Species of Aegean Region of Turkey'. *ANADOLU, J. of AARI ISSN:* 1300 – 0225, 27 (2) 2017, 1–8

Notes

1   This case study is based on already published studies on the BFN website. Find them here: www.b4fn.org/case-studies/case-studies/students-in-nature-in-the-garden-and-in-the-kitchen/, www.b4fn.org/case-studies/case-studies/improving-diets-with-wild-edibles-in-rural-lebanese-schools/.
2   Evidence is shared in different platforms including the B4FN Species database: http://www.b4fn.org/resources/species-database/, TürKomp (Turkish Food Composition Database): http://www.turkomp.gov.tr/main, and FAO/INFOODS Food Composition Database for Biodiversity – Version 4.0 (BioFoodComp4.0: http://www.fao.org/3/a-i7364e.pdf.

References

Batal, M. and Hunter, E. (2007) 'Traditional Lebanese recipes based on wild plants: an answer to diet simplification?', *Food and Nutrition Bulletin* 28 (2 Suppl): S303–S311.

Batal, M., Al-Hakimi, A. and Pelat, F. (2012) 'Chapter 6 Dietary diversity in Lebanon and Yemen: a tale of two countries'. In D.F. Charron (ed.), 'Ecohealth Research in Practice: Innovative Applications 69 of an Ecosystem Approach to Health', *Insight and Innovation in International Development 1*, DOI 10.1007/978-1-4614-0517-7_6, International Development Research Centre, 2012.

Dogan, Y. 2012. 'Traditionally used wild edible greens in the Aegean region of Turkey'. *Acta Societatis Botanicorum Poloniae* 81, 4.

Erem, C. (2015) 'Prevalence of overweight and obesity in Turkey'. *IJC Metabolic & Endocrine* 8, 38–41.

Ertug, F. (2014) 'Yenen Bitkiler' (Edible Plants). In: Güner, A and Ekim, T. (Eds.) 'Resimli Türkiye Florası' (İllustrated Flora of Turkey). Vol. 1. Ali Nihat Gökyiğit Vakfı, Flora Araştırmaları Derneği and Türkiye İş bankası Kültür Yayınları, İstanbul.

FAO (2017) 'The future of food and agriculture – Trends and challenges'. Rome, Italy.

Güzelsoy, N.A., Ucurum, Ö., Tokat, E., Tan, A., Tuğrul Ay, S. and Özbek, K. (2017) 'Nutritional properties of some wild edible species in Turkey'. *ANADOLU, Journal of AARI* ISSN: 1300–0225, 27 (2), 39–45.

Güner, A. et al. (edlr.) (2012) 'Türkiye Bitkileri Listesi (Damarlı Bitkiler)' (List of Turkish Plants (vascular plant)). Nezahat Gökyiğit Botanik Bahçesi ve Flora Araştırmaları Derneği Yayını. İstanbul.

Heywood, V. (1999) 'Use and potential of wild plants in farm households'. *FAO Farm systems management series* 15, Rome, Italy.

Łuczaj, L., Pieroni, A., Tardío, J., Pardo-de-Santayana, M., Sõukand, R., Svanberg, I. and Kalle, R. (2012) 'Wild food plant use in 21st century Europe: the disappearance of old traditions and the search for new cuisines involving wild edibles', *Acta Societatis Botanicorum Poloniae,* 81 (4).

Nasreddine, L., Naja, F., Chamieh, M.C., Adra, N., Sibai, A.M. and Hwalla, N. (2012) 'Trends in overweight and obesity in Lebanon: evidence from two national cross-sectional surveys (1997 and 2009)'. *BMC Public Health* 12, 798.

MoE/UNEP/GEF (2016). 'Lebanon's National Biodiversity Strategy and Action Plan' – NBSAP. Ministry of Environment, Lebanon.

Sekercioglu, C. H., Anderson, S. S., Akcay, E. Bilgin, R., Emre Can, O., Semiz, G., Tavsanoglu, C., Yokeş, M.B., Soyumert, A., Ipekdal, K., Sağlam, I.K., Yucel, M. and Dalfes, H.N. (2011) 'Turkey's globally important biodiversity in crisis', *Biological Conservation* 144, 2752–2769.

Tan, A., Adanacioğlu, N., Karabak, S., Aykas, L., Tas, N. and Taylan, T. (2017) 'Biodiversity for Food and Nutrition: Edible Wild Plant Species of Aegean Region of Turkey', *ANADOLU, Journal of AARI* ISSN: 1300–0225, 27 (2), 1–8.

CASE STUDY 14

SLOW FOOD 10,000 GARDENS – CULTIVATING THE FUTURE OF AFRICA

Reguli Damas Marandu, John Kariuki Mwangi, Samson Kiiru Ngugi, and Edward Mukiibi

In 2011, Slow Food launched the 1,000 Gardens in Africa project. The original objective was to create a thousand good, clean, and fair food gardens in schools, villages and urban areas to ensure that communities had access to high-quality, healthy and sustainable food. This included promoting a positive perspective on food, agriculture and the environment to young people, raising awareness of the threats to their food sovereignty and empowering them to reject the corporate takeover of the African food system. Thanks to the hard work of the Slow Food network worldwide, this objective was achieved in 2013 and was then scaled up with a new target of 10,000 gardens.

The project

The 10,000 gardens project in Africa, promoted by the *Slow Food Foundation for Biodiversity*, supports the establishment of either community gardens or school gardens, designed, created, and run by the local communities. Slow Food Foundation for Biodiversity is the operational body for the protection of food biodiversity within Slow Food. The organization is active in over 100 countries, involving thousands of small-scale producers in its projects, providing technical assistance, training, facilitating producer exchanges and advocating for a sustainable food production system. With the gardens, Slow Food is promoting an idea of agriculture based on knowledge of the landscape and respect for biodiversity and local cultures. The belief is that sustainable agriculture has the potential to meet the nutritional requirements of African communities without distorting social relations and destroying the environment, while also giving value to cultural heritage and traditional knowledge.

The primary purpose of a school garden is its educational function. The students gain hands-on experience in sustainable gardening and environment and learn about different crops and their adaptability to different climatic conditions. The garden is used to teach children and youth about local foods and recipes for vegetables and fruits. The school garden serves as an open-air classroom which gives children the tools for improving the quality of life of their families. Many parents replicate at home what their children have learned in the school garden. Additionally, thanks to its interdisciplinary value, many subjects can be studied in the school garden such as: history, through the spread of gastronomic traditions and crops; geography, through the origin of products; mathematics and geometry, indispensable to planning the garden and calculating the expected value of its produce.

The vegetables grown in the school gardens are also used for school meals, but the gardens are usually not big enough to provide a regular supply. Instead they provide vegetables to accompany rice or millet for a few weeks or served at festive events. The harvest from school gardens can also sometimes be sold at the local market and the income used, for example, to buy school materials or equipment for the garden thus contributing to the project's sustainability (Figure C14.1).

Each garden has its own coordinator, helping to organize and plan the garden, and each country has its own project coordinators, responsible for national and regional organization. The coordinators are usually agronomists, local agricultural experts or young people who have returned to their home country after education from the University of Gastronomic Sciences in Italy or other schools and universities. The main office is located in Italy at the Slow Food International headquarters, working closely together with the African country

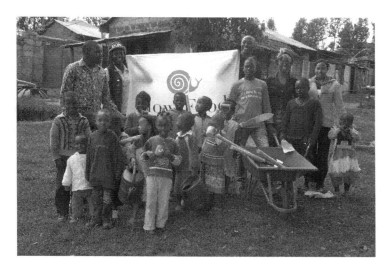

FIGURE C14.1 Molo Street Children Community Garden in Nakuru county, Kenya. Credit: Slow Food International Archive.

The benefit of agricultural biodiversity

Agroecology is essential in Slow Food's African gardens project and is the key to ensuring access to nutrient-rich diets, preserving biodiversity and natural resources, adapting to climate change, respecting traditional knowledge and local cultures and re-establishing the central role of agriculture and farmers in African food systems.

The gardens always contain a vast diversity of different species for various purposes: vegetables, legumes, tubers and fruit trees for eating, medicinal herbs, dye-producing plants, ornamental plants, soil-restoring plants, plants that help repel parasites and trees for wood production. The idea is to create gardens with the use of sustainable management practices that accommodate livelihoods and are useful on as many aspects as possible. Cultivating many different crops and other plant products adds to the conservation of biodiversity while guaranteeing a nutritionally varied and healthy diet. Thereby the gardens contribute to food security and sovereignty while constructing a more resilient agroecological system. Agricultural activities are also well integrated with animal husbandry. The vegetable scraps are used to feed the animals, while manure is used to fertilize the soil.

In the school gardens, and the Slow Food gardens in general, traditional varieties of the plant species are chosen and local plant varieties are often more resilient to pest and diseases and require fewer inputs. As such, using traditional varieties is both more environmental and economically sustainable.

The exchange between traditional and innovative knowledge

According to Slow Food, traditional knowledge is an important source of wisdom and the basis of technical and scientific knowledge. This knowledge can contribute to the spread of ecological methods both of production and of food consumption. Knowledge from the elder generation must therefore be preserved but in a dynamic exchange between generations, between communities or countries and between different disciplines. Especially the dialogue between traditional and new knowledge holders is fundamental for conserving traditional knowledge. This is accommodated by the involvement of youth in the garden communities, happening in Slow Food gardens in general but especially through the school gardens. Teaching children about the importance of biodiversity and encouraging them to be proud of cultivating foods is an important component to create awareness about the value of their land and their culture and to ensure a renewed exchange between traditional and innovative knowledge (Figure C14.2).

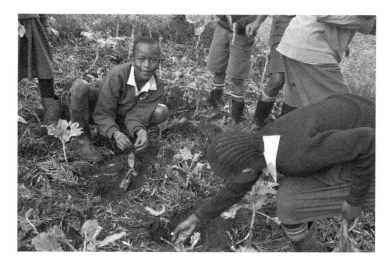

FIGURE C14.2 Planting seedlings in the Kibubuti Primary School Garden in Kiambu county, Kenya. Credit: Slow Food International Archive.

What characterizes a slow food garden?

A Slow Food garden supports and regenerates itself. It needs few external resources to get started. The critical factor for its launch and success is the community's eagerness and willingness to participate. After a year or two, the garden become autonomous and start generating resources such as producing seeds and compost, which can be used to create other gardens.

As already mentioned, a Slow Food garden is based on local, traditional seeds which can be sourced locally by talking to the community, particularly the women. During the first year, seeds will be obtained from local sources, then from the second year on, seeds has to be selected from the previous harvest. To accommodate this a seedbed or nursery is created where the plants can be germinated. Soil management is integrated in the gardens, but only natural methods are used to solve problems of nutrient loss, erosion and salinization. These include crop rotation, compost, green manuring and mulching. Such types of management maintain the soils health and biodiversity in terms of bacteria, insects and other organisms. Rainwater is collected, used for a variety of different irrigation systems that help the plants survive the dry periods and extended droughts.

Impact

- 1,623 school gardens in 35 countries have been established until now (July 2019) involving around 305,000 students, parents and teachers;
- School gardens change children's negative perception of farming as a profession. Some children, after their experience with the garden, go on to proudly pursue a career in farming;

- Students in the school gardens are encouraged to go home and teach their parents how to apply the garden techniques that they have learned in school, spreading knowledge on sustainable cultivation technics more broadly to the community;
- Students gain knowledge on local agrobiodiversity and on how to safeguard it, thus contributing to raising awareness on the importance of preserving the local ecosystem;
- School gardens produce a variety of vegetables used in school meals to supplement already existing lunches (Figure C14.3);
- In some places, gardens have been reported to increase the variety of local crops for food security. For example, in Uganda the amount of local edible vegetable species out of total crops cultivated in community gardens increased from 53% to 78% in three years between 2015 and 2018.

> The agroecological food gardens that Slow Food has created in 35 African countries are now a small but significant contribution to addressing the problem of malnutrition, a positive model of community participation and organisation coming from the grassroots level. Above all, it is an easily replicable model: with our own strengths - relatively few compared to those of institutions and governments - we have managed to create over 3,000 gardens. Each of these gardens contributes in many cases to preventing individuals from adding to the already dramatic figures on malnutrition that today the UN has given us.
> —*Edward Mukiibi, Slow Food International Vice President.*

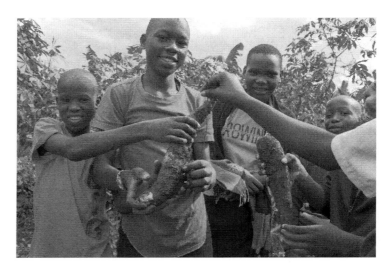

FIGURE C14.3 Schoolchildren with yams in the Nkosi Memorial School Garden in Mukono district, Uganda. Credit: Aimie Eliots.

Scaling up

Since 2011, the 'Thousand Gardens in Africa' project has involved over 340,000 people in 35 African countries, as well as tens of thousands of members and activists around the world. After the original target for the project (1,000 gardens) was reached at the end of 2013, Slow Food decided to relaunch the initiative in 2014 with the new aim to create 10,000 gardens across the continent. For now, (July 2019) 3,215 gardens have been established of which more than a half (1,623) is school gardens.

Creating school gardens in African schools means teaching young people about the importance of food biodiversity and about access to fresh and healthy food. It also creates a network of young people who are aware of the value of their own land and culture. This network can give rise to agents of change across all continents: a change based on the liberation of traditional foods and knowledge, in a social economy linked to the land and environment.

Lessons learned

Slow Food has established gardens in 35 different African countries. The situation in terms of climate, terrain, ecology, traditions and culture is highly diverse between and even within the countries. Therefore, each garden must be based on observations of the contextual situation and carefully planned with each community in accordance to the local conditions deciding what to cultivate, how and when.

The community should be included as much as possible in the school gardens such as the teachers, the principal, the parents and the villages near the school. Only by involving all of these people is it possible to manage the garden even during holidays, to source seeds and manure for fertilizing. The more people that supervise the garden, the greater chance there is for success and strong community ownership around a garden.

In 2016, a study was launched with the University of Turin to evaluate the environmental, social and economic sustainability of the project. A questionnaire was compiled with 58 questions on various aspects connected to the garden: the type of products grown, how they are processed, the number of people involved, the type of work done with the groups and so on. This tool was used to analyze 83 gardens in seven countries (Kenya, Rwanda, Tanzania, Burkina Faso, Uganda, Ghana, Madagascar). According to the study's results, 'The Slow Food Gardens in Africa project can fully be included in the dynamics of socio-ecological innovation [...] The involvement of various subjects in the creation and management of the gardens allows the development and/or strengthening of social networks in various countries and makes it possible to tackle issues like food security and nutrition, but most of all themes around so-called "hidden hunger," caused by the lack of micronutrients, typical of poor-quality food and/or poor differentiation of the food being consumed'.

Read more

- The Slow Food Foundation website: https://www.fondazioneslowfood.com/en/
- Slow Food for Africa – 10,000 gardens to cultivate the future: www.fondazioneslowfood.com/en/categorie-pubblicazioni/handbook-en/
- 10,000 Gardens in Africa – Handbook: www.fondazioneslowfood.com/en/categorie-pubblicazioni/vademecum-en/
- 'Annual report 2017'. The Slow Food Foundation https://www.slowfood.com/wp-content/uploads/2018/09/ENG_annual_report_2017_b-1.pdf

CASE STUDY 15

THE INTEGRATION OF FOOD BIODIVERSITY IN SCHOOL CURRICULA THROUGH SCHOOL GARDENS AND GASTRONOMY IN BRAZIL

Ana Rosa Domingues dos Santos, Nádia Lúcia Almeida Nunes, Alessandra Santos dos Santos, Camila Neves Soares Oliveira, Lidio Coradin, Daniela Moura de Oliveira Beltrame, and Neio Lúcio de Oliveira Campos

Introduction

Brazil is a country of superlatives in almost every way. Being the largest tropical country, it occupies roughly half of the South American continent. One of its main features is its distinct biodiversity, consisting of 15–20% of the Earth's total number of species, with various biogeographic zones or biomes: the Amazon Rainforest, the world's largest rainforest; the Pantanal, the largest floodplain; the Cerrado of savannah; the Caatinga of semi-arid forests; the fields of the Pampas; and the rain forest of the Atlantic Forest. Brazil is considered the most megadiverse country on earth, being almost always at the top of the global list for every group of organisms (Mittermeier et al., 1997).

In addition, it figures among the world's largest in area, population, gross domestic product and many other indices. Brazil has also the second-largest national school feeding program in the world, the *Programa Nacional de Alimentação Escolar* – PNAE (National School Feeding Program), providing daily meals to more than 43 million students (Drake et al., 2016). Implemented since 1955, PNAE is the largest and the oldest social policy in food and nutrition in Brazil and one of the few continuous policies that has endured throughout different governments. This programme reaches different audiences and realities, from nursery and pre-schools to high schools and young and adult education, from both urban and rural areas, including those in land reform settlements, and indigenous and 'quilombola' (slave-descendant) communities, across all the 5,570 municipalities of Brazil.

PNAE is coordinated by the National Fund for the Development of Education (*Fundo Nacional para o Desenvolvimento da Educação* – FNDE), linked to Brazil's Ministry of Education, based on the following guiding principles: food and nutritional education, social development and community participation, human right to adequate food, local food purchases, and respect for regional food habits and traditions.[1] As a part of the actions to fulfil its educational framework and pedagogical objective, FNDE established a partnership with the Centre for Excellence in Tourism of the University of Brasília (CET-UnB), resulting in the 'Educating with School Gardens and Gastronomy' project (in Portuguese: *Projeto Educando com a Horta Escolar e a Gastronomia* – PEHEG), which was partially based on a previous FAO/FNDE project called 'Educating with School Gardens' (*Projeto Educando com a Horta Escolar*, in Portuguese).

The essence of both projects was the continued education of stakeholders (for instance, school feeding coordinators, nutritionists, pedagogical coordinators, specialists on environment and school gardens, and representatives of the local school feeding councils) in all the core areas: pedagogy and education, environment and school gardens, nutrition, and, in the case of PEHEG, gastronomy. The participants were expected to act as multipliers, passing on the acquired knowledge for other public agents and stakeholders at local levels. These projects promoted the use of school gardens (and gastronomy, in PEHEG) as tools for pedagogical practices and to develop actions on healthy and sustainable habits towards the environment, diets, local food cultures and heritage.

'Educating with School Gardens and Gastronomy' (PEHEG) – an overview

The 'Educating with School Gardens and Gastronomy' project (PEHEG) sought to empower stakeholders to promote healthy eating and stimulate the appreciation of regional foods and cuisines, and sustainable food production processes, among students and the surrounding school community. School gardens and gastronomy worked as entry points for a dynamic and transdisciplinary pedagogical practice, which paved the way for Food and Nutrition education, as well as environmental education, recognition of cultural heritage and local products, in addition to the greater involvement of the community in school activities.

PEHEG's continued education strategy was implemented through in-class courses and online learning, with the support of materials made available on the online platform (Moodle) and as printouts. The course design and materials were developed by an interdisciplinary team of professionals from the University of Brasília, including all the core areas of the project: education, environment, nutrition, and gastronomy. PEHEG was implemented from 2011 to 2016, during three successful editions, totalling 541 municipalities and state participants.

To take part in this experience, each municipality or states needed only to formally indicate their interest and establish and empower a coordinating group (future multipliers), assuring the necessary means and ways to incorporate the indicated activities in the plans and programs of the local Education Secretary.

The team of multipliers (Local Coordination Unit) needed to be composed of at least one specialist in education, a nutritionist, and an environment professional, generating cooperation in a transdisciplinary atmosphere. Other professionals could be part of the team, such as municipal school feeding or pedagogical coordinators, project managers, teachers, and psychologists, public agents from health, agriculture, and/or environment departments, social workers and advisers from the school feeding council.

These local units were responsible for the implementation of the project in their municipality or state, which included the development of a customized workplan; allocation of necessary resources; selection of schools; engagement of policy makers and decision makers (governor or mayor, municipal or state secretaries, school directors, etc.); and, along with the principle of network learning and as part of their roles as multipliers, the mobilization and training of the various social actors in the school communities.

The Local Coordination Units were also responsible for monitoring and evaluation of the implementation and maintenance of school gardens and gastronomy activities, besides the dissemination of the results and experiences. Creative ideas were encouraged to advertise the Project, such as invitations to authorities and press members for key moments like the launch of the local project, the first planting, harvests, and other celebrations. The integration of the Project's activities with municipal events, like competitions, commemorative dates and civic parades also turned out to be a helpful strategy. The importance of keeping records of the actions and outputs through portfolios and reports was also emphasized, along with the organization of local seminars in which progress and results were presented.

Each local unit customized the implementation of the Project according to their local realities, including a lot of opportunities and flexibility to generate creativity. In most instances, schools implemented both the school garden and activities related to gastronomy, however, some schools implemented only gastronomy activities, due to inadequate conditions to build a school garden, such as the lack of space and materials or due to environmental constraints such as locations in permanent flooded or polluted areas.

Some school 'gardens' might only consist of a couple of edible species, or a school tree nursery, a permaculture mandala vegetable garden, a mixed chicken-vegetable garden, or a worm farm (or a combination of some of those). One of the key aspects of PEHEG was its open methodology and flexibility to accommodate to local realities. In this sense, the 'school garden' could be even small animals or fish farms, since the objective of the vegetable gardens is not only the harvesting in itself but the cultivation of living beings and respect to local reality. These aspects provided several opportunities for debates and reflections on contents of the school curriculum, including principles, responsibilities and commitment to nature, to the school environment, to the community life, to the sustainability of the planet and to the appreciation and valuing of native and traditional species.

There were also situations in which the pedagogical gardens were not located inside the school and turned out being a community vegetable garden, which boosted even further the results. Despite the different forms of implementation, the Project's goals were always present, promoting social development capable of transforming the natural and constructed environment while strengthening cultural heritage and valuing regional cuisines, as well as creating a collective sense of responsibility and belonging, fostering human well-being and a balanced environment.

Pathways for integrating Brazilian food biodiversity in school gardens

As explained above, the main goal of the school gardens was to enable debates and generate dynamic ways of learning and creating behavioural changes towards a healthier way of life. The planning, maintenance and harvesting of the production of the school gardens were rich tools for learning the programmatic contents for each level and different classes (Figure C15.1).

The schools were encouraged to make impactful interventions in favour of the environment, such as selective waste collection, which also enabled the students to reflect on their history, environment and everyday life. To set the baseline, one important activity conducted by PEHEG was to understand the history and social characteristics of the community in which the school was inserted, its topography and climate, endemic and regional species, and many other aspects that generated data used to create innovations and to help with the planning of several activities of the Project.

The multipliers were trained on techniques that enabled the implementation of the school gardens, including basic notions of agriculture for structuring and maintaining the gardens, and to plan the production. Other important contents of the trainings were selective waste collection to produce organic fertilizers;

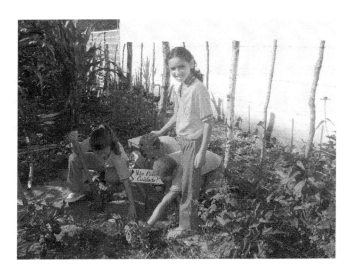

FIGURE C15.1 Students working at the vegetable garden.
Source: Municipality of Zabelê, Paraíba.

production of seedlings of vegetables and medicinal plants; rational use of water for irrigation of the gardens; and alternative techniques for planting in school gardens, such as vertical planting using recycled materials like plastic bottles, milk packages, and plastic containers.

One relevant impact was the promotion of significant debates conducted by the stakeholders on the importance of organic and agroecological production, biodiverse production systems, regional foods and habits, traditional and unconventional vegetables, friends and foes plants, and natural control of pests and diseases.

PEHEG also worked to promote the value and use of Brazilian biodiversity during the in-class and online courses, and also featured in the technical material an entire section with recommendations of the periods for planting and harvesting, ways of propagation, cultivation, spacing, and uses of some regional vegetables (Figure C15.2). A chapter for implementing nurseries of native trees in schools was also included in the material. One important partnership in this process was the Biodiversity for Food and Nutrition Project (BFN), implemented by the Ministry of the Environment, who conducted a specific training module for the University of Brasília's coordination team, about the importance of biodiversity for food and nutrition and how this recognition promotes biodiversity conservation and use.

The vegetable gardens were rich pedagogical tools used in different kinds of classes, not only in biology and geography, as initially expected, but also in arts, math, and languages. Creative ideas were developed and generated activities such as the design of posters and signs to raise awareness of the community about environmental issues, mathematics involving the calculation of the perimeters and areas, poetry writing, and even learning the names of certain foods in a second language and tagging the species in the garden with multi-lingual signs.

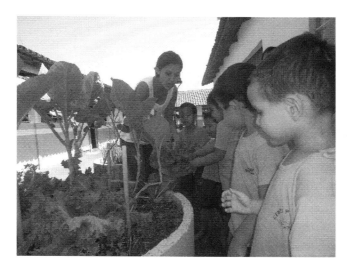

FIGURE C15.2 Example of a tiny space consortium vegetable production.
Source: Municipality of Jaraguá, Goiás.

Pathways for integrating Brazilian food biodiversity in gastronomy activities and in school feeding

The gastronomy area focussed on two core aspects: one oriented to cultural and regional food habits and the other related to the techniques and sensorial features of food.

To address the cultural and regional habits, activities were developed to generate appreciation of regional ingredients, products and recipes, and the recognition and respect of the seasonality of the foods, traditional preparation methods and techniques, taking into consideration the environmental aspects and valuing of local production and family farmers. In addition, attention was given to practical and symbolic aspects of food, including reflection on what is eaten, how it is eaten, how the food is cultivated, prepared, and presented, and, above all, the reasons for each one of these stages. Such an approach was important for the recognition of aspects related to heritage, but also for the comprehension that both malnutrition and obesity can only be understood as effects of a set of practices which emerge from a broader socio-cultural system; and that the choices of some foods over others in different groups reflect food classification systems that are based on socioeconomic and cultural values (Brasil. Ministério da Saúde, 2005).

As for the technical and sensorial aspects of gastronomy, the stakeholders were instructed in the basics of culinary techniques, to use kitchen utensils and equipment to improve the presentation and taste of meals, and to avoid loss and wastage (Figure C15.3). One of the first challenges was to contest the general misconception of gastronomy as the exclusive domain of elites and privileged people, or a chef-made food, or even a habit of other countries.

Just like with the school gardens, the gastronomy activities became rich and innovative tools for learning and generated a more participatory pedagogical practice that made the school curriculum more dynamic. Some schools included assignments

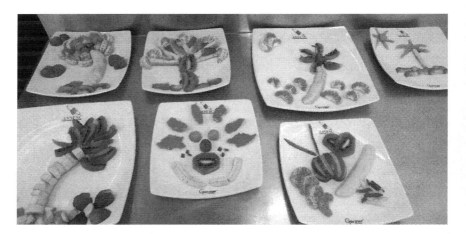

FIGURE C15.3 Food presentation activity.
Source: Municipality of Florianópolis, Santa Catarina.

involving the whole family in which students had to interview older relatives or to participate actively in the choices and purchases of groceries for the whole household. The most recurring activities were cooking workshops and the development of recipe books with traditional recipes and/or local biodiversity products, which were to be used at the school and by families (Figures C15.4 and C15.5). Some remarkable examples included a school musical play focussed on fruits and vegetables, the creation of a sticker album and a school fair of natural spices and jams.

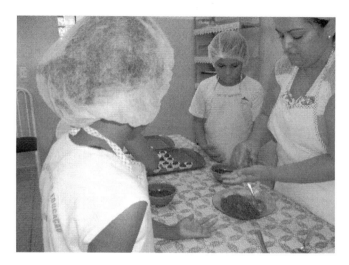

FIGURE C15.4 Traditional recipes cooking workshop.
Source: Municipality of Presidente Prudente, São Paulo.

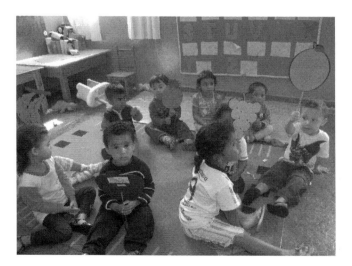

FIGURE C15.5 Toddlers learning about the benefits of fruits.
Source: Municipality of Rio Branco, Acre.

Gastronomy was also used as a pedagogical tool in different classes, from history and sociology, to math and geography. Among the successful examples were research topics on the history and food habits of the family and community, health classes, mathematics using fractions and multiplication for the recipes, debates on food crisis, famine and migration in Brazil and globally, as well as environmental sustainability of current food systems.

Besides the pedagogical aspects mentioned above, the multipliers within PEHEG promoted new possibilities for school feeding practices and to increase acceptance by students, such as:

- the development of new recipes, adaptation of old preparations, and revision of the school menus;
- a boost in the nutritional quality, flavours and appearance of the school meals, with the use of appropriate techniques that favour the sensorial quality and nutritional value of foods;
- the decrease in the use of processed seasoned spices, ready-to-use sauces, fats, sugar, and salt, promoting the use of natural broths and aromatics with appropriate techniques instead;
- the appreciation of the school cooks and recognition of their role as Food and Nutrition educators, along with teachers and other school staff;
- the development of different recipes with the integral use of ingredients that used to be discarded, such as leaves, peels, and seeds, in addition to the greater use of Brazilian food biodiversity ingredients in the school meals.

PEHEG – one step towards mainstreaming Brazilian food biodiversity in schools

Biodiversity is the natural and essential basis for the maintenance and reproduction of livelihoods and culture of social groups, especially traditional peoples and communities. By tasting regional foods, through their own flavours, techniques, and rituals, an immediate interaction with those peoples and places, with their culture and environment, is established.

Despite the wide diversity of plant species in nature, only a very small portion of this variety is used in some way by humans, and this is reflected, for example, in the low diversification of ingredients. This is largely due to the choices countries have made regarding food production. In Brazil, the current agricultural modernization technological package, adopted in the late 1960s, has resulted in a growing reduction in agricultural and food biodiversity. That model, based on the cultivation of high yielding genetic varieties, use of chemical-synthetic inputs, mechanization, and use of non-renewable energy sources, reduces biodiversity, generates environmental imbalances, and significantly alters landscapes and local identities.

On the other hand, local species and crops are the food base for hundreds of millions of people and can be potentially nourishing for countless others. Many of these species are of utmost importance to local communities and exploiting the potential of these species is crucial to achieving food security.

The inclusion of Brazilian food biodiversity in school feeding and school curricula represents a cultural appreciation of local resources and food practices, raising awareness and recognition of traditional knowledges and techniques of cultivation, rational extraction, production, and transformation. In addition, it contributes to the food and nutrition security of the involved communities, as those foods are rich in micro and macronutrients.

The PEHEG contributed to the process of educating, empowering, and engaging the educators and public agents, as well as the members of the school communities about those themes, through the implementation of school gardens and activities related to gastronomy as pedagogical tools for environmental and food and nutrition education. In short, the project helped to create awareness about healthy eating and environmental issues, encouraging the students and communities to promote the necessary transformations to build a more sustainable society.

Note

1 For more information about the PNAE programme, please consult the corresponding chapter at Global School Feeding Sourcebook Lessons from 14 countries (Drake et al., 2016), available at https://documents.wfp.org/stellent/groups/public/documents/communications/wfp284904.pdf.

References

Brasil. Ministério da Saúde (2005) 'Guia alimentar para crianças menores de 2 anos', Ministério da Saúde, Brasília.

Drake, L.J., Woolnough, A., Burbano, C. and Bundy, D. (Eds.) (2016) 'Global school feeding sourcebook: lessons from 14 countries', Imperial College Press, London.

Mittermeier, R.A., Mittermeier, C.G. and Gil, P.R. (1997) 'Megadiversity: Earth's biologically wealthiest nations', CEMEX/Agrupación Sierra Madre, Mexico City.

INDEX

Note: **Bold** page numbers refer to tables; *italic* page numbers refer to figures and page numbers followed by "n" denote endnotes.

Aboriginal culture 200–202; *see also* Australia
Accelerated Hunger-Mitigation Program (Philippines) 142
Action Aid Arab Region 219
Action Plan for Strengthening the Link between Education and Employment (IMEIGEP) 272
Adansonia digitata (baobab fruit) 90, 107
Africa: Slow Food Foundation for Biodiversity project 276–281; 10,000 gardens project 276–281
African leafy vegetables (ALVs) 28, 209, *209*; potential of 210; and school gardens 210–212
Africans for Africa (PAA Africa) programme 40
Afzelia quanzensis 106
aghdmi (*Armeria alliacea*) 189
agricultural and livelihood skills: development of 4–7
agricultural biodiversity 4, 13, 278; Agro-Biodiversity Initiative (TABI) 29, 246, 249–256, 256n1; benefits of 187–189; conservation of local 11–14; curriculum in Laos 249–256; East Khasi Hills District 234, *235*; education in Xiengkhouang Province, Laos 246–256; and Hawaiian culture 173–175; role in Vietnam's school gardens programme 180–181; school garden foods 174; sustainable use of local 11–14

agricultural practices education, and Moroccan High Atlas women 186–187
agrobiodiversity *see* agricultural biodiversity
agro-ecological scaling *see* agroecology
agroecology 233, 238–239, 242, 278; Mexico 238–244; through food-based education 238–244; through garden-based education 238–244
agroforestry 87; role for diversified production, diets and improved health 87–91
'Aina Pono Farm to School Program 175
Amazigh (or Berber) communities 185; medicinal plants 189
Amazon Rainforest 283
Anacardium occidentale 88
Angat Buhay programme 155
Anthropocene 105
AOG World Relief Vietnam 27, 178, 179, 182, 183
Arnhem Land Progress Aboriginal Corporation Aboriginal (ALPA) 203, 205, 206n8
Asian Development Bank 152
Association of Southeast Asian Nations (ASEAN) 24, 48, 50
Atlantic Forest 283
Australia 13–14; agrobiodiversity initiatives 195; Arnhem Land Progress Aboriginal Corporation Aboriginal (ALPA) 203, 205, 206n8; Australian Centre for International Agricultural Research

294 Index

(ACIAR) 209; Close the Gap and National Reconciliation 194; European colonization 196; First Peoples 194–196; Stephanie Alexander Kitchen Garden Foundation (SAKGF) 26, 160–170; traditional food gardens in schools 193–194, *194*
Australian Centre for International Agricultural Research (ACIAR) 209
Azanza garckeana (azanza) 100
azuka (*Tetraclinis articulata*) 189

Balanites aegyptiaca (desert dates) 100
Baraem El Moustaqbal education centre, Bar Elias, Beqaa Valley 216
Basella alba 27
behaviours: change communication 8; promotion of healthy diets by influencing 9–11; promotion of healthy eating habits by influencing 9–11
Benincasa hispida 27
Berchemia discolor (bird cherry) 100
Bhutan: current evidence for school garden programmes 116–117; impact of school garden intervention on nutrition outcomes in **120**
Bidens pilosa 107
Bill & Melinda Gates Foundation 122
biodiversity: agricultural 278; Brazil 283–291; Brazilian food 288–290; conservation, Dar Taliba 187–189; losses in Laos 246, 247; *see also* agricultural biodiversity
Biodiversity for Food and Nutrition (BFN) 28, 40, 209–213, 287; Brazil Ministry of Environment 287; African leafy vegetables (ALVs) 209; in Turkey 268, 269, *270*
bio-intensive garden (BIG), in Philippines 7, 53, 66–68, *67*, 75, 142
botanic gardens 108–109
Brazil 40; biodiversity 283–291; Centre for Excellence in Tourism of the University of Brasília (CET-UnB) 284; moringa trees improving diets in 107–108; moringa trees improving environmental awareness in 107–108; national school feeding program 283; overview 283
Burkina Faso: current evidence for school garden programmes 116–117; impact of school garden intervention on nutrition outcomes in **120**
Busia County, Kenya *212*, 212–213
Buzuruna Juzuruna (NGO in Lebanon) 216, 218, 219

California Thursdays 9
Campaign on Healthy Diet 153
Canadian International Development Agency 20
Canvasback Wellness Centre of Majuro 258
Centre for Ecoliteracy 9
Chiapas (Mexico): agro-ecological scaling 238–244; food-based education 238–244; garden-based education 238–244
children: anaemic, percentage in Meghalaya 232; consumption of vegetables and 136; improvement in nutrition status of undernourished 73–74; knowledge about indigenous food 235–236; and NESFAS programme 235; nutritional gains among undernourished 133; nutrition education for 68–69; stunting 7
Citrus sinensis (orange) 90
Civil Society in Development (CISU) 219
Cleome gynandra 90
climate change: and malnourished children 14; manifestations of 139; school gardens to increase awareness of 14–16; sustainability of gardens and 16
Climate Change Fund 15
Close the Gap and National Reconciliation 194
Collingwood College 160–162
Commission on Genetic Resources for Food and Agriculture (FAO) 91
Committee on Economic, Social and Cultural Rights 35
Committee on the Rights of the Child 35
conservation: of indigenous vegetables 73; of local agrobiodiversity 11–14
copra cake 262, *262*
Cornell University 10, 11
costs, of school-based nutrition interventions 43–44
Council of Agriculture and Rural Development (CARD) 53
crop museums 11, 12, 24, 64; lighthouse schools as 145; role of 148–150; seed exchange 150
crop portfolios, in school gardens 98–99

Dark Emu: Black Seeds: Agriculture or Accident? (Pascoe) 195
Dar Taliba 27, 186; agricultural education for girls 186–187; biodiversity conservation 187–189; ethnobotanical garden 187–188; future 190–191; impact of 190; organic food production 189; self-sufficiency 189; traditional plant knowledge *188*, 188–189

Deakin University 169–170
Department of Agriculture (Philippines) 143, 155
Department of Agriculture Bureau of Plant and Industry (Philippines) 151, 155
Department of Social Welfare and Development (DSWD) 143, 151
Department of Social Welfare and Development Region IV-A (DSWD IV-A) 155
dietary habits problem: in Lebanon 267–268; and obesity 258; Republic of the Marshall Islands (RMI) 258–259; in Turkey 267–268
diets: diversity through garden diversity 135; linking appreciation of trees to better 106–108
Disease Control Priorities 3rd Edition 34
Driver Primary School, and Stephanie Alexander Kitchen Garden Program 165–167
Drivers of Food Choice Competitive Grants Program 122

Ecohealth Program 269
Edible Schoolyards 17; in Leith, Scotland 14–15
'Educating with School Gardens and Gastronomy' project (PEHEG) 284–286, 287; education strategy 284; implementation of 285
education: educational aspects of school gardens 134–135; *Education for all - Global monitoring report* 48; as entry point for leveraging production diversity to consumption diversity 94–100; food-based *see* food-based education; formal nutrition 154; garden-based *see* garden-based education; non-formal nutrition 154; *see also* food and nutrition education (FNE)
EduGrow 193; award themes 204; and healthy food 205–206; 'Healthy Food Enterprise Projects' 204; overview 205; and Remote Indigenous Gardens Network 203; School Garden Awards 202–206, 206n8
Elton B. Stephens Co. (EBSCO) research database 49
Enterprise School Garden Innovation Project (Ghana) 41
environmental disposition 16
Ethiopia 40–41, 100
'ETIOBE Mates' online game 55
Euclea divinorum (magic gwarra) 100

Expanded National Nutrition Survey (ENNS) (Philippines) 156
extension services, in Philippines: for farmers 132; from government units 132

Facebook, and digital communication 58
farm-to-school movement: in Brazil 244; in the United States 244
Federal Bureau of Education, in the United States 3
Feed the Children, Kenya 95
The Field Alliance (TFA) 248
First World War 29
food: for better nutrition and health 86–87; project accomplishments in improving children's access to food in Laguna 133–135
Food and Agriculture Organization of United Nations (FAO) 10, 40, 238; Regional Training of Trainers on Integrating Nutrition in Primary Education Curriculum 52
food and nutrition education (FNE) 34; challenges 57–58; curriculum approach 51–53; customized 99; formal nutrition education 154; health and nutrition problems among schoolchildren 49–50; PEHEG and 284; parental involvement 55–56; school feeding programmes 56–57; school gardening 53–54; in schools 42–43; strategies for integrating in primary school curriculum 48–58; strategies in nutrition education 50–51; technology/web-based approach 54–55; training tools 99
Food and Nutrition Research Institute (FNRI), Philippines 126
Food and Nutrition Research Institute of the Department of Science and Technology (FNRI-DOST) Philippines 64–65, 73, 143, 156
food-based education: agro-ecological scaling through 238–244; Mexico 238–244
FoodCorps Hawai'i 175
FoodCorps movement 3, 10
Food Heritage Foundation, Lebanon 216, 219
Food Plant Solutions 27, 179
food tree: location-specific 98–99; nutritional contributions of 88–91
Food Tree and Crop Portfolios 91; development of 91–94; filling harvest and nutrient 'gaps' through local species 91–94

forest genetic resources 108–111
Fostering Education & Environment for Development (FEED), Philippines 155
4H Ghana 42
FRESH Initiative (Focussing Resources on Effective School Health), Philippines 33
fruit trees: artificial cross-breeding of *112*; school gardens and conservation of genetic resources in central Asia 111

garden-based education: agro-ecological scaling through 238–244; learning from 242–244; Mexico 238–44
garden-based learning 53–54
garden diversity 73; diet diversity and 135; garden functionality and sustainability and 73
Garden to Cafeteria Program, Hawai'i 175
Garo community, Meghalaya (India) 29, 232
gastronomy activities: examples 289, *289*; integrating Brazilian food biodiversity in 288–290
George Putnam School in Massachusetts 3
Ghana 40–42
Global Diversity Foundation 27, 186, 190; Dar Taliba *see* Dar Taliba
Global Environment Facility (GEF) 209
Global Panel Foresight Report (GLOPAN) 39
Google Scholar 49
GPP *see* Gulayan sa Paaralan (Vegetable Gardens in School) Program
Green Peace 153
Green School Program, Nepal 84, 122
Gulayan sa Paaralan (Vegetable Gardens in School) Program (GPP) 62, 126, 142, 152

Halim Foçali Anatolian Vocational and Technical College (Halim Foçali VTAH) 269–270, 272
hauhake 226
Hawai'ian Islands: culture and agrobiodiversity 173–175; food system problem 171–172; Hawai'i Island School Gardening Network (HISGN) 172–173; local food systems in 171–177
Hawai'i Farm to School Bill (Act 218) 175
Hawai'i Farm to School Hui 175, 176
Hawai'i Island School Gardening Network (HISGN) 26, 172–173, *172–173*; Hawai'i School Garden Curriculum Map 172–173; Ku 'Aina Pa teacher training programme 172; scaling up school gardens initiative 175–176; stakeholder and policy maker involvement 176
health: food and agriculture systems for better 86–87; problems among schoolchildren 49–50
healthy diets: described 37; promotion of, by influencing behaviours 9–11; WHO *Healthy Diets Factsheet* on 37
healthy eating habits: promotion of, by influencing behaviours 9–11
Healthy Kitchen 269, 272
Helen Keller International (HKI) 37
Heritage Seed Library 110
High Atlas Morocco: and female illiteracy rates 186; local species conservation 187–188; overview 185–186; and primary school education 186; traditional plant knowledge 188–189
home gardens/gardening: assured supply of nutritious vegetables from 135; benefits from and challenges faced in participating in **137–138**; experience of respondent households **130–131**; extending school gardening to 134; and other reserves of forest genetic resources 108–111; role for enhancing connectivity with 108–111
home-grown school feeding (HGSF) 39–41
horizontal scaling: and ISNM 145; lighthouse schools (LSs) 148
horizontal scaling up 144
human rights: rights of the child 35–37; right to adequate food and right to health 35–37; steps towards healthy school environment and 35–37

indigenous vegetables: chemical-free 66; conservation of 73; recipes with 64; supplementary feeding with 68
innovations: and formal nutrition education 154; and integrated school nutrition model 154; and non-formal nutrition education 154
integrated school nutrition model (ISNM) 8, 66, *66*, 142–143; broad-based partnership for 151–152; and innovations 154; and investment 155–156; and media 154; overview 143; in Philippines 142–156; scaling 144–156; school nutrition 145; and social media 154
International Development and Research Centre (IDRC) 8, 143; Ecohealth Program 269
International Green Academy 21

International Institute of Rural
  Reconstruction (IIRR) 15, 53, 62,
  152–153; research conceptual and
  theoretical framework *146*; scaling up
  framework *144*
International Nutrition Conference
  (ICN2) 91
Iowa State University 10
Ipomoea aquatica 27
iron-fortified rice: supplementary feeding
  with 68

Jaintia community 232
Jikin kallib ilo jikuul (RMI School Learning
  Garden Program) 29, 259, 260–261;
  adaptations 261–264; Curriculum
  Map 263; findings 261–264; impacts
  261–264; overview 259–260; role of
  communication and transportation
  264–265; scaling up 264–265; themes 260

Ka Hikitia 228
Kaupapa Māori 228
Kenya: African leafy vegetables (ALVs) *209*,
  209–212; Amagoro Primary School 211;
  Biodiversity for Food and Nutrition
  (BFN) 209–213; food tree and crop
  portfolios project sites in *93*, *94*; Kenyan
  students and 'planetary health' diet 96;
  Mundika Special Needs School 211;
  overview 208–209; school gardens in
  208–213
Khasi community 232
Kū 'Āina Pā: Standing Firmly in Knowledge
  Upon the Land (KAP) 260
Kohala Center 26
Kohanga Reo 226
Kura Kaupapa children *225*

Laboratorios para la Vida (LabVida) 29, 238;
  certificate programme modules **240**;
  educators in *241*; food- and
  garden-based education 239–242; pilot
  training programme 239–242
La Dieta Mesoamericana: Orígenes 241
La Jornada del Campo on *quelites* 241
Laos: overview 247; reasons for biodiversity
  losses in 246, 247
learning: aptitude, enhancing 16–17; linking
  appreciation of trees to 106–108
Lebanon: dietary habits problems
  267–268; food aid for refugee camps
  219; integration of wild edible
  species into schools and educational
  programmes 271–272; permaculture
  education 216–218; Syrian refugee
  population in 215; wild edible plants to
  enhance agrobiodiversity in 271
lighthouse schools (LSs) 64, 142; as crop
  museums 145; example of *65*; garden
  use as platform for learning and sharing
  nutrition and environment information
  in **74**; horizontal scaling 148; integration
  of garden visitation in learning areas
  of **75**
livelihoods: linking appreciation of trees to
  106–108
local food, growing 197–200; *see also*
  self-sufficiency
local species conservation 187–188
location-specific food tree: in school
  gardens 98–99
low-income countries: current evidence
  for school garden programmes 116–117;
  impact of school gardens on nutrition
  outcomes in 115–123

Machakos and Laikipia Counties, Kenya
  95–100
Malaak 219
malnutrition: and school garden
  programmes 179–180; in Vietnam
  178–179
Mana (Māori society) 28, 227
Manihot esculenta 90
maramataka 226
McGill University 232
media: and integrated school nutrition
  model 154; social media 154, 227, 244
medicinal plants 189; garden *252*,
  252–253
Meghalaya (India): anaemic population
  percentage in 232; children knowledge
  about indigenous food 235–236;
  indigenous communities 232; literacy
  rate 232; overview 231–233; school
  gardens in 231–237
Mexico: agro-ecological scaling 238–244;
  food-based education 238–244; garden-
  based education 238–244
milpa 239–242, **240**
mkhinza (*Dysphania ambrosoides*) 189
Māori 228; *Māra* 222–224
Moringa oleifera see moringa trees
moringa trees: improving diets in Brazil
  107–108; improving environmental
  awareness in Brazil 107–108
Moroccan Biodiversity and Livelihoods
  Association (MBLA) 186
Moroccan High Atlas 185–191

Moville Community College in County Donegal, Ireland 6
māra 222–224; importance of 226–227; plants of 224; *Tahuri Whenua* 223, 225–229; *see also* school gardens
māra kai 222–223
multipurpose trees 15
multi-scalar approach to scaling 145–146, *147*

National Dietary Guidelines for Healthy Nutrition in Kindergartens, Slovenia 38
National Fund for the Development of Education (*Fundo Nacional para o Desenvolvimento da Educação*–FNDE) 283–284
National Greening Program, Philippines 62
National Māori Horticultural Collective (New Zealand) 28, 222
National Nutrition Council of the Department of Health (Philippines) 143, 151–152
National Nutrition Policy and Strategy (Government of Nepal) 77
National School Health and Nutrition Strategy (Government of Nepal) 77
National School Meals Programme (NSMP), Slovenia 38
Native Hawaiian and Other Pacific Island (NHOPI) populations 171
Nature Conservation Center of the American University of Beirut 269
Nepal: current evidence for school garden programmes 116–117; impact of school garden intervention on nutrition outcomes in **120**; Multisector Nutrition Plan 77; Nepal Agricultural Research Council (NARC) 78, 81; pilot in Sindhupalchok district 83; pilots in Dolakha and Ramechhap districts 81–83; school garden components 79–81; school gardening activities in Ramechhap district of *82*; school gardens in 77–85; school selection 78–79; standard cropping calendar used for Nepal school gardens **80**; standard garden design with crop calendar *79*; training and follow-up 81
New Zealand Ministry of Education 228
non-formal nutrition education 154
non-governmental organizations (NGOs) 63, 146, 147, 153, 195; and Syrian refugee population 216–218; *see also* specific NGOs
North Eastern Region of India, and school gardens 231–237

North East Slow Food and Agrobiodiversity Society (NESFAS) 28–29, 231–236; children knowledge about indigenous food 235–236; improving diets with vegetables 235; Indigenous Food System (IFS) Curriculum 234; mid-day meal 235; purpose of 233
nutrition: contributions of tree foods 88–91; food and agriculture systems for better 86–87; gains among undernourished children 133; project accomplishments in improving children's access to 133–135
Nutrition Center of the Philippines (NCP) 55
nutrition education: for children and their parents 68–69; in the Philippines 62–76; and school feeding link 72; strategies in 50–51
Nutrition-Friendly Schools Initiative (NFSI) 37
Nutrition Goes to School (NGTS) programme (UAE) 50
Nutrition Month, in Philippines 52
nutrition-sensitive agriculture 87
Nutrition Sensitive Food Systems 153

Oh My Gulay! (Oh, my vegetable) campaign, Angara 63
1,000 Gardens in Africa project 30, 276
organic food production 189

Pantanal, Brazil 283
Papatūānuku (Māori society) 224
parents: food and nutrition education 55–56; nutrition education for 68–69; parent-teacher associations (PTA) 132
Partnership for Child Development 7
Partnership with the Educating through School Gardens and Gastronomy (PEHEG) initiative, in Brazil 40
People's Garden School Pilot Project, Arkansas, United States 10
permaculture 216–218, *217*; Permaculture Association; movement 7; plant and seed selection 218
Philippines 37; action research methodology 64–65; BIG approach 66–68; conservation of indigenous vegetables 73; Department of Agriculture 143; Department of Social Welfare and Development 143, 152; diversification of school gardens 73; gardens and nutrition and environment information 74–75; improvement in soil quality in school gardens 72–73; improving children's

access to food and nutrition 133–135; integrated school nutrition model 66; integrated school nutrition model in 142–156; mechanisms to enhance integration of components 69–72; National Nutrition Council of the Department of Health 143; nutrition education for children and their parents 68–69; nutrition education in 62–76; nutrition education-school feeding link 72; nutrition status of undernourished children 73–74; overview 62–64; Philippine Association of Nutrition Convention 152; Philippine Coalition of Advocates for Nutrition Security 153; Philippine Institute for Development Studies (PIDS) 127; Philippine Plan of Action for Nutrition (PPAN) 152; profile of families of undernourished students 129–131; project outcomes enhanced by parent engagement in S+HGP 135–139; school feeding in 62–76; school garden-education link 71–72; school gardening in 62–76; school garden-school feeding link 69–71; School Plus Home Gardens Project (S+HGP) 127–129; strategies to engage and sustain parents' participation 131–133; supplementary feeding with iron-fortified rice and indigenous vegetables 68

Philippines Department of Education (DepEd) 37, 142; Bureau of Learner Support Services 152; capacity-building programme 150; crop museums and 150; Memorandum Order 156; school-based feeding programme 142, 145

Philippines ISNM 8

Philippine Society of Nutritionist-Dietitians, Inc. Convention 152

Philippines' Republic Act 11037 58

Plant for the Planet campaign (UNEP) 110

pleasurable food education 164

primary school curriculum: strategies for integrating food in 48–58; strategies for integrating nutrition in 48–58

Programa Nacional de Alimentação Escolar– PNAE (National School Feeding Program), Brazil 283–284

Project Oidag (Arizona, United States)19

Psidium guajava 107

Radiant Design, and premaculture trainings 186

Rangatiratanga 228

rau muong 27

Red Chiapaneca de Huertos Educativos (RCHE), Mexico 242, 244

Red Internacional de Huertos Educativos (RIHE), Mexico 242, 244

Regional Institute of Public Health (IRSP) 37

Reiby Aboriginal Community Consultative Committee (RACCC), Australia 200

Reiby Juvenile Justice Centre, Australia 200

Remind, and digital communication 58

Remote Indigenous Gardens Network, Australia 203

Republic of the Marshall Islands (RMI): dietary habits problem 258–259; Ministry of Health 258; overview 257–258; seawater problem of 258

Rhus natalensis (wild berry) 100

Right of Children to Free and Compulsory Education Act 232

Robert Wood Johnson Foundation (RWJF) 10

Rocky Mountain Institute 172

Rotarian Action Group (Food Plant Solutions) 178, 179, 182–183

Royal Botanic Garden's Youth Community Greening (YCG) programme, Australia 193, 200–201

Sawa for Development and Aid (SDAID), Lebanon 216

scaling: building grassroots movements 144; defined 144–5; enabling environment for 147–8; horizontal 144; implementing at scale 145–7; influencing policy reform 144; integrated school nutrition model 144–7; *Jikin kallib ilo jikuul* 264–5; learning about 146–7; multi-scalar approach to 145–6; out 144; project replication 144; scaling up 144–5; school gardens initiative by HISGN 175–6; Spud-in-abucket 228; 10,000 gardens project 281; vertical 146; Vietnam school gardens programme 182–3; wild edible species in Lebanon and Turkey 272

school-based feeding programme (SBFP) 126; in Brazil 283; expanded coverage of 133; integrating Brazilian food biodiversity in 290; in Philippines 142; trends in percentage of SBFP repeaters *136*

school-based nutrition interventions: agents of change 43; benefits and costs of 43; food and nutrition education in schools 42–43; home-grown school

feeding 39–42; human rights and 35–37; overview 33–35; school meals and social protection 37–39
schoolchildren: health and nutrition problems among 49–50; training module on tree planting and management and 97
school feeding 56–57; in the Philippines 62–76; reduced number of repeaters in 135–136
school gardening 53–54; activities in Ramechhap district of Nepal 82; home gardening and 134; in the Philippines 62–76
school gardens: activity with children from Khasi community in Meghalaya 18; agrobiodiversity, in Naxaithong Village School 252–253; as an inspirational pocket landscape 129; application of Food Tree and Crop Portfolios in 95–100; assured supply of nutritious vegetables from 135; and awareness of climate change 14–16; benefits derived from participating in **137–138**; and better diets, livelihoods, and learning 106–108; challenges faced in participating in **137–138**; as conservation networks for tree genetic resources 105–113; and conservation of fruit tree genetic resources 111; crop museums and *12*; development of agricultural and livelihood skills and 4–7; diversification of 73; in the East Coast–Australia 13–14; educational aspects of 134–135; education and 94–100; and education link 71–72; enhancing academic skills and 16–17; enhancing learning aptitude and academic performance 16–17; establishing location-specific food tree and crop portfolios in 98–99; establishing location-specific portfolios in 99; establishment of 98–99; example in Vietnam *181*; foods and agrobiodiversity 174; impact on community *236*, 236–237; improvement in soil quality in 72–73; initiative by HISGN 175–176; integrating Brazilian food biodiversity in 286–287, *286–287*; in Kenya 208–213; key issues for future of 22–23; as a learning garden 129; lessons learned 183–184; and local agrobiodiversity 11–14; Māori 222–229; in Meghalaya (India) 231–237; multiple benefits of 2, 4–21; in North Eastern Region of India 231–237; other benefits of school gardens 18–21; overview 1–2; practical 'hands-on' agricultural activities in 94–100; programme impact in Vietnam 181–182; promotion of healthy diets by influencing behaviours 9–11; promotion of healthy eating habits by influencing behaviours 9–11; role for enhancing connectivity with 108–111; role in complementing school feeding 7–9; and school feeding link 69–71; short history 3–4; training and 94–100; in Vietnam 178–184; and women's empowerment 20–21
school gardens in Nepal: challenges encountered 83; lessons learnt 84; overview 77–78; piloting 81–83; scaling up 84; school garden components 79–81; school garden design 78–83; school selection 78–79; training and follow-up 81
School Gardens Project (SGP), Laguna 128
School Learning Garden Programme, Republic of Marshall Islands 29
school meals and social protection 37–39
'School Meals Planning' tool 41
School Peace Gardens, Hawai'i 175
School-Plus-Home Gardens Project (S+HGP) 127–129; benefits realized and challenges encountered 137–139; contests, awards, and recognition 133; diet diversity through garden diversity 135; educational aspects of school gardens 134–135; engaging and sustaining parents' participation 131–133; expanded coverage of SBFP 133; extending school gardening to home gardening 134; extension services and supporting policies 132; families of undernourished students 129–131; improving children's consumption of vegetables 136; nutritional gains among undernourished children 133; operational model of 128; and parent-teacher associations (PTA) 132; participatory development approaches 131; project outcomes enhanced by parent engagement in 135–139; reduced number of repeaters in feeding programme 135–136; school savings and income generation 134; stepwise capacity building of key stakeholders 131–132; supply of nutritious vegetables from home gardens 135; supply of nutritious vegetables from school 135
schools: food and nutrition education in 42–43; harvesting produce in Meghalaya 235; mainstreaming Brazilian food biodiversity in 290–291; programmes and

wild edible species 271–272; savings and income generation 134; and traditional food gardens benefits 193–194, *194*
Sclerocarya birrea (marula fruit) 90
SDG 2–Zero Hunger 87
SEAMEO INNOTECH, Philippines 49
SEAMEO-RECFON, Philippines 49, 50
Second World War 28
seed exchange 150
seeds, and nutrition 95–100
Seed: The Untold Story 241
Seesaw, and digital communication 58
self-sufficiency: benefits of 199; Dar Taliba 189; Torres Webb 197–200
sentinel schools: children benefit from garden produce shared to SBFP in **71**; results of soil analysis in **73**; savings on expenses in 120-day feeding cycle in **70**; savings on expenses in 200-day feeding cycle in **70**; use of gardens as learning venues **75**
Shepherdson College *205*, 205–206
Slovenian School Meals Act of 2010 38
Slow Food Foundation for Biodiversity, Tanzania 30; and agricultural biodiversity 278; overview 276; 10,000 gardens project 276–281; traditional and innovative knowledge exchange 278, *279*
Socially Useful Productive Work (SUPW) course (India) 233
social media 227, 244; and integrated school nutrition model 154
SOILS (Lebanon NGOs) 216, 218
Soils for Life (Australian NGO) 5
Sorindeia madagascariensis 90
Southeast Asian Ministers of Education Organization-Southeast Asian Regional Center for Graduate Study and Research in Agriculture (SEAMEO- SEARCA), Philippines 153
Southeast Asian Regional Center for Graduate Study and Research in Agriculture (SEARCA), Philippines 53, 127
South Korea, and free meal schools 56
Spud-in-a-bucket (New Zealand) 225–227; scaling up 228
Stephanie Alexander Kitchen Garden Foundation (SAKGF) Australia 26, 161; beginning of 160–161; and Driver Primary School 165–167; membership 163; overview 159; as part of school curriculum 161–162; pleasurable food education 164; programme models 162; reason for starting 159–160; University of Melbourne/Deakin University evaluation 169–170; University of Wollongong evaluation 168–169
student learning 16, 55
supplementary feeding: with indigenous vegetables 68; with iron-fortified rice 68
supplementary school feeding 142, 143
Sustainable Development Goals (SDGs) 87, 152
sustainable food systems 4–7
Sustainable Income Generating Investment (SINGI), Kenya 209
sustainable use of local agrobiodiversity 11–14
Swiss Agency for Development and Cooperation (SDC) 24, 29, 78, 117, 246
Syrian refugee population: food aid for 219; in Lebanon 215; and NGOs 216–218; value of learning gardens for 218–219

taewa (Maori society) 225
tafleyout (*Mentha gatefossei*) 189
Tagai State College School Community, Torres Strait 198
Tahuri Whenua 28, 223, 225–227, 228–229
Tamarindus indica (tamarind) 100
tarubi (*Rubia peregrina*) 189
Technical and Vocational Education and Training (TVET) programmes, Turkey 272
technology: food and nutrition education 54–55
10,000 gardens project: in Africa 276–281; agricultural biodiversity benefits 278; characteristics of 279; impact 279–280, *280*; purpose of 276–277; scaling up 281; structure of 277–278; traditional and innovative knowledge exchange 278, *279*
Tharawal Aboriginal Corporation, Australia 200, 201
Tisch Center for Food Education and Policy, United States 10
Tohono O'odham Community Action (TOCA), Arizona, United States 19
Tohono O'odham Nation 19
traditional food gardens: and learning settings 193–194; multi-functional benefits of 193–194; in schools 193–194, *194*
traditional plant knowledge 188–189
training: consumption diversity and 94–100; production diversity and 94–100
Training of Trainers (ToTs) 209
tree-based agroforestry systems 87
tree foods: nutrient composition of selected **89**; nutritional contributions of 88–91
tree genetic resources: school gardens as conservation networks for 105–113

trees: and agroforestry 87–91; diets and 106–108; education and school gardens 94–100; fill harvest and nutrient 'gaps' 91–94; food and agriculture systems for nutrition and health 86–87; Food Tree and Crop Portfolios 91–94; Food Tree and Crop Portfolios in school gardens 95–100; learning and 106–108; livelihoods and 106–108; nutritional contributions of tree foods 88–91; overview 86; planting seeds for nutrition 95–100; practical 'hands-on' agricultural activities in school gardens 94–100; training and school gardens 94–100
Trees for the Future (TREES) 107–108
Turkey: BFN Project in 268, 269, *270*; dietary habits problems 267–268; integration of wild edible species into schools and educational programmes 272

UK Garden Organisation 110
Uncle Dean Kelly 200, 202
Uncle Ivan Wellington 200, 201
UNESCO 48
United Nations Children's Funds (UNICEF) 258
United Nation's International Year of Indigenous Languages 195
United Nations System Standing Committee on Nutrition (UNSCN) 23, 33
United States Department of Agriculture (USDA): Fresh Fruit and Vegetable Program 175
University of Arkansas 10
University of Melbourne 169–170
University of Montreal 37, 269
University of Ottawa 269
University of the Philippines Los Baños (UPLB) 127
University of Wollongong 168–169
Urtica massaica 107
U.S. Department of Agriculture (USDA) 3; People's Garden *Healthy Gardens, Healthy Youth* project 10
'U.S. Garden Armies' 3

Vangueria madagascariensis (common wild medlar) 100
vegetables: conservation of indigenous 73; improving children's consumption of 136; supplementary feeding with indigenous 68

'Vegetables Go to School: Improving Nutrition by Agricultural Diversification' project, Nepal 117–118
Vegetables Go to School (VGtS) project 24, 25, 78, 122
vertical scaling 146
Victory Gardens, Massachusetts, United States 3
Vietnam: Department of Labour, Invalids, and Social Affairs (DOLISA) 183; malnourishment in 178–179; nutritional standards in 178–179; role of agrobiodiversity 180–181; school gardens in 178–184; stakeholder and policy maker involvement 183
Vigna unguiculata 88, 90
Vitellaria paradoxa 88
Vitex payos (chocolate berries) 100

Washington State University 10
Web-based approach: food and nutrition education 54–55
whakapapa (genealogy) 224, 227, 228
wild edible plants 268; to enhance agrobiodiversity in Lebanon 271; species in Lebanon 269–272; species in Turkey 269–272; testimonials from Turkish beneficiaries 273
women: agricultural practices education in Moroccan High Atlas 186–187; anaemic, percentage in Meghalaya 232; illiteracy rates and High Atlas Mountains 186; school gardens and empowerment of 20–21
World Agroforestry Centre (ICRAF) 88, 91; Food Trees Project 95; Fruit Tree Portfolio *91*; ICRAF programmes 88, 90
World Bank (WB) 7
World Food Day 52, 153
World Food Programme (WFP) 7, 40, 41
World Health Organization (WHO) 127, 140n1; *Healthy Diets Factsheet* 37; Nutrition-Friendly Schools Initiative (NFSI) 37
World Vegetable Center 78, 118
World Wars 3

Xiengkhouang Province, Laos: ABD curriculum 249–251, 253–255, **254**; ABD school garden and medicinal plants garden 252–253; agrobiodiversity education in 246–256; map *247*; Office of Education and Sports (POES) 248

Zaher – Grow to Learn 216, 218, 220
Zimbabwe 106, 111